Mindfulness in Behavioral Health

Series Editor
Nirbhay N. Singh
Medical College of Georgia,
Georgia Regents University,
Augusta, Georgia, USA

Mindfulness-based therapy is one of the fastest evolving treatment approaches in psychology and related fields. It has been used to treat many forms of psychological and psychiatric distress and medical conditions as well as to foster health and wellness. Early empirical studies and meta-analyses of current research suggest that mindfulness-based therapies are effective and long lasting, but much more data from research and training studies are needed to fully understand its nature and effective practice. The Mindfulness in Behavioral Health series aims to foster this understanding by aggregating this knowledge in a series of high-quality books that will encourage and enhance dialogue among clinicians, researchers, theorists, philosophers, and practitioners in the fields of psychology, medicine, social work, counseling, and allied disciplines. The books in the series are appropriate for upper level undergraduate and graduate courses. Each book targets a core audience, but also appeals to others interested in behavior change and personal transformation.

More information about this series at http://www.springer.com/series/8678

Edo Shonin • William Van Gordon •
Nirbhay N. Singh
Editors

Buddhist Foundations of Mindfulness

Springer

Editors
Edo Shonin
Awake to Wisdom, Centre for Meditation and Mindfulness Research
Nottingham
United Kingdom

William Van Gordon
Awake to Wisdom, Centre for Meditation and Mindfulness Research
Nottingham
United Kingdom

Nirbhay N. Singh
Dept. Psychiatry and Health Behavior
Medical College of Georgia
Georgia Regents University
Augusta
Georgia
USA

ISSN 2195-9579
ISSN 2195-9587 (electronic)
Mindfulness in Behavioral Health
ISBN 978-3-319-18590-3
ISBN 978-3-319-18591-0 (eBook)
DOI 10.1007/978-3-319-18591-0

Library of Congress Control Number: 2015939420

Springer Cham Heidelberg New York Dordrecht London

Printed on acid-free paper

Springer International Publishing AG Switzerland is part of Springer Science+Business Media (www.springer.com)

To my stubborn but dear friend, Jacqi Sein

E.S.

To the simple monk, Ven Edo Shonin

W.VG.

To my granddaughters, Anicca Singh and Priya Joy

N.N.S.

Preface

Mindfulness was taught and practiced by the historical Buddha some 2500 years ago and is a fundamental aspect of Buddhist practice. Teachers from diverse Buddhist traditions consistently convey the message that mindfulness is essential for cultivating meditative awareness and lasting psycho-spiritual wellbeing. In this sense, mindfulness can be viewed as a prerequisite for entering the advanced stages of spiritual practice and for perceiving the ultimate mode in which phenomena exist. The Buddha taught that when mindfulness is used as a basis for apprehending this ultimate aspect of reality, all forms of suffering and ignorance are transmuted.

Although there are different interpretations of mindfulness in Buddhism, there are a number of constants that unite these interpretations and point towards certain inborn characteristics of mindfulness. For example, a more exoteric Buddhist interpretation might describe mindfulness as the practice of being fully aware of the present moment, while a more esoteric Buddhist interpretation might describe it, in the words of Dudjom Rinpoche, as the *simple recollection of the recognition of your own nature*. Although these delineations allude to different perceptual referents that should be adopted as the object of mindful awareness, they both imply that mindfulness entails being fully aware of what is unfolding in the here and now. Depending upon an individual's meditative experience and the particular spiritual path that they are following, this awareness could relate to simply acknowledging the existence and/or gross properties of the various bodily, affective, and cognitive processes that are present in any given moment, or it could relate to directly perceiving the underlying and ultimate nature of these same phenomena.

Thus, despite the different ways in which Buddhist traditions describe mindfulness, there appears to be a degree of consensus in Buddhism that mindfulness involves being fully aware of the gross and/or ultimate properties of phenomena at the moment they enter into the attentional sphere. There is also consensus in Buddhism that mindfulness should be cultivated at all stages of an individual's meditative journey. In this respect, the Buddhist delineation of mindfulness is of a simple yet spiritually profound practice that is good at the beginning, good in the middle, and good at the end.

In recent decades, there has been growing scientific and public interest in the health benefits of mindfulness as well as its applications in various applied settings.

For example, initiatives are underway and/or research has been conducted that supports the use of mindfulness as a tool for: (i) treating psychological and somatic illness, (ii) reducing reoffending and regulating anger in forensic populations, (iii) improving work-related wellbeing, job satisfaction, and job performance in occupational and commercial settings, (iv) improving academic performance, knowledge acquisition, cognitive functioning, and quality of learning environment in schools and other education establishments, and (v) helping athletes and sports professionals enhance situational awareness, task focus, and competitive performance more generally.

Understandably and in many cases, mindfulness has been introduced to the non-Buddhist Westerner in a manner that filters out many of the contextual factors that connect it with its Buddhist origins. To a large extent, this has been a successful strategy and has meant that individuals who might otherwise be deterred from practicing mindfulness (i.e., due to it being an explicitly Buddhist practice) have been willing to explore its potential merits. Indeed, it is our personal belief that had mindfulness not been operationalized in this manner, it would not have experienced the same popularity or been assigned the same level of scientific value that it currently enjoys.

However, it is for this exact same reason—the apparent watering-down of mindfulness—that there have been growing concerns amongst academicians, clinicians, and Buddhist teachers that secular mindfulness has become estranged from the traditional Buddhist model to such an extent that it can no longer be accurately described as "mindfulness." We have previously explicated the implications of these concerns as follows:

1. If it is the case that secular mindfulness approaches are incongruent with the Buddhist model, then it is ethically inappropriate and potentially misleading (e.g., to participants and service-users) to describe them as being grounded in Buddhist principles.
2. Since secular mindfulness approaches have been shown to be efficacious for various clinical and nonclinical population groups, research is warranted to investigate whether there are additional benefits associated with utilizing an approach that more closely accords with the traditional Buddhist construction of mindfulness.
3. There may be risks associated with teaching mindfulness in isolation of the principles and practices that are traditionally assumed to underlie the effective development of mindful awareness (e.g., ethical awareness, compassionate outlook, insight into nonself, etc.). This remains an important future direction for mindfulness research because empirical enquiry specifically assessing whether secular mindfulness can induce nonsalutatory health outcomes is currently underdeveloped.

One valid argument in response to these concerns is that if secular mindfulness approaches can be shown to be efficacious for a given application, then it is of little relevance whether they embody a traditional Buddhist construction. A further counter-argument is that the abovementioned concerns appear to be based on the assumption that compared to secular mindfulness modalities, present-day Buddhist teachers and traditions necessarily embody a more ethically wholesome and spiritually potent approach. Although it is comparatively easier for mainstream Buddhist teachers and traditions to claim a spiritual connection (i.e., lineage) to the historical Buddha's teachings on mindfulness, this does not, by default, mean that they are any more or less "superficial" than secular mindfulness approaches.

Irrespective of an individual's perspective on the above debate, what is certain is that the more they understand the Buddhist theory and principles that underlie the practice of mindfulness, the better positioned they will be to study, practice, and/or teach mindfulness effectively. This, in short, reflects the provenance for the current volume on the *Buddhist Foundations of Mindfulness*. This book provides a comprehensive overview of the Buddhist fundamentals of mindfulness, and discusses the relationship of mindfulness to core Buddhist practices and teachings. It is intended to be an essential guide for academics, clinicians, Buddhist scholars, mindfulness and Buddhist teachers, university students, and Buddhist and mindfulness practitioners wishing to consolidate and expand their understanding of mindfulness.

As discussed further in the introductory chapter, the current volume includes contributions from some of the world's leading scholars, Buddhist teachers, clinicians, and scientists in the field of mindfulness practice and research. In addition to ensuring a complete coverage of relevant topics, the contributors were selected in order to introduce diversity in respect of professional background, meditation experience, and scholarly interpretation of the Buddhist teachings. In Part One of the book, mindfulness is discussed in the context of core Buddhist teachings such as the *Four Noble Truths*, ethics, *Samatha* and *Vipassanā* meditation, and emptiness. Part One also includes separate chapters on the *Ānāpānasati Sutta* and the *Satipaṭṭhāna Sutta*—two key Buddhist teachings of mindfulness. The dialogue progresses in Part Two with an examination of how to effectively integrate and utilize the core Buddhist principles relating to mindfulness in research and applied settings. In Part Three, mindfulness is then discussed in relation to a broader selection of Buddhist themes and modes of practice.

Chapters follow a logical sequence such that earlier chapters provide the necessary foundations to understand and analyze the additional layers of Buddhist theory and teachings that are presented in subsequent chapters. However, although earlier chapters focus on core Buddhist teachings, they invariably do so in a way that introduces original ideas and/or clarifies areas of confusion in relation to Buddhist thought. Consequently, all chapters make an important contribution to improving understanding regarding the Buddhist principles that underlie effective mindfulness practice and they can be read in sequential order or as standalone entities.

We hope that this volume on the *Buddhist Foundations of Mindfulness* will help to establish robust foundations for the ongoing integration of mindfulness into Western clinical and scientific settings. We also hope the volume will make a valuable contribution to the mainstream Buddhist literature on mindfulness and on Buddhist practice more generally. Finally, we hope that the volume will inspire readers of both Buddhist and non-Buddhist backgrounds to seek guidance from an authentic teacher and take up a personal practice of mindfulness so that they can encounter the mindfulness teachings directly for themselves.

Edo Shonin
William Van Gordon
Nirbhay N. Singh

Contents

Part II Integrating Mindfulness into Research and Applied Settings

Part III Further Buddhist Perspectives on Mindfulness

About the Editors

Venerable Edo Shonin has been a Buddhist monk for 30 years and is Spiritual Director of the international Mahayana Bodhayati School of Buddhism. He is Research Director of the Awake to Wisdom Centre for Meditation and Mindfulness Research and a research psychologist at the Nottingham Trent University (UK). He sits on the International Advisory Board for the journal *Mindfulness* and is an editorial board member of the *International Journal of Mental Health and Addiction.* He is internationally known for his work and has more than 100 academic publications relating to the scientific study of mindfulness and Buddhist practice. He runs the *Meditation Practice and Research Blog* at www.edoshonin.com.

Venerable William Van Gordon has been a Buddhist monk for 10 years and is Operations Director of the international Mahayana Bodhayati School of Buddhism. He is co-founder of the Awake to Wisdom Centre for Meditation and Mindfulness Research and is a research psychologist based at the Nottingham Trent University (UK). He is currently Principal Investigator on a number of randomized controlled trials investigating the applications of an intervention known as Meditation Awareness Training (MAT) in clinical and occupational settings. He sits on the editorial board for the *International Journal of Buddhism* and has more than 100 academic publications relating to the scientific study of Buddhism and associated meditative approaches.

Nirbhay N. Singh is Clinical Professor of Psychiatry and Health Behavior at the Medical College of Georgia, Georgia Regents University, Augusta, Georgia, USA. Prior to his current appointment, he was a Professor of Psychiatry, Pediatrics and Psychology at the Virginia Commonwealth University School of Medicine and Director of the Commonwealth Institute for Family Studies, Richmond, Virginia. His research interests include mindfulness, behavioral and psychopharmacological treatments of individuals with disabilities, and assistive technology for supporting individuals with severe/profound and multiple disabilities. He is the Editor-in-Chief of two journals: *Journal of Child and Family Studies* and *Mindfulness;* and Editor of three book series: *Mindfulness in Behavioral Health, Evidence-based Practice in Behavioral Health*, and *Children and Families*.

List of Contributors

Bhikkhu Anālayo Numata Center for Buddhist Studies, University of Hamburg, Hamburg, Germany

James B Apple Department of Classics and Religion, University of Calgary, Calgary, AB, Canada

Mark D. Griffiths Division of Psychology, Nottingham Trent University, Nottingham, Chaucer Building, Burton Street, UK

Peter Harvey University of Sunderland, York, UK

Malcolm Huxter Westminster Centre for Resilience, University of Westminster, London, UK

Jnanavaca London Buddhist Centre, London, UK

G. T. Maurits Kwee Karma Transformation by Conversation & Meditation, Bentveld, The Netherlands

Tse-fu Kuan College of General Studies, Yuan Ze University, Taoyuan City, Taiwan

Tim Lomas School of Psychology, The University of East London, London, UK

Spencer A. McWilliams Psychology Department, California State University San Marcos, San Marcos, CA, USA

Lynette M. Monteiro Ottawa Mindfulness Clinic, Ottawa, ON,Canada

Edo Shonin Division of Psychology, Nottingham Trent University, Nottingham, Chaucer Building, Burton Street, UK

Kaisa Puhakka Department of Clinical Psychology, California Institute of Integral Studies, San Francisco, CA, USA

Nirbhay N. Singh Medical College of Georgia, Georgia Regents University, Augusta, GA, USA

Steven Stanley School of Social Sciences, Cardiff University, Cardiff, Wales, UK

Karma Lekshe Tsomo Department of Theology and Religious Studies,University of San Diego, San Diego CA, USA

William Van Gordon Division of Psychology, Nottingham Trent University, Nottingham, Chaucer Building, Burton Street, UK

Chapter 1
Mindfulness and Buddhist Practice

Edo Shonin, William Van Gordon and Nirbhay N. Singh

1.1 Introduction

According to historical sources, Shakyamuni Buddha, who lived and expounded spiritual teachings in India, is understood to have been born approximately 2500 years ago (Gombrich 2009). Historical sources also suggest that as part of growing into an adult, he played with other children, received an education, explored feelings of a sexual nature, and developed various interests and skills. At some point in early adult life, it appears that he experienced a yearning to embrace spirituality. At the point this desire first arose in the Buddha, he probably did not fully understand it. Although it is likely that the Buddha had been exposed to religion during his upbringing, we suspect the longing he experienced went far beyond the type of interest expressed by most religious/spiritual teachers and scholars. Consistent with the accounts of other reportedly enlightened spiritual practitioners (e.g. Milarepa 1999), it is likely that the Buddha's wish to permanently transmute suffering arose from deep within and was the result of a long-standing connection with the spiritual teachings.

The Buddha chose not to ignore the urge to spiritually awaken, and he made spiritual development his primary life objective. Consistent with the experiences of other Buddhist and non-Buddhist spiritual adepts, in the course of living and pursuing this objective, the Buddha encountered numerous adversities. However, because the Buddha's intentions were "right" (Pāli: *sammā sankappa*, Sanskrit:

E. Shonin (✉) · W. Van Gordon
Awake to Wisdom, Centre for Meditation and Mindfulness Research, Nottingham, UK
e-mail: e.shonin@awaketowisdom.co.uk

Bodhayati School of Buddhism, Nottingham, UK

Division of Psychology, Nottingham Trent University, Chaucer Building, Burton Street, Nottingham, UK

N. N. Singh
Medical College of Georgia, Georgia Regents University, Augusta, GA, USA

E. Shonin et al. (eds.), *Buddhist Foundations of Mindfulness*,
Mindfulness in Behavioral Health, DOI 10.1007/978-3-319-18591-0_1

samyak-saṃkalpa), rather than deter him these challenges only cemented his spiritual competencies and convictions (Shonin and Van Gordon 2015). At some point in his life, the Buddha's commitment and efforts began to yield results. He encountered—within himself—an unremitting wealth of wisdom, spiritual energy, and love for all beings, and he eventually realised his enlightened nature.

Although the Buddha was an enlightened being, whilst he remained alive, he was also a human being. He ate, slept, walked, talked, bathed, defecated, laughed, and cried. Although not bound by his feelings, he felt happy when others were kind to each other and felt sad when he observed people behaving in a hurtful manner. He was approachable to individuals from all remits of society, and it is almost certain that he was neither aloof, clinical, nor overly solemn in the way he interacted with others.

Whilst attempting to guide individuals towards embracing the truth (Pāli: *Dhamma,* Sanskrit: *Dharma*), and whilst recollecting the condition of his own mind prior to realising its (inherent) enlightened nature, it seems that the Buddha recognised that the human mind has a propensity to be eternally distracted. Consistent with empirical research findings and contemporary clinical opinion, thought rumination and a distracted mind are not conducive for the cultivation of psychological wellbeing and invariably play a role in the onset and maintenance of mental illness (Davey 2008). Consequently, the Buddha required a method—that was easily digestible for individuals from a broad range of socioeconomic and educational backgrounds—which he could teach in order to help individuals regulate maladaptive thinking patterns and introduce spiritual awareness, calm, and focus into their minds.

Based on the importance assigned to it in the canonical record of the Buddha's teachings, it appears that he deemed mindfulness (Pāli: *sati*, Sanskrit: *smṛti*) to be such a method. Mindfulness was taught by the Buddha as a core aspect of the path to awakening and as a competency to be developed and practised throughout the lifespan of the spiritual journey. The Buddha described mindfulness as the spiritual process of being fully aware of *that which is,* as opposed to *that which was* or *that which might be* (Shonin et al. 2014). The Buddha taught that when suitably developed, the concentration-regulating faculty of mindfulness: (i) gives rise to a pervasive and enduring feeling of calm and spiritual wellness, and (ii) brings the mind into a state of meditative focus that is conducive for examining and gaining insight into the nonself or empty nature of self and reality (Van Gordon et al. 2015).

This book provides a comprehensive and scholarly examination of the Buddha's teachings on mindfulness, and how they can be used to traverse the various stages and obstacles of the Buddhist spiritual path. The dialogue extends outward from an examination of the Buddhist foundational principles of mindfulness in Part One, to the application of these principles in applied and research settings in Part Two, and then in Part Three to a discussion of mindfulness in relation to a broader collection of Buddhist themes and practice traditions.

1.2 Part One

Part One of the book focusses on the relationship of mindfulness to core Buddhist teachings and principles. In the first chapter of this section (Chap. 2), William Van Gordon, Edo Shonin, Mark Griffiths, and Nirbhay Singh explore the relationship between mindfulness and the *Four Noble Truths*. The *Four Noble Truths* are recorded as being the first teaching given by the Buddha after he attained enlightenment, and they represent the foundations for the entire collection of teachings that the Buddha subsequently expounded. Chapter 2 employs logical deductive analysis in order to examine the validity and logical soundness of the *Four Noble Truths* and then discusses the relationship of mindfulness to the Four Noble Truths as a collective, and to each truth individually.

Following the dialogue on mindfulness and the *Four Noble Truths* in Chap. 2, the obvious direction for Chap. 3 is to discuss how mindfulness fits into the framework of the *Noble Eightfold Path* (which is the spiritual path referred to in the fourth of the *Four Noble Truths*). This task is undertaken by Malcolm Huxter who analyses mindfulness in relation to each aspect of the *Noble Eightfold Path,* and then discusses in-depth the meaning of *right mindfulness* (Pāli: *sammā-sati*, Sanskrit: *samyak-smrti*) which appears as the seventh aspect of the *Noble Eightfold Path.*

The next two chapters (Chaps. 4 and 5) are written by Anālayo who examines the instructions recorded in the *Ānāpānasati Sutta* and *Satipaṭṭhāna Sutta*—two core Buddhist teachings on mindfulness. These chapters compare the version of the *suttas* as recorded in the Pāli canon with parallel versions preserved in Chinese translation. The chapters demonstrate that by comparing and drawing on multiple historical records of these teachings, a collective and reliable wisdom emerges in terms of how to cultivate mindfulness effectively and use it as a means for traversing the path to awakening.

In Chap. 6, Steven Stanley explores the relationship between mindfulness and Buddhist ethics. He examines the ethical psychology of early Buddhism and discusses how this understanding can help inform the development of ethically sensitive mindfulness-based approaches in modern-day society. The chapter also includes a discussion of *wrong mindfulness* (Pāli: *micchā sati*, Sanskrit: *mithyā smṛti*) and shows how an understanding of the "wrong" way to practise can help prevent the development of misconceptions relating to mindfulness.

Peter Harvey undertakes the task in Chap. 7 of examining the role of mindfulness in calm (Pāli*: samatha, Sanskrit: shamatha*) and insight (Pāli*: vipassanā,* Sanskrit: *vipaśyanā*) meditation. The theme of Chap. 7 is particularly timely given the confusion that exists in the academic literature regarding the meaning of these different forms of Buddhist meditation. The chapter emphasises the importance and benefits of utilizing both *samatha* and *vipassanā* meditation, and explicates the various functions that mindfulness performs as part of the effective practice of these different meditative modes.

The *six perfections,* which assume a central role in Mahayana Buddhist practice, are the subject of Chap. 8. Here, Karma Lekshe Tsomo examines the role of mindfulness in the cultivation of the *six perfections,* and she explicates how mindful practice of the *six perfections* facilitates an individual's progression through the various stages of the path to enlightenment.

Part One concludes with a contribution by Edo Shonin, William Van Gordon, Nirbhay Singh, and Mark Griffiths that examines the relationship between mindfulness and emptiness (Pāli: *suññatā,* Sanskrit: *śūnyatā*), and how these two fundamental aspects of Buddhist practice interact in order to foster spiritual awakening. In addition to elucidating the practice of *mindfulness of emptiness*, Chap. 9 introduces the idea that mindfulness is empty of intrinsic existence, and that there are risks associated with developing attachments to the practice and construct of mindfulness.

1.3 Part Two

The chapters in Part Two of the book examine how to utilise the core Buddhist principles discussed in Part One and effectively integrate them into research and applied settings. In the first chapter of Part Two (Chap. 10), Lynette Monteiro makes use of key teachings from the *Ānāpānasati* and *Satipaṭṭhāna Suttas,* as well as meditation principles underlying a number of Buddhist practice modalities, and demonstrates how these Buddhist teachings and principles can inform and enrich the content and development of secular mindfulness-based approaches.

The next chapter is written by Kaisa Puhakka who explores whether the potency of Buddhist mindfulness practice diminishes when it is adapted into forms suitable for psychological research and evidence-supported clinical practice. Chapter 11 also examines the limitations inherent within contemporary research designs and assumptions, and it discusses how these limitations often result in the various subtleties and profound aspects of Buddhist practice being overlooked.

1.4 Part Three

Part Three of the book discusses mindfulness in relation to a wider selection of Buddhist themes and modes of practice. The first chapter in Part Three (Chap. 12) examines the role of mindfulness and vigilance in Tsong-kha-pa's *Great Treatise on the Stages of Path to Enlightenment.* Tsong-kha-pa (1357–1419) was a highly acclaimed Tibetan Buddhist saint and founding figure of what became the Gelukpa tradition of Tibetan Buddhism. In this chapter, James Apple comments on Tsong-kha-pa's treatise and explicates how mindfulness and vigilance help to regulate mental excitement and laxity—two primary hindrances in the development of meditative serenity.

In Chap. 13, Tse-fu Kuan examines how the Buddha provided instructions on mindfulness through the use of similes. Similes were frequently employed by the

Buddha as a didactic strategy, and the chapter focuses on four different types of similes: (i) prevention, (ii) healing, (iii) binding, and (iv) altruism. The discussion focusses on the early Buddhist literature, including the *suttas* in the Pāli *Nikāyas* and the *Āgamas* extant in Chinese translation. The challenges associated with reading some of the early Buddhist texts are also appraised.

In Chap. 14, Tim Lomas and Jnanavaca identify three different types of mindfulness that emphasise elements of recollection, ethical care, and spiritual development, respectively. The chapter then discusses the relationship of this threefold model of mindfulness to the law of conditionality and Sangharakshita's five-stage model of the Buddhist spiritual path.

The following chapter is written by Spencer McWilliams who examines mindfulness from the Zen Buddhist perspective—with a particular focus on Hubert Benoit's Zen writings and Charlotte Jōko Beck's Ordinary Mind School of Zen. Chapter 15 discusses how applying these teachings and practising mindful awareness of self-centred thoughts and feelings can lead to an awakened and transformed experience of life.

Part Three concludes with a chapter by Maurits Kwee that outlines a mode of practice that he devised called Pristine Mindfulness. Pristine Mindfulness is an eight-step process that draws upon teachings from numerous traditional and contemporary Buddhist movements. Chapter 16 examines the differences between Pristine Mindfulness and established secular mindfulness-based interventions.

The scholarly interpretations featured in this volume bring the reader into contact with teachings that have been practiced for thousands of years and that represent a diverse selection of Buddhist practice traditions. The volume is intended to help advance both theoretical understanding and mindfulness practice competency. However, although the current volume focusses on the Buddhist principles that underlie effective mindfulness practice, we hope that readers will derive benefit and knowledge from the broad selection of Buddhist practices, themes, and teachings that are traversed throughout the book.

References

Davey, G. C. (2008). *Psychopathology: Research, assessment and treatment in clinical psychology*. Chichester: Wiley-Blackwell.

Gombrich, R., (2009). Early Buddhist historiography: The need for authentication. In B. Ray (Ed.), *History of science, philosophy and culture in Indian civilization. v.XIV, Part 4: Different types of history* (pp. 43–58). Delhi: Pearson Longman.

Milarepa. (1999). *The hundred thousand songs of Milarepa: The life-story and teaching of the greatest poet-saint ever to appear in the history of Buddhism* (Chang, G. C. C., Trans.). Boston: Shambala.

Shonin, E., & Van Gordon, W. (2015). The lineage of mindfulness. *Mindfulness, 6,* 141–145.

Shonin, E., Van Gordon W., & Griffiths, M. D. (2014). The emerging role of Buddhism in clinical psychology: Toward effective integration. *Psychology of Religion and Spirituality, 6,* 123–137.

Van Gordon, W., Shonin, E., Griffiths, M. D., & Singh, N. N. (2015). There is only one mindfulness: Why science and Buddhism need to work together. *Mindfulness, 6,* 49–56.

Edo Shonin has been a Buddhist monk for 30 years and is spiritual director of the International Mahayana Bodhayati School of Buddhism. He is research director of the Awake to Wisdom Centre for Meditation and Mindfulness Research and a research psychologist at the Nottingham Trent University (UK). He sits on the International Advisory Board for the journal *Mindfulness* and is an editorial board member of the *International Journal of Mental Health and Addiction*. He is internationally known for his work and has more than 100 academic publications relating to the scientific study of mindfulness and Buddhist practice. He runs the *Meditation Practice and Research Blog* at www.edoshonin.com.

William Van Gordon has been a Buddhist monk for 10 years and is operations director of the International Mahayana Bodhayati School of Buddhism. He is cofounder of the Awake to Wisdom Centre for Meditation and Mindfulness Research and is a research psychologist based at the Nottingham Trent University (UK). He is currently principal investigator on a number of randomised controlled trials investigating the applications of an intervention known as meditation awareness training (MAT) in clinical and occupational settings. He sits on the editorial board for the *International Journal of Buddhism* and has more than 100 academic publications relating to the scientific study of Buddhism and associated meditative approaches.

Nirbhay N. Singh is a clinical professor of psychiatry and health behaviour at the Medical College of Georgia, Georgia Regents University, Augusta, Georgia, USA. Prior to his current appointment, he was a professor of psychiatry, pediatrics and psychology at the Virginia Commonwealth University School of Medicine and director of the Commonwealth Institute for Family Studies, Richmond, Virginia. His research interests include mindfulness, behavioural and psychopharmacological treatments of individuals with disabilities, and assistive technology for supporting individuals with severe/profound and multiple disabilities. He is the editor-in-chief of two journals: *Journal of Child and Family Studies* and *Mindfulness* and editor of three book series: *Mindfulness in Behavioral Health, Evidence-Based Practice in Behavioral Health*, and *Children and Families.*

Part I
Mindfulness and Its Relationship to Core Buddhist Teachings

Chapter 2
Mindfulness and the Four Noble Truths

William Van Gordon, Edo Shonin, Mark D. Griffiths and Nirbhay N. Singh

2.1 Introduction

The teaching of the Four Noble Truths is recorded as being the first teaching given by the Buddha after he attained enlightenment. It is arguably the most important of all Buddhist teachings and provides the foundation for the entire collection of discourses that the Buddha subsequently provided. Without exception, every aspect of Buddhist practice is somehow encompassed by this simple yet profound teaching, and no study or practice of any component of the Buddha's teachings—including mindfulness—is complete without a thorough comprehension of how it relates to the Four Noble Truths. In this chapter, we examine the significance and meaning of the Four Noble Truths and then discuss their individual and collective implications for understanding, practising, and working with mindfulness.

2.2 The Four Noble Truths

In the *Discourse that Sets the Wheel of Dharma in Motion* (*Dhammacakkappavattana Sutta,* Saṃyutta Nikāya, 56:11) that forms part of the *Connected Discourses on the Truths* (*Saccasamyutta,* Saṃyutta Nikāya, 56), the Buddha is recorded as expounding the Four Noble Truths as follows (Bodhi 2000, p. 1844):

W. V. Gordon (✉) · E. Shonin
Awake to Wisdom, Centre for Meditation and Mindfulness Research, Nottingham, UK
e-mail: william@awaketowisdom.co.uk

Bodhayati School of Buddhism, Nottingham, UK

W. V. Gordon · E. Shonin · M. D. Griffiths
Division of Psychology, Nottingham Trent University,
Chaucer Building, Burton Street, Nottingham, UK

N. N. Singh
Medical College of Georgia, Georgia Regents University, Augusta, GA, USA

E. Shonin et al. (eds.), *Buddhist Foundations of Mindfulness,*
Mindfulness in Behavioral Health, DOI 10.1007/978-3-319-18591-0_2

1. Now this, bhikkhus, is the noble truth of suffering: birth is suffering, aging is suffering, illness is suffering, death is suffering; union with what is displeasing is suffering; separation from what is pleasing is suffering; not to get what one wants is suffering; in brief, the five aggregates subject to clinging are suffering.
2. Now this, bhikkhus, is the noble truth of the origin of suffering: it is this craving which leads to renewed existence, accompanied by delight and lust, seeking delight here and there; that is, craving for sensual pleasures, craving for existence, craving for extermination.
3. Now this, bhikkhus, is the noble truth of the cessation of suffering: it is the remainderless fading away and cessation of that same craving, the giving up and relinquishing of it, freedom from it, nonreliance on it.
4. Now this, bhikkhus, is the noble truth of the way leading to the cessation of suffering: it is this noble eightfold path; that is, right view… right concentration.

During subsequent teachings, the Buddha provided additional accounts and explanations of the Four Noble Truths (e.g. *Saccavibhanga Sutta* (The Exposition of the Truths Sutta), Majimma Nikāya, 141 (MN 141)). However, consistent with the generally accepted abbreviated form of the Four Noble Truths, for the purposes of this chapter, we will summarise and refer to them as follows:

1. Suffering exists
2. There is a cause of suffering
3. There is cessation of suffering
4. There is a path that leads to the cessation of suffering

The *Dhammacakkappavattana Sutta* records that on the occasion when the Buddha first taught the Four Noble Truths (an event referred to as the "first turning of the wheel of Dharma") at the Deer Park in Sarnath near Varanasi, the primary recipients of the teaching were the five aesthetics (the Buddha's first disciples). However, a frequently overlooked observation concerning the *Dhammacakkappavattana Sutta* is that the *sutta* also records that the earth-dwelling devas were recipients of this teaching. The inclusion within the audience of two very different types of being—those in human form and those of the deva realm—has important implications for understanding the significance of Four Noble Truths and of the Buddha's teaching more generally. Most importantly, it implies that there are both outer and inner (or hidden) aspects to the Buddhist teachings that can be interpreted and transmitted on both exoteric and esoteric levels (Gampopa 1998).

Understanding that the Buddhist teachings are multilayered in their meaning and profundity is an essential take-home message for anybody wishing to comprehend, practice, or work with any aspect of the Buddhadharma. In fact, as illustrated and discussed in the section below that utilises deductive logical analysis (DLA) in order to investigate the theoretical and spiritual validity of the Four Noble Truths, each individual teaching given by the Buddha embodies the meaning and potency of the entire spectrum of the Buddha's wisdom and knowledge (Gampopa 1998). It is probably for this reason that there exist reports of some of the Buddha's followers directly ascending to liberation simply upon hearing the Buddha utter the

Four Noble Truths. Some examples are (i) the Venerable Añña Kondañña (one of the five aesthetics) who awoke to the "dust-free, stainless vision of the dhamma" (Bodhi 2000, p. 1846; the prefix Añña before the name Kondañña denotes "one who has understood" or "one who has realised"), and (ii) the householder Upāli who "saw the Dhamma, understood the Dhamma, fathomed the Dhamma, attained the Dhamma; he crossed beyond doubt, did away with perplexity, gained intrepidity, and became independent of others in the teacher's dispensation" (Nanamoli and Bodhi 2009, p. 485).

In addition to appreciating the spiritual significance and potency of the Four Noble Truths, a further essential take-home message concerning this teaching is that the statements that comprise the Four Noble Truths were never intended to be ambiguous. Indeed, not only were the noble truths intended to represent the Buddha's experiential understanding and expression of the truth but they were also intended to represent statements of fact. For example, the Buddha's statement that suffering exists does not just mean that there is the potential for suffering to exist, it means that with the exception of those beings that have realised the third noble truth (i.e. the cessation of suffering), all beings suffer (Shonin et al. 2015). Likewise, the noble truth of suffering does not mean that sentient beings suffer at certain times but not at other times, it means that sentient beings that have not ascended to liberation are continuously immersed in suffering.

2.3 Suffering Exists

In Western culture, suffering is generally construed as the experience of either somatic or psychological pain. Therefore, in the absence of such pain and whilst experiencing favourable socio-environmental conditions, individuals are generally not categorised as suffering or ill according to Western medical conventions (e.g. as defined by the World Health Organization). However, within Buddhism, the term "suffering" takes on a much more encompassing meaning. Irrespective of whether a sentient being is currently experiencing psychological or somatic pain, and irrespective of whether a sentient being considers itself to be suffering, Buddhism asserts that the very fact an unenlightened being exists means it suffers (Shonin et al. 2015).

This type of enduring latent suffering referred to above is known in Buddhism as *all-pervasive suffering* (Gampopa 1998). In essence, it is the suffering that arises due to an individual's ignorance as to the ultimate nature of self and reality. Given that unenlightened beings have a distorted perception of reality, Buddhism asserts that they are deluded (Tsong-Kha-pa 2004). Accordingly, within Buddhism and to a large extent, the terms "suffering", "deluded", and "ignorant" can all be used interchangeably.

One means of conceptualising the Buddhist interpretation of suffering as a form of delusion (or ignorance) is by drawing parallels between the two conditions of mindlessness and hallucination. Mindlessness refers to a lack of present moment awareness, whereby the mind is preoccupied with future (i.e. fantasised) conjectures, or past (i.e. bygone) occurrences (Shonin et al. 2014a). Therefore, an individual afflicted by mindlessness might be said to be engaging in the *non-perceiving of that which is*. Hallucination, on the other hand, can be described as being *the perceiving of that which is not*. Thus, given that both states involve an erroneous perception of the here and now, some of the current authors have previously argued that mindlessness is actually a form of inverted hallucination (Shonin et al. 2014a).

According to Buddhist thought, the overwhelming majority of people are deemed to be delusional (i.e. suffering) and in a permanent inverted hallucinatory state (Shonin et al. 2014a). However, as the twelfth century Tibetan Buddhist Gampopa (1998, p. 96) aptly pointed out, although all unenlightened beings (human or otherwise) experience all-pervasive suffering, they are generally ignorant of this fact:

> Ordinary people will not feel the all-pervasive suffering as, for example, when one is stricken with a serious plague and a small pain in the ears and so forth is not noticeable. But the saintly beings—the noble ones beyond samsara such as the stream enterers and so forth—will see the all-pervasive suffering as suffering ….

In addition to all-pervasive suffering that might be described as a more subtle form of suffering, Buddhism recognises two other primary forms of suffering that are much more tangible. The first is known as the *suffering of change* and refers to the fact that whatever temporary happiness there might be, it simply cannot endure. As stated by the Buddha in his explication of the first noble truth, birth leads to the suffering of sickness and old age, and sickness and old age lead to the suffering of death. Being in love leads to the suffering of separation, and having possessions (e.g. wealth, health, reputation, family, friends) leads to suffering when one is ultimately parted from such favourable circumstances. In short, suffering is ubiquitous to the human condition, and the principle of impermanence means that just as with all phenomena and experiences, favourable circumstances are transient and are subject to dissolution (Dalai Lama 1995).

The third primary form of suffering recognised in the Buddhist teachings is that of the *suffering of suffering*. This is the most palpable form of suffering and is typified by experiences such as somatic pain, psychological distress, illness, hunger or starvation, thirst or dehydration, being too hot, and being too cold. Buddhism asserts that the human being comprises five aggregates (i.e. form, feelings, perceptions, mental formations, and consciousness; Sanskrit: *skandhas;* Pali: *khandha*s) and that each individual aggregate is likewise composite (Dalai Lama and Berzin 1997). For example, the first aggregate of form (or the body) in turn comprises the five elements of water, wind (i.e. air), earth (i.e. food), sun (i.e. heat/energy), and space (i.e. in the bodily cavities, between molecules, and so on; Shonin et al. 2014b). Due to the fact that the human body exists in reliance upon a delicate balance of innumerable causes, components, and conditions, Buddhism teaches that even a slight imbalance in these elements and components results in both the suffering of suffering (e.g. pain and discomfort) and, ultimately, the suffering of change (e.g. illness and death; Gampopa 1998).

2.4 The Cause of Suffering

As a means of operationalising (within Western psychological and scientific domains) Buddhism's position concerning the aetiology of suffering, we recently formulated the concept of *ontological addiction* (Shonin et al. 2013). Ontological addiction can effectively be considered a new category of addiction (i.e. in addition to chemical addiction and behavioural addiction) and is defined as "the unwillingness to relinquish an erroneous and deep-rooted belief in an inherently existing 'self' or 'I' as well as the 'impaired functionality' that arises from such a belief" (Shonin et al. 2013, p. 64). Due to a firmly embedded, yet scientifically and logically implausible belief that the self is an inherent and independently existing entity, Buddhism teaches that afflictive mental states arise as a result of the imputed "self" incessantly craving after objects it considers to be attractive or harbouring aversion towards objects it considers to be unattractive (Shonin et al. 2014a). Put simply, Buddhism asserts that because sentient beings believe they inherently exist, they constantly crave after objects and/or situations that they deem will better their predicament (Dalai and Berzin 1997). Not only is this craving itself a form of suffering but as explained by the Buddha, it also causes an unending torrent of sorrows to ensue:

> Whoever is overcome by this wretched and sticky craving, his sorrows grow like grass after the rains. (*Dhammapada*, 24, 335; Buddharakkhita 1986, p. 113)

In Buddhist terminology, the word craving has very similar connotations to the meaning of the word attachment, which is deemed to be an undesirable quality that leads to the reification of the ego-self. We have previously defined attachment as "the over-allocation of cognitive and emotional resources towards a particular object, construct, or idea to the extent that the object is assigned an attractive quality that is unrealistic and that exceeds its intrinsic worth" (Shonin et al. 2014a, p. 4). Thus, attachment takes on a different meaning in Buddhism vis-a-vis its construction in Western psychology where attachment (i.e. in the context of relationships) is generally considered to exert a protective influence over psychopathology (Shonin et al. 2014a, b). Based on a Buddhist construction of attachment, lower levels of attachment have been shown to predict greater levels of mindfulness, acceptance, non-reactivity, self-compassion, subjective wellbeing, and eudemonic wellbeing (Sahdra et al. 2010). Furthermore, the Buddhist attachment construct is positively correlated with avoidance (i.e. of intimacy), dissociation, fatalistic outlook, and alexithymia (i.e. an impaired capacity to identify or describe feelings; Sahdra et al. 2010).

It is important to understand that although there are many similarities between the Buddhist notion of craving/attachment and the connotation of these terms in, for example, substance misuse and behavioural addiction contexts, additional levels of meaning are implied by the Buddhist construction. Indeed, the type of craving referred to in the Buddhist model of suffering is incredibly deep-rooted and stems from a wrong view that has been developed and cemented over innumerable lifetimes of samsaric wandering (Tsong-Kha-pa 2004). Therefore, as stated by the

Buddha, sentient beings have a propensity for craving, and any path that does not facilitate the severing of craving at its roots will only result in a short-term reduction in suffering:

> Just as a tree, though cut down, sprouts up again if its roots remain uncut and firm, even so, until the craving that lies dormant is rooted out, suffering springs up again and again. (*Dhammapada*, 24, 338; Buddharakkhita 1986, p. 133)

2.5 The Cessation of Suffering

There is debate amongst Buddhist schools as to exactly what constitutes liberation (i.e. the cessation of suffering) and whether it represents the conclusion of the spiritual journey. For example, some Buddhist systems contend that liberation and enlightenment are two distinct conditions, whereby liberation signifies the removal of obscurations caused by emotional defilements (Sanskrit: *klesavarana*), but not of all obscurations to knowledge (Sanskrit: *jneyavarana*). However, despite the slight variations in how different Buddhist approaches interpret the meaning of the term "liberation", all Buddhist schools agree that spiritual liberation implies breaking free of samsaric wandering.

Within Buddhism, beings are said to be samsaric if they are bound to the cycle of birth, death, and rebirth. Buddhism contends that the particular category (i.e. hell being, preta, animal, human, demigod, god) and quality (i.e. attractive/ugly, rich/poor, healthy/unhealthy) of an individual's rebirth are directly influenced by their karmic baggage (Tsong-Kha-pa 2004). In this context, karmic baggage refers to the imprint that each individual's thoughts, words, and deeds leaves upon their mind and this, in turn, determines how they react to and perceive the conditions and occurrences around them.

Although we would argue that a being—including those that have attained Buddhahood—never actually concludes its spiritual journey, the Buddha's statement that there is cessation of suffering implies that liberation from suffering is not a half-way stage on the path to enlightenment. The reason for this is because it is logically implausible to assert that there exists a state in which suffering has completely ceased, but that in this state, a being is still subject to a subtle class of ignorance (i.e. suffering) due to still not having awoken to complete omniscience and enlightenment. Therefore, we would argue that to experience the cessation of suffering means to have fully actualised: (i) omniscience, (ii) deathlessness, (iii) emptiness, (iv) unconditional blissful abiding, (iv) freedom to take rebirth in any realm according to the needs of beings, (v) great compassion (Sanskrit: *maha karuna*), and (vi) command over animate and inanimate phenomena.

Implicit as part of advancing on the path towards liberation is the accumulation of spiritual wisdom. There are numerous delineations of the term "wisdom" in Buddhism, but we would define it as "the extent to which an individual accurately apprehends both themselves and reality". In other words, the Buddhist notion of wisdom refers to the gradual (or in some cases instantaneous) development of insight that permits an individual to undergo recovery from ontological addiction by reconstructing their erroneous view of self and reality (Shonin et al. 2014a). Therefore, the Buddhist interpretation of wisdom contrasts with the Western psychological depiction where wisdom is generally measured against indices of knowledge, adaptive psychological functioning, and socio-environmental mastery (Baltes and Staudinger 2000).

Consistent with Buddhist thought, the degree of respect awarded to a particular Buddhist practitioner or teacher is (or should be) based on the amount of spiritual wisdom they have accumulated (Shonin and Van Gordon 2015). Indeed, for all intents and purposes, Buddhism assigns a similar meaning to the word wisdom (Sanskrit: *prajna*) as it does to the word enlightenment (i.e. the wiser a person is, the closer they are to enlightenment and vice versa). Shonin and Van Gordon (2014a, p. 1) described the Buddhist construction of wisdom as follows:

> A wise person knows every inch of their mind. They know why it exists, where it exists, and how it exists. Not only do they know their mind, but they also know that part of them that knows that it knows the mind. They appreciate fully that they are both the observed mind as well as the mind that observes. Because they know their own minds, they also know every inch of everybody else's minds and they are fully aware that all minds are interconnected. They are aware that their mind is without limitations and they know that all other sentient beings also have the potential to have a mind without limitations. In short, their outlook is vast and unconditionally compassionate—everything is encompassed in it.
>
> Although the wise person has realised the full potential of their mind, they are in no way conceited or boastful about this. In fact, the wiser a person is, the more humble they are. Wise people don't have goals or agendas *per se*, and they place no importance on being recognised for their efforts or successes. Their main objective is to simply be, and from this state of simply being, profound tranquillity and lucidity arises that allows them to act in a way that is inconceivably skilful yet completely uncontrived.

A noteworthy observation concerning the Buddhist construction of wisdom is that intelligence is not a prerequisite for being wise. Obviously, there are numerous categories (e.g. emotional, social, logical, linguistic, and so on) and interpretations of intelligence, but here, we are using the term according to its popular definition of the ability to acquire and apply knowledge and skills. Thus, based on a Buddhist view, it is probable that a wise person will be intelligent in the conventional sense, but it is also conceivably possible that they will not be. Buddhism regards intelligence as a tool that wise people can cultivate and make use of as required, but it also asserts that wise people appreciate the need to handle intelligence carefully. This is because in the absence of wisdom, intelligence can become an obstacle to enlightenment and therefore an obstacle to the development of a dynamic and fluid wisdom (Shonin and Van Gordon 2014a).

2.6 The Path

The fourth noble truth that there is a path that leads to the cessation of suffering principally refers to the Noble Eightfold Path that comprises the elements of (i) right view, (ii) right intention, (iii) right speech, (iv) right action, (v) right livelihood,

(vi) right effort, (vii) right mindfulness, and (viii) right concentration. A more detailed discussion of the eightfold path and its relationship to mindfulness is provided in Chap. 2, so here we briefly outline three considerations concerning the eightfold path that we deem to be pertinent in the context of the current discussion:

1. *The Noble Eightfold Path Is One Path:* As inferred by the Buddha's teachings on the noble eightfold path in the *Mahācattārisaka Sutta* (*The Great Forty Sutta*; MN 117), although the eightfold path comprises eight individual elements, these elements should be considered as the individual strands that comprise a single rope. A rope is at its strongest when all of the strands are wound together, and it is only when practised and embodied as a single path that the noble eightfold path provides all of the factors necessary to attain liberation. In fact, the same principle applies to the entire collection of Buddhist teachings. Irrespective of the complexity, aspect (i.e. esoteric or exoteric), and intended audience of a particular strand of teachings, all authentic Dharma teachings take their place as part of a cohesive whole, and they originate from a single source. In effect, there is only one path to liberation, but it manifests in various guises in order to appeal to the differing needs, dispositions, and capacities of suffering beings.
2. *Treading the Path Requires Right Effort:* In order to realise their corresponding outcomes, Dharma teachings require continuous effort on behalf of the practitioner. This may seem like an obvious statement, but what is perhaps less obvious is the type of effort that is required. An individual can only be said to be making the "right effort" when they adhere to each of the following sets of advice provided by the Buddha:

    a. Understand and accept that nobody but themselves can eliminate their suffering:

    > You yourselves must strive; the Buddhas only point the way. Those meditative ones who tread the path are released from the bonds of Māra. (*Dhammapada*, 20, 276; Buddharakkhita 1986, p. 109)

    b. Make nothing less than complete liberation the object of their practice:

    > He whose cankers are destroyed…whose object is the void, the unconditioned freedom—his path cannot be traced, like that of birds in the air. (*Dhammapada*, 7, 93; Buddharakkhita 1986, p. 37)

    c. Adopt the middle way between extremes (e.g. of trying too hard and not trying hard enough, of being attached to possessions/material comforts and of being averse to having possessions/material comforts):

    > He who holds aloof from house holders and ascetics alike…him do I call a holy man. (*Dhammapada*, 26, 404; Buddharakkhita 1986, p. 159)

    d. At all times, hold the teacher and teachings as dear to their heart:

    > Of all the paths the eightfold path is the best; of all the truths the four noble truths are the best; of all things passionlessness is the best; of men the Seeing One (the Buddha) is the best. (*Dhammapada*, 20, 273; Buddharakkhita 1986, p. 109)

e. View their life as a practice ground and persevere at all times:

> Ever grows the glory of him who is energetic, mindful and pure in conduct, discerning and self-controlled, righteous and heedful. By effort and heedfulness, discipline and self-mastery, let the wise one make for himself an island which no flood can overwhelm. (*Dhammapada*, 2, 24–25; Buddharakkhita 1986, p. 11)

f. Offer loving-kindness and compassion unconditionally to all suffering beings:

> Come bhikkhus, abide pervading one quarter [of directional space] with a mind imbued with loving-kindness, likewise the second, likewise the third, likewise the fourth; so above, below, around and everywhere, and to all as to yourselves, abide pervading the all-encompassing world with a mind imbued with loving-kindness, abundant, exalted, immeasurable, without hostility and ill will. Abide pervading one quarter with a mind imbued with compassion, likewise the second, likewise the third, likewise the fourth; so above, below, around and everywhere and to all as to yourselves, abide pervading the all-encompassing world with a mind imbued with compassion, abundant, exalted, immeasurable, without hostility and ill will. (Nanamoli and Bodhi 2009, p. 434; MN 50)

3. *Any Attachment to A Path Must Be Relinquished:* In essence, walking the path is the practice of simply being and allowing the mind to relax into its natural state. Striving to do something other than this is an example of attachment and serves only to obscure pure perception:

> Whoever meditates on me will not encounter me precisely on account of that meditation. As I am the manifestation of the fundamental nature, [in my state] suffering does not arise, and consequently, there is no need to try to eliminate it [by walking a path]. (Norbu and Clemente 1999, p. 187)

2.7 Deductive Logical Analysis of the Four Noble Truths

Robust empirical investigation permits the credible testing of hypotheses that involve observable variables. However, the utility of empiricism comes into question when attempting to investigate subtle spiritual phenomena or metaphysical propositions (Puhakka 2015). For example, to date, no scientifically credible empirical study has been conducted that allows reliable conclusions to be drawn regarding the claim made in the third noble truth that sentient beings can transcend to a state of spiritual liberation in which suffering has completely ceased. However, as far as Buddhism is concerned, the absence of scientific evidence in support of a given theory or assertion does not necessarily present a cause for concern. This is not to say that Buddhism does not recognise or value empirical findings, because it most certainly does. Indeed, what in our opinion constitutes a particular strength of Buddhist doctrine is that if robust scientific evidence comes to light that invalidates a particular aspect of Buddhist thought, then Buddhism is dynamic and humble enough to re-evaluate its spiritual and philosophical outlook accordingly.

However, although Buddhism recognises the importance of empirical evidence, the value it assigns to different forms of scientific evidence arguably proceeds in the reverse direction compared with contemporary research paradigms. For example, the research and scientific community generally places experimental evidence (particularly from randomised controlled trials) much higher up the hierarchical-evidence pyramid than it does expert opinion. Buddhism, on the other hand, places much greater value on the opinion of spiritual adepts who are deemed to have directly tasted and penetrated the truth of existence. However, rather than some religious systems where followers are required or encouraged to accept claims made by the spiritually inspired as "the gospel truth", the emphasis in Buddhism is for practitioners to adopt such claims as hypotheses to be accepted or rejected based on their own meditative and spiritual experience.

In conjunction with the investigating of spiritual hypotheses on the personal and experiential level, a key technique utilised in Buddhist practice is the examining of a given proposition via the use of DLA. DLA lends itself to the testing of hypotheses or theoretical assumptions that involve non-observable variables. In essence, the technique makes use of top-down (i.e. deductive) logical principles (e.g. detachment, syllogism, contraposition) such that reliable conclusions can be drawn from a given starting premise. Of course, any conclusions reached by using DLA are only as reliable as the soundness of the original premise. However, where the assumptions of logical validity and scientific soundness are not violated throughout a given deductive logical sequence, then the final outcome can be regarded as being necessarily true. In this section, we use DLA in order to test the logical validity of the Four Noble Truths and, in particular, to assess whether those aspects of the Four Noble Truths that relate to non-observable phenomena represent logically plausible assertions.

Taken at face value, the Buddha's Four Noble Truths do not follow a coherent logical sequence. In the first noble truth, the Buddha states that "there is suffering", but in the third noble truth, he states that "there is non-suffering" (i.e. cessation). Thus, the third noble truth negates the first noble truth, and the second noble truth does not provide a plausible or logical explanation of why this is so. However, Buddhism (and contemporary science) accepts the principle of causality (i.e. effects rely on causes) and so by factoring this premise into a deductive logical sequence, the link between the first and third noble truths becomes apparent:

Sequence 1 (taking the first noble truth as a starting premise; P premise, C conclusion):

P1: There is suffering
P2: Phenomena exist in reliance upon causes
C: Therefore, there is a cause to suffering

Sequence 2 (taking the conclusion of sequence 1 as the starting premise):

P1: There is a cause to suffering
P2: Phenomena exist in reliance upon causes
C2: Therefore, removal of the causes of suffering leads to the removal of suffering

Sequence 1 above validates from a logical perspective both the first and second of the Buddha's noble truths (i.e. that suffering exists, and it has a cause). Taking the outcome of sequence 1 as the stating premise, sequence 2 then provides the logical validation for both the third and fourth noble truths (i.e. that there is the cessation of suffering which also has a cause—the cause of the end of suffering is treading the path that eradicates suffering).

Thus, in a single-sentence format, the Four Noble Truths could be rendered as follows: "There is suffering which has a cause and there is liberation which has a cause". However, because Buddhism accepts the principle of causality, even the above sentence could be condensed to a simpler form. For example, in stating that there is suffering, there is no requirement to then state that there is a cause to suffering because this is already implied. Likewise, since the statement "there is suffering" infers that suffering relies for its existence on certain causes (i.e. ignorance, attachment, and aversion), then it is already implied that the removal of these causes will lead to the eradication of suffering. In other words, the entire meaning of the Four Noble Truths can be captured by simply stating that "there is suffering" or "suffering exists" (or for want of being less pessimistic, the statement that "there is liberation" likewise implies each of the other noble truths).

However, although the statement "there is suffering" implies that suffering has a cause and that removal of the cause will lead to the cessation of suffering, it could be argued that this statement does not, by logical default, imply the existence of a path that can eradicate this suffering (i.e. the fourth noble truth). However, as demonstrated by sequence 3 below, such an objection can be easily overcome because upon stating that "there is suffering", the existence of "non-suffering" (i.e. liberation) is automatically established. In other words, at the same time as positing the existence of a relative phenomenon, the existence of its opposite is also posited. For example, if it is accepted that the "left" exists, then it must also be accepted that the "right" exists. The "left" only exists because there is "right"—if "right" is eliminated, then "left" no longer exists.

Sequence 3 (taking the conclusion of sequence 1 as the starting premise):

P1: There is suffering (which is diametrically opposed to liberation)
P2: The law of duality governs the existence of relative phenomena
C1: Therefore, there is liberation
P3: Phenomena exist in reliance upon causes
C2: There is a cause to liberation

Accordingly, the statement that "suffering exists" also implies that "liberation exists" and vice versa. Based on the principle of causality, having accepted that liberation exists, it now follows logically that liberation has a cause. The cause of liberation is none other than the path (i.e. the fourth truth), and it must now be accepted that (i) there exists a state of existence in which suffering has completely ceased and (ii) the meaning and essence of all four of the Buddha's noble truths are implicit within each truth individually.

2.8 Mindfulness of Suffering and Its Causes

The *Satipaṭṭhāna Sutta* (Sanskrit: *Smṛtyupasthāna Sūtra*; MN, 10) teaches that mindfulness should be developed across the following four frames of reference: (i) body, (ii) feelings, (iii) mind, and (iv) phenomena (collectively known as the "four establishments of mindfulness" or the "four foundations of mindfulness"). One of the principal reasons for this is because these four frames of reference are the precise locality where suffering abides. Outside of the body, feelings, mind, and (their perception of) phenomena, sentient beings do not experience suffering. As previously discussed, for a sentient being that has not attained liberation, suffering continuously manifests in each of these four domains. Therefore, to practice mindfulness correctly means to be fully aware of the suffering within the body, feelings, mind, and phenomena at any given point in time. This includes both the suffering that is currently manifest (i.e. the suffering of suffering) and the suffering that lies dormant and is yet to manifest (i.e. the suffering of change).

Consistent with the advice provided in the *Mindfulness of Breathing In and Out Sutta* (Pali: *Ānāpānasati Sutta*; Sanskrit: *Ānāpānasmṛti Sūtra;* MN 118), mindfulness of the suffering of suffering can be cultivated by using the breath to "tie the mind" to the present moment whilst awareness is directed to any palpable suffering present in the above-mentioned focal points (i.e. body, feelings, mind, and phenomena; Shonin et al. 2014a). For example, the third exercise of the *Ānāpānasati Sutta* simply involves resting awareness on the body, and the next exercise involves observing the body becoming calm and tranquil as a natural consequence of it being mindfully observed. The same process of attending mindfully to a particular focal point and then observing it calm and tranquilise (of its own accord) occurs again in the seventh and eighth exercises (which relate to calming mental formations), and once more in the ninth and tenth exercises (which relate to calming the mind).

Despite the above technique being taught by the Buddha for calming and introducing rapture into the body and mind, it is important to understand that contrary to the intent of some contemporary approaches to mindfulness practice, Buddhism does not promote the utilisation of mindfulness for the treatment of medical ailments and/or for the short-term relief of pain. According to Buddhist theory, a condition of their existence is that in one way or another (unenlightened) sentient beings must experience the consequences of their ego-driven actions (i.e. karma), and will continue to experience suffering until the point they attain enlightenment (Gampopa 1998). Of course, this is not to say that Buddhism does not support the use of medical or pharmacological intervention in order to minimise an individual's discomfort or pain. To advocate such an approach would run contrary to a central theme of Buddhist practice, which is the offering of loving-kindness and compassion towards all life forms. However, the point is that arresting a particular course of suffering at one point in time inevitably serves as the cause for an episode of suffering at a future point. Consequently, rather than striving to provide sentient beings with temporary relief from their (self-created) problems, Buddhism is concerned with equipping individuals with the knowledge, means, and motivation to permanently eradicate suffering at its roots (Dalai Lama 1995).

Thus, the practice of mindfulness of suffering is not about seeking a rapid recovery from a particular somatic or psychological problem. Rather, it is about developing a spiritual relationship with suffering so that the individual perceives and works with suffering in such a manner that suffering itself becomes a principal cause of liberation. Accordingly, the following are based on a synthesis of key Buddhist discourses and principles for working with suffering and outline what we believe to be essential requirements for practising mindfulness of the suffering of suffering effectively:

1. Accept the presence and inevitability of suffering for the duration of the spiritual journey.
2. Understand that the causes of suffering can be permanently eradicated.
3. Objectify suffering by adopting it as a meditative object.
4. Perceive that suffering continuously changes in both severity and variety.
5. Recognise that the intensity of suffering is inversely associated with the degree of tranquillity in the mind that experiences it.
6. Understand that suffering provides the raw material that the spiritual practitioner works with in order to attain liberation (without experiencing the starkness and unyielding nature of suffering, it is unlikely that sentient beings would choose to strive towards enlightenment).
7. Understand that ultimately, suffering is a relative phenomenon, and it relies for its existence on a "self" that can experience it.
8. Instinctively understand that the perceiver of suffering lacks inherent existence and, as such, suffering is a creation of the mind.

As referred to earlier in this chapter, unlike the suffering of suffering which is difficult for individuals not to notice, the suffering of change requires a deeper insight. Therefore, adopting it as the object of mindful awareness requires slightly more effort and intuition on behalf of the practitioner. Accordingly, in order to cultivate mindfulness of the suffering of change, the practitioner should aim to maintain a continuous awareness—to the point that it pervades all thought processes and arises automatically—of what are collectively known as the Four Summaries of the Dhamma (Nanamoli and Bodhi 2009, pp. 686–687; MN 82):

1. Life in any world is unstable; it is swept away.
2. Life in any world has no shelter and no protector.
3. Life in any world has nothing of its own; one has to leave all and pass on.
4. Life in any world is incomplete, insatiate, the slave of craving.

As implied by the Four Summaries of the Dhamma, the practise of mindfulness of the suffering of change requires perspectiv and clarity of vision on behalf of the practitioner. It also requires a full understanding of the principle and law of impermanence. Phenomena are born, they live, and they pass away. There are no exceptions to this rule—it is a mark of existence. The very fact that an individual enjoys good health serves as a cause for poor health at a future point. The fact that an individual is alive serves as the cause for death.

Mindfulness of the suffering of change requires the practitioner to have internalised and embodied the truth of impermanence to such a degree that it changes the way they interpret and process sensory information around them. The change we are referring to here could, in effect, be described as a form of metacognitive reappraisal. Instead of apprehending objects and situations as fixed or even existing, by practising mindfulness of the suffering of change, the meditation practitioner begins to perceive and instinctively understand that reality is completely fluid, transient, and ephemeral (Norbu and Clemente 1999). As such, the extent to which they crave after objects or experiences significantly diminishes, and in this manner, they no longer create the causes of suffering. Shonin and Van Gordon (2013, p. 107) have referred to this stage of realisation as "piercing through the present moment", and it gives rise to an awareness that transcends the constraints of thinking in terms of past, present, and future. The Buddha described this ability to non-conceptually observe and accept the coming and going of phenomena as follows:

> But let be the past, Udāyin, let be the future. I shall teach you the Dhamma: When this exists, that comes to be; with the arising of this, that arises. When this does not exist, that does not come to be; with the cessation of this, that ceases. (Nanamoli and Bodhi 2009, p. 655; MN 79)

Thus, attending with present moment awareness to the suffering that lies latent in every situation—including within (so-called) favourable circumstances—ultimately leads to the development of pure perception. In other words, practising mindfulness of suffering has the effect of honing an individual's perceptive faculties to the point that the practitioner is effectively forced to apprehend reality in its true form and render suffering as a cause for liberation.

A further and final consideration concerning the practice of mindfulness of suffering is developing an awareness of the suffering of others. Included in this awareness should be an appreciation of the suffering that others are currently experiencing, as well as the suffering that might arise in others due to unskilful thoughts, words, and deeds on behalf of the practitioner. Accordingly, the Dalai Lama (1995) has taught that spiritual practitioners have a responsibility for ensuring that their speech, writing, and general behaviour are infused with gentleness, wisdom, and awareness. In this respect, Buddhism asserts that all human beings are creators with the difference between the everyday person and the realised practitioner being that the latter is fully aware of their inherent creative potency:

> The realized being is like a master artist who uses the tools of insight, compassion, and skilful means to create a dynamic masterpiece of interwoven mind and matter upon the canvas of all-pervasive emptiness … Each of our thoughts, words, and actions dictate who we are now and who we will be in the future. Those same thoughts, words, and deeds also influence who others will be in the future. (Shonin and Van Gordon 2014b, p. 346)

In fact, the practitioner's responsibility for the effects of their actions does not stop at how they will influence other sentient being's happiness or suffering but also includes how they might introduce disorder into the ambient and natural environment around them. For example, based on the principle of interconnectedness, Shonin and Van Gordon (2014b) asserted that the mind directly influences the natural environment and that natural disasters such as tsunamis, earthquakes, and volcanic eruptions can be attributed to growing levels of negativity, selfishness, and ignorance in the hearts and minds of the population. Therefore, the type of awareness required to practise mindfulness of suffering effectively is not only incredibly encompassing but also it is unconditionally compassionate and extends well beyond the interests of the self.

2.9 Mindfulness of Cessation and Its Causes

Mindfulness of cessation and its causes principally involves maintaining a continuous meditative awareness of the practitioner's inherent potential for spiritual awakening. Buddhism asserts that practising mindfulness with the full knowledge and understanding that liberation is a real possibility—including within this lifetime—adds a new dimension to an individual's mindfulness practice and nourishes them with spiritual and meditative energy (Shonin and Van Gordon 2015). This "right intention" facilitates a broadening of perspective as well as the arising of a firm resolve to overcome any obstacles to complete spiritual awakening. According to Shonin and Van Gordon (2015, p. 144), by practising mindfulness with a firm intention to actualise their potential for liberation, the practitioner is able to tap into the lineage blessings that lie latent within them:

> The lineage we are referring to here is the universal Dharma lineage—or you can call it the lineage of mindfulness if you prefer. It belongs to nobody yet everybody can access it. It exists within every sentient being but only reveals itself to those that choose to live in awareness. In order to acquire this universal lineage, we do not need anybody's permission. We do not need to be empowered by another person and we do not need to attend any initiation ceremonies. We empower ourselves simply by being sincere and diligent in our practice. In fact, if you are sincere in your mindfulness practice—if your intentions are pure and wholesome—then progress and results will follow naturally. At this point, it doesn't matter in the slightest whether you belong to a religion or a meditation tradition, nor does it matter whether you have undergone an extensive study of the spiritual texts. You can take your place as an authentic heir to the mindfulness lineage.

The Buddha's third noble truth that there is cessation or liberation represents the primary goal of Buddhist practice. Consequently, every moment that spiritual practitioners apply themselves to spiritual development should be infused with both a firm belief in the truth of liberation and the knowledge that they are already innately liberated. This absolute conviction that liberation is a realistic eventuality avails to the practitioner hidden spiritual resources (Khyentse 2007). Put simply, by having complete faith that enlightenment comes from within and not without, practitioners cease to be bound by the idea of walking a path and of seeing themselves as separate from their goal. As long as the mind—which is already innately enlightened and inseparable from the realm of liberation—seeks to find liberation outside of itself, there is no alternative other than for it to remain trapped in the domain of dualistic perception. Indeed, Buddhism asserts that everything the mind perceives is already liberated and of the nature of mind (Shonin et al. 2014a). A mind that separates its single entity into both a subject and an object and then as a subject attempts to search for its object self, is destined to fail. Maintaining mindfulness of the fact that experience unfolds within the expanse of mind means that an individual is liberated, not being mindful of this means that they are deluded. Other than this, there is not a hair's breadth of difference between a Buddha and an ignorant being (Norbu and Clemente 1999).

Therefore, ultimately, there is no ascending to liberation, and grasping after liberation or any of the fruits of spiritual practice only serves as a cause of attachment and further suffering. Mindfulness of the causes of cessation/liberation means remaining aware of this fact and of the need to abandon clinging—no matter how subtle:

> Here Ānanda, a bhikkhu is practising thus … What exists, what has come to be, that I am abandoning. Thus he obtains equanimity. He delights in that equanimity, welcomes it, and remains holding to it. As he does so, his consciousness becomes dependant on it and clings to it. A bhikkhu with clinging, Ānanda, does not attain Nibbāna. (Nanamoli and Bodhi 2009, p. 872; MN 106)

The same principle applies to being attached to the idea of being a spiritual practitioner or of being a recipient of the lineage of mindfulness:

> Along with being a holder of the lineage of mindfulness comes a tremendous responsibility to keep the lineage teachings alive and authentic. However, the way to do this is not by trying to own or protect the lineage, but by letting go of it. This is because lineage is, and has to be, completely dynamic. As you grow in awareness, the teachings that are all around and within you change and present themselves in different ways. Therefore, if you want the lineage to endure and remain effective, then you have to allow it to evolve—and you have to evolve with it. The way to allow things to evolve is to simply be and allow experience to unfold without clinging to it. You have to understand that the moment you become attached to the lineage of mindfulness, it slips through your fingers and you cease being an authentic lineage holder. (Shonin and Van Gordon 2015, p. 144)

By not attaching themselves to situations, achievements, or experiences, Buddhism asserts that mindfulness practitioners remain unbound to any time or place. In other words, they establish as their home the present moment and enjoy freedom and refuge wherever they find themselves:

> The mindful ones exert themselves. They are not attached to any home; like swans that abandon the lake, they leave home after home behind. (*Dhammapada*, 7, 91; Buddharakkhita 1986, p. 37)

In essence, the final four insight exercises of the *Ānāpānasati Sutta* provide a means of practising and establishing mindfulness of cessation and its causes. There are differing views amongst Buddhist scholars and traditions as to whether the experiences/realisations referred to in the final tetrad of the 16 *Ānāpānasati Sutta* exercises arise of their own accord (i.e. as a natural consequence of practising the foregoing 12 exercises) or whether they require a deliberate and subtle shift in meditative mode. It is our view (and experience) that the latter scenario is the case, but ultimately such differing opinions are of limited consequence. The key point is that having first calmed and immersed the body, feelings, and mind in mindful awareness, the mind is then suitably disposed for insight into manifest. In order of appearance (i.e. beginning with exercise 13 and finishing with exercise 16), the insights that the *Ānāpānasati Sutta* refers to are a spiritual comprehension of impermanence, fading away, cessation, relinquishment. These spiritual realisations essentially describe the practitioner's passage from the relative to the absolute realm, and the inclusion of cessation and relinquishment in the 15th and 16th *Ānāpānasati Sutta* exercises refers, precisely, to the cessation and relinquishment of self and therefore of suffering that the practitioner experiences as they relax progressively further into their intrinsic wakeful state.

2.10 Conclusion

As with all Buddhist practices, mindfulness is deeply connected to the Buddha's teaching of the Four Noble Truths. The quintessential message of the Four Noble Truths is that until a sentient being attains spiritual liberation (the third truth), it will suffer (the first truth), and the only way to end this suffering is to walk the path (the fourth truth) that acts upon the causes of suffering (the second truth). A mindfulness practice that does not encompass and remain attentive to these four truths of existence cannot be said to embody the authentic Dharma. Suffering is a mark of existence, but by incorporating suffering into the sphere of mindful awareness, Buddhism asserts that suffering itself can become a causal agent of liberation. In other words, as demonstrated by the outcome of the DLA performed earlier in this chapter, within the truth of suffering exists the truth of liberation—and for that matter, the truth of the entire collection of the Buddha's teachings.

From a Buddhist perspective, practising mindfulness with a firmly embedded understanding of the principles implied and outlined by the Four Noble Truths helps the individual to remain acutely aware of why they are practising mindfulness as well as the severity of their predicament. Without such awareness, and without an unshakeable resolve to permanently uproot the causes of suffering, there is a distinct possibility that the mindfulness practitioner's efforts will be in vain, and their practice will remain at the superficial level. From a Buddhist perspective, this is the same as abandoning the spiritual path—a fate that we would argue is worse than death itself:

> For it is death in the Discipline of the Noble One, Sunakkhatta, when one abandons the training to the low life. (Nanamoli and Bodhi 2009, p. 866; MN 105)

Acknowledgments Some parts of this chapter significantly expand upon and adapt content or themes that originally appeared in the following publications: Shonin et al. (2014a, b) and Shonin and Van Gordon (2014a). Meditation Practice and Research Blog. Available at www.edoshonin.com.

References

Baltes, P. B., & Staudinger, U. M. (2000). Wisdom: A metaheuristic (pragmatic) to orchestrate mind and virtue toward excellence. *American Psychologist, 55,* 122–136.
Bodhi, B. (2000). *The connected discourses of the Buddha: A new translation of the Samyutta Nikaya.* Massachusetts: Wisdom.
Buddharakkhita. (1986). *Dhammapada: A practical guide to right living.* Bangalore: Maha Bodhi Society.
Dalai Lama. (1995). *Essential teachings.* London: Souvenir.
Dalai Lama., & Berzin, A. (1997). *The Gelug/Kagyu tradition of mahamudra.* New York: Snow Lion.
Gampopa. (1998). *The jewel ornament of liberation: The wish-fulfilling gem of the noble teachings.* New York: Snow Lion.
Khyentse, D. (2007). *The heart of compassion: The thirty-seven verses on the practice of a bodhisattva.* Boston: Shambhala.
Nanamoli B., & Bodhi, B. (2009). *Majjhima Nikaya: The middle length discourses of the Buddha* (4th ed.). Massachusetts: Wisdom.
Norbu, C., & Clemente, A. (1999). *The supreme source. The fundamental tantra of the Dzogchen Semde.* New York: Snow Lion.
Puhakka, K. (2015). *Encountering the psychological research paradigm: How Buddhist practice has fared in the most recent phase of its western migration.* In E. Shonin, W. Van Gordon, & N. N. Singh (Eds.), *Buddhist foundations of mindfulness.* New York: Springer.
Sahdra, B. K., Shaver, P. R., & Brown, K. W. (2010). A scale to measure non-attachment: A Buddhist complement to Western research on attachment and adaptive functioning. *Journal of Personality Assessment, 92,* 116–127.
Shonin, E., & Van Gordon, W. (2013). Searching for the present moment. *Mindfulness, 5,* 105–107.
Shonin, E., & Van Gordon, W. (2014a). Can a person be Ignorant and Intelligent at the same time? Located at http://edoshonin.com/2014/06/11/can-a-person-be-ignorant-and-intelligent-at-the-same-time/. Accessed 11 June 2011.
Shonin, E., & Van Gordon, W. (2014b). The consuming mind. *Mindfulness, 5,* 345–347.
Shonin, E., & Van Gordon, W. (2015). The lineage of mindfulness. *Mindfulness, 6,* 141–145.
Shonin, E., Van Gordon W., & Griffiths, M. D. (2013). Buddhist philosophy for the treatment of problem gambling. *Journal of Behavioural Addictions, 2,* 63–71.
Shonin, E., Van Gordon W., & Griffiths, M. D. (2014a). The emerging role of Buddhism in clinical psychology: Toward effective integration. *Psychology of Religion and Spirituality, 6,* 123–137.
Shonin, E., Van Gordon, W., & Griffiths, M. D. (2014b). Changing paradigms: Buddhist insight in western psychological treatments. *Psy-PAG Quarterly, 92,* 35–39.
Shonin, E., Van Gordon, W., Compare, A., Zangeneh, M., & Griffiths, M. D. (2015). Buddhist-derived loving-kindness and compassion meditation for the treatment of psychopathology: A systematic review. *Mindfulness.* doi:10.1007/s12671–014-0368–1.
Tsong-Kha-pa. (2004). *The great treatise on the stages of the path to enlightenment* (Vol. 1). New York: Snow Lion.

William Van Gordon has been a Buddhist monk for 10 years and is operations director of the International Mahayana Bodhayati School of Buddhism. He is co-founder of the Awake to Wisdom Centre for Meditation and Mindfulness Research and is a research psychologist based at the Nottingham Trent University (UK). He is currently principal investigator on a number of randomised controlled trials investigating the applications of an intervention known as meditation awareness training (MAT) in clinical and occupational settings. He sits on the editorial board for the *International Journal of Buddhism* and has more than 100 academic publications relating to the scientific study of Buddhism and associated meditative approaches.

Edo Shonin has been a Buddhist monk for 30 years and is spiritual director of the International Mahayana Bodhayati School of Buddhism. He is research director of the Awake to Wisdom Centre for Meditation and Mindfulness Research and a research psychologist at the Nottingham Trent University (UK). He sits on the International Advisory Board for the journal *Mindfulness* and is an editorial board member of the *International Journal of Mental Health and Addiction*. He is internationally known for his work and has more than 100 academic publications relating to the scientific study of mindfulness and Buddhist practice. He runs the *Meditation Practice and Research Blog* at www.edoshonin.com.

Mark D. Griffiths is a chartered psychologist and professor of gambling studies at the Nottingham Trent University and director of the International Gaming Research Unit. He has spent almost 30 years in the field and is internationally known for his work into gambling, gaming, and other behavioural addictions. More recently, he has published many papers on the practical applications of mindfulness with Edo Shonin and William Van Gordon. He has published over 500 refereed research papers, four books, 120+ book chapters, and over 1000 other articles. He has won 14 national and international awards for his work including the *John Rosecrance Prize* (1994), *CELEJ Prize* (1998), *Joseph Lister Prize* (2004), and the US *National Council on Problem Gambling Lifetime Research Award* (2013). He also does a lot of freelance journalism and has appeared on over 2500 radio and television programmes.

Nirbhay N. Singh is a clinical professor of psychiatry and health behaviour at the Medical College of Georgia, Georgia Regents University, Augusta, Georgia, USA. Prior to his current appointment, he was a professor of psychiatry, pediatrics, and psychology at the Virginia Commonwealth University School of Medicine and director of the Commonwealth Institute for Family Studies, Richmond, Virginia. His research interests include mindfulness, behavioural and psychopharmacological treatments of individuals with disabilities, and assistive technology for supporting individuals with severe/profound and multiple disabilities. He is the editor-in-chief of two journals: *Journal of Child and Family Studies and Mindfulness* and editor of three book series: *Mindfulness in Behavioral Health, Evidence-based Practice in Behavioral Health*, and *Children and Families*.

Chapter 3
Mindfulness and the Buddha's Noble Eightfold Path

Malcolm Huxter

3.1 Introduction

In the late 1970s, Kabat-Zinn, an immunologist, was on a Buddhist meditation retreat practicing mindfulness meditation. Inspired by the personal benefits, he developed a strong intention to share these skills with those who would not normally attend retreats or wish to practice meditation. Kabat-Zinn developed and began conducting mindfulness-based stress reduction (MBSR) in 1979. He defined mindfulness as, "the awareness that emerges through paying attention on purpose, in the present moment, and non-judgmentally to the unfolding of experience moment to moment" (Kabat-Zinn 2003, p. 145). Since the establishment of MBSR, thousands of individuals have reduced psychological and physical suffering by attending these programs (see www.unmassmed.edu/cfm/mbsr/). Furthermore, the research into and popularity of mindfulness and mindfulness-based programs in medical and psychological settings has grown exponentially (Kabat-Zinn 2009).

Kabat-Zinn (1990) deliberately detached the language and practice of mindfulness from its Buddhist origins so that it would be more readily acceptable in Western health settings (Kabat-Zinn 1990). Despite a lack of consensus about the finer details (Singh et al. 2008), Kabat-Zinn's operational definition of mindfulness remains possibly the most referred to in the field. Dozens of empirically validated mindfulness-based programs have emerged in the past three decades. However, the most acknowledged approaches include: MBSR (Kabat-Zinn 1990), dialectical behavior therapy (DBT; Linehan 1993), acceptance and commitment therapy (ACT; Hayes et al. 1999), and mindfulness-based cognitive therapy (MBCT; Segal et al. 2002).

In its appropriation into the scientific community, mindfulness has had to, understandably, be free from many of the religious and cultural additions that these

M. Huxter (✉)
Westminster Centre for Resilience, University of Westminster, 115 New Cavendish St, London W1W 6UW, UK
e-mail: malhuxter@gmail.com

E. Shonin et al. (eds.), *Buddhist Foundations of Mindfulness*,
Mindfulness in Behavioral Health, DOI 10.1007/978-3-319-18591-0_3

teachings had acquired over the centuries. Unfortunately, the timely and appropriate distillation of mindfulness from a Buddhist framework in the early 1980s continued over the following decades, and for many it became the accepted protocol. When Baer (2003) wrote a well-read and cited empirical review of mindfulness training as a clinical intervention, the Buddhist framework hardly received a mention. Currently, the importance of Buddhist psychology in the therapeutic endeavor is beginning to be recognized and acknowledged (e.g., Didonna 2009; Williams and Kabat-Zinn 2013). Up until very recently, however, mindfulness in contemporary psychology has usually been taught in a manner that is absent of any particular philosophical, cultural tradition, or vocabulary (Allen et al. 2006). According to some Buddhist psychotherapists, the practices

> have become dislodged from their ethical and philosophical frames and redefined in ways intelligible to secular, scientific minds. (Dawson and Turnbull 2006, p. 60)

In the twenty-first century, the interest in and benefits of mindfulness have moved beyond the domains of health and psychotherapy to include neuroscience, education, the military, the justice system, and the corporate sector (e.g., Carroll 2011; Davidson et al. 2003; Stone 2014; Wilson 2014). No longer on the fringe of society as an alternative activity, mindfulness has become a mainstream interest. Lifestyle magazines regularly feature articles about mindfulness, and according to one major advertising company it is one of ten trends that will shape our world in 2014 and beyond (http://www.jwt.com/blog/consumer_insights/10-trends-that-will-shape-our-world-in-2014-and-beyond/). Mindfulness is now a commodity with a growing market value (Wilson 2014). We can find on the shelves of our Internet supermarket products such as "mindful mayonnaise" (e.g., http://earthbalancenatural.com/product/original-mayo/), indicating that mere associations with the word are a selling point. As the contemporary world embraces mindfulness, the meaning and details of the practice that originally inspired Kabat-Zinn, in 1979, seem to have drifted away. Currently, mindfulness can mean many different things.

Long-term Buddhist meditation practitioners have mixed feelings about the popularization and commodification of mindfulness. On the one hand, we celebrate such a powerful healing tool being readily available, albeit at a price, to the world. On the other hand, some of us feel discomfort about how the public perception of mindfulness sometimes seems superficial, confused, and naïve (Huxter 2013). The meaning of what is to the long-term meditation practitioner a profoundly liberating practice seems to have become diluted, obscured, and presented in a manner that is tangential to the Buddha's original descriptions.

In 2014, 35 years after Kabat-Zinn launched MBSR into a world cautious about the influence of Eastern religions, it is perhaps timely to fully remove the camouflage hiding the Buddhist origins of this practice. Perhaps it is timely to unreservedly clarify the details of this practice in accordance with its foundations. In this chapter, I highlight the Theravada Buddhist understanding of mindfulness. Then, in order to connect mindfulness to a context of wisdom, ethics, and meditation, I discuss mindfulness in the relation to the Buddha's eightfold path.

3.2 Mindfulness: The Buddha's Perspective

Despite the lack of consensus, most contemporary psychologists describe mindfulness in a way that is roughly similar to Kabat-Zinn's operational definition cited earlier. This definition, however, describes only part of what is known in the Buddhist traditions as mindfulness. The contemporary definitions of mindfulness are more consistent with what modern Buddhist meditation teachers call "bare attention."

According to Wallace (2008, p. 60), "bare attention corresponds most closely to the Pali term *manasikara,* which is commonly translated as "attention" or "mental engagement." This word refers to the initial split seconds of the bare cognizing of an object before one begins to recognize, identify, and conceptualize." Bare attention may be an aspect of Buddhist mindfulness. However, according to the traditional perspectives, mindfulness is much more than just nonjudgmentally being aware. Mindfulness was the word that an English-born Pali scholar used in 1881 to translate the term *sati. Sati* literally means "memory". *Sati* involves *remembering* to be attentive. The opposite of *sati* is forgetfulness. With forgetfulness, we forget to be present, forget our purpose, and forget the lessons from the past. *Sati* is the type of memory that can be trained and cultivated. According to the ancient texts on Buddhist psychology, *sati,* is a form of recollecting or calling back to mind or bearing in mind (Narada 1956).

Wallace (2008, p. 60) wrote that mindfulness *(sati):* "includes retrospective memory of things in the past, prospectively remembering to do something in the future, and present-centered recollection in the sense of maintaining unwavering attention to a present reality." In resonance with Wallace, mindfulness has also been described as remembering where we are, what we are doing, and who we are with (Hanh 1975, 1998) as well as the presence of mind (Bodhi 2000b).

In possibly the most authoritative text on Buddhist meditation, the *Visuddhimagga* written by Buddhaghosa in 412 AC, other features of mindfulness are highlighted as follows:

> Its characteristic is not floating; its property is not losing; its manifestation is guarding or the state of being face to face with an object; its basis is strong noting or the close applications of mindfulness of the body and so on. It should be seen as like a post due to its state of being set in the object, and as like a gatekeeper [preventing the unwholesome from entering the mind and allowing the wholesome to enter] because it guards the gate of the eye and so on. (Nanamoli 1956, p. 524)

The practice of mindfulness may include bare attention or *manasikara,* but it is not limited to it. With bare attention, judgments and interpretations are suspended in favor of noting experience as it is, here now, not lost in proliferative elaboration and embellishment. When the remembering aspect of mindfulness is combined with bare attention, it connects the many moments of experience in a way that brings understanding. The connection of distinct and separate moments of attention is analogous to a child's dot-to-dot drawing. When the child makes the effort to connect the dots together, a coherent picture emerges and one sees the big picture. Understanding takes into account the big and broad picture of the stream of consciousness as it meanders and flows through the moment-to-moment, week-to-week, year-to-year experience called life. The application of mindfulness provides a way to connect the moments, weeks, months, and years so that there is insight and a coherent picture of our lives.

Sati is often coupled with another mental factor called *sampajanya* as *sati-sampajanya.* This coupling points to the strength of the connections between these two mental factors. *Sampajanya* translates as clear comprehension or introspection. *Sampajanya* involves understanding the purpose, timeliness, and suitability of what one is doing. In relation to meditation, it is a form of meta-awareness and quality control. When meditation involves focusing on an object, mindfulness remembers to prevent attention straying from the object, while *sampajanya* recognizes that attention has strayed (Wallace 2008).

Sati in combination with other helpful factors such as *sampajanya* leads to the development of wisdom. In Buddhism, wisdom *(punya)* can refer to reason, logic, and intuitive knowing. It can involve the coherent picture, mentioned above, of our own and other lives so that we can make decisions about what is helpful and what is not helpful on our journey towards what is meaningful for us. Wisdom involves understanding the picture of our lives in combination with intentions to act skillfully. When we can remember the purpose of our actions, what we are doing and where we are going, we are more able to live in alignment with wisely chosen life directions. From a Buddhist perspective, skillful mindfulness cannot be separated from the context of wise discernment and acting in accordance with principles of harmlessness, which are integral aspects of the Buddha's the eightfold path leading to awakening.

3.3 Awakening to the Four Noble Truths

Synonymous with the term "enlightenment," awakening can refer to radical transformations of consciousness where individuals wake up to the truths of existence. Systems of practice that lead to awakening have been called the consciousness disciplines (Walsh 1980). The contemplative traditions of Theravada Buddhism, Tibetan Buddhism, and Hindu Yoga are examples of consciousness disciplines that may lead to awakening (Brown 1986). According to Brown (1986), scholars have different ideas about how the different traditions perceive the path of practice and ultimate reality. Despite differences, all traditions agree that awakening "produces two major changes: the view of external reality is permanently altered and the internal experience of suffering is alleviated" (Brown 1986, p. 268). Thus, the results of awakening are that suffering is released and there are radical transformations of perceptions and consciousness. The honorific term "Buddha" comes from the Pali verb root "*budh,*" which means "to understand" or "to awaken." Historically, Siddhartha Gotama became a Buddha about 2560 years ago, and he taught ways to understand or awaken to the four noble truths. In essence, the four noble truths are two cause–effect relationships: suffering and its causes, freedom from suffering, and the causes for this. The first noble truth in Pali is termed *dukkha.* Though *dukkha* is often translated as suffering, the words "discontent" or "unsatisfactoriness" may more accurately capture the meaning of this term. The extent of *dukkha* can range from the gross and obvious such as severe illness and death to the subtle and obscure, such as not getting what we want exactly how we want it. The main aim of the Buddha's teachings is freedom from *dukkha* via the realization of the four noble truths.

The term "noble" is used to describe profoundly awakened realizations and impeccable behaviors that result from these realizations. The relationships evident in the four noble truths can also be applied to the patterns evident in more basic human issues including psychological disorders and ways to work with these disorders. At this basic level, the four truths could be described as "ennobling" (Bodhi 2000a) because, though not yet signifying profound realizations, they are nonetheless reducing the severity of suffering. According to Huxter (2009), the four ennobling truths could be described from a cognitive behavioral therapy perspective as follows:

1. There are presenting problems or disorders *(dukkha)*.
2. There are causative factors leading to the development of disorders and psychological patterns maintaining them *(the causes of dukkha)*.
3. It is possible to reduce the level of suffering or completely resolve the problem (freedom from *dukkha*).
4. There are treatments using cognitive, behavioral, and affective strategies that address both the causative and maintaining factors (the causes for freedom from *dukkha*).

3.4 The Fourth Truth: The Buddha's Eightfold Path

The eightfold path is also called the middle way because it is balanced with moderation and does not incline to extremes of self-indulgence or self-denial. The Buddha's eight-factored path is a way to balance any imbalances of connotation, attention, cognition, and affect (Wallace and Shapiro 2006). It contains factors that are in opposition to the patterns driven by what Buddhists call the root causes of *dukkha:* craving/clinging, aversion/hatred, and confusion/ignorance. The eightfold path is a general framework which has within it numerous subsystems, all of which work together in a manner that inhibits or uproots the types of mental, emotional, and behavioral patterns that cause and perpetuate psychological suffering. This path and its subsystems also nurture what is best by cultivating optimal, compassionate, and wise ways of perceiving, being, and understanding.

According to some scholars, the path has two levels, ennobling and noble (Bodhi 2000a; Thanissaro 1996). The first, fundamental or ennobling level leads to the alleviation of severity of *dukkha.* Most contemporary psychotherapies utilize strategies consistent with the ennobling eightfold path. When the ennobling path has been travelled and there is an alleviation of *dukkha* with some stress reduction, the conditions for a vision of Nirvana are more likely. With even just a glimpse of Nirvana, major psychological transformations occur and a more refined and noble level of the path can be followed, leading to complete liberation.

The Buddha's eightfold path is divided into three basic trainings, which are: wisdom with two factors (right understanding, view, or conceptualization and right intention, resolve, thought, or vision), ethics or a wholesome lifestyle with three factors (right action, speech, and livelihood, or upkeep), and meditation with another three factors (right effort, mindfulness, and concentration). Each factor on the path starts with the word right. Right is the usual translation of the Pali term *samma*. Other ways *samma* could be understood include: complete, authentic, fully, skillful, appropriate, or correct. The eight factors support each other to collectively lead towards freedom from *dukkha*. These interdependent factors are "comparable to the intertwining strands of a single cable that requires the contributions of all the strands for maximum strength" (Bodhi 2000a, p. 13).

At a basic ennobling level, right view is the understanding that actions have consequences and that unhelpful actions often lead to things not working out for the best. Right view leads to making skillful decisions and commitments to act in ways that are harmless, kind, and liberating (right intention). When one acts in a manner that is wise (right speech, action, and livelihood), there is a level of mental composure that is conducive to motivation and focused attention. Looking at oneself honestly (mindfulness) often requires courageous effort. The combination of effort, remembering to be attentive, and seeing deeply with focused attention gives rise to understanding. When understanding arises, this leads to right intentions, then right actions and the path of liberation continues. In essence, this eight-factored pathway describes a process for changing or releasing unhelpful habits and behaviors and developing, instead, what is helpful to reach desired goals that are beneficial for self and others.

3.5 Wisdom Training

According to Thanissaro (2006), "the Buddha had a simple test for measuring wisdom. You're wise, he said, to the extent that you can get yourself to do things you don't like doing but know will result in happiness, and to refrain from things you like doing but know will result in pain and harm." A Buddhist perspective of wisdom is that it is manifold and includes the factors of view and intention, seeing, and volition. Wisdom guides strategies to abandon the thinking and emotional and behavioral patterns that lead to being bound up in *dukkha.* The seeing aspect of wisdom can refer to knowledge, understanding, or insight about how suffering arises and how it is abandoned. The intentional aspects of wisdom include the interpersonal and intrapersonal correlates of insight, which are loving-kindness, compassion, and letting go. Wisdom can arise from meditation (effort, mindfulness, and concentration). It can also arise from hearing or reading wise words and reflection or thinking clearly and realistically. Thus, wisdom may include the helpful thinking processes encouraged by therapies such as cognitive therapy (Beck 1976). However, wisdom is not limited to this type of verbal and logical thought as it can include a nonverbal knowing that is described by some as intuitive (Pandita 1992).

Intuitive knowing involves being able to remember, know, and plan for what could be the best course of action for any particular situation. What is remembered may not be readily available in conscious verbal memory, but is readily available in the form of intuitive nonverbal knowing. An intuitive medical practitioner in an emergency, for example, may have a sense that something is not quite right in their patient and know, intuitively, that a particular course of intervention is needed. At the time of the emergency, this particular medical practitioner may not be able to articulate or consciously access verbal and rational information about the problem. However, she knows from experience and this knowledge has been stored in the unconscious so that it is retrieved intuitively. In this case, the doctor has clinical wisdom and it is accessed nonverbally. Wisdom about life can result from remembering to be attentive to experience (mindfulness). Such wisdom may be able to be articulated verbally or it may be simply a silent knowing.

3.6 Right View

Right view is the first stage of the path and the first aspect of wisdom. Without a clear perspective on where to go it is easy to get lost. Right view is also the result of the path. That is, when we begin to make wise decisions to act in a way that avoids harm it helps us see clearly, which circles back to shape our attitudes, the ways we think and further decisions we make about life. With a clear view, our perception of things is no longer distorted by ideas that are unhelpful. One fundamental distortion, according to the Buddha's discourses, is the view that things are permanent, independent, and able to be controlled. The belief that actions do not have consequences and that we can behave unethically without consequences, is another mistaken view according to the teachings of the Buddha. Such a view means that individuals do not see that the way they behave in the world has an impact. At a more subtle level, this view means that people do not see how everything is, somehow or other, connected to everything else, and that what we do affects others and the environment around us. The ennobling level of right view has already been mentioned. At the noble level, right view refers to seeing the four noble truths, completely. It also entails the profound perspectives on consciousness and the world that these realization produce.

When we are able to see clearly with insight that specific actions may lead to specific consequences, we may be more willing to act in ways that produce less suffering. The Pali term for insight is *vipassana.* According to scholars, the *vi* of *vipassana* denotes separate, intense, or distinct and the *passana* refers to seeing. Therefore, *vipassana* literally translates as seeing separately and seeing distinctly (Kearney 1995). In resonance with this meaning, Goleman (1988, p. 123) wrote that insight can refer to "the clear perception of the object as it really is." Insight directly counters ignorance and it is a key factor in being able to bring an end to *dukkha.* Insight is the realization of the four truths and knowing, at an experiential level, three universal characteristics of existence.

3.7 Three Universal Characteristics of Existence

Also called the three marks of existence, the three universal characteristics of existence according to Buddhism are:

1. *Annica:* impermanence or change
2. *Dukkha:* discontent, unreliability, ambiguity, uncertainty, or not a source of genuine happiness
3. *Anatta:* interdependence, no-thing-ness, no self-ness, insubstantiality, contingency, or emptiness (Huxter 2007)

These three universal characteristics of existence, each linked, describe the nature of things from three angles. Everything changes *(annica)* and because it does, nothing is reliable or certain *(dukkha)*. *Dukkha* when it is described as a characteristic of existence is slightly different to how it is described as the first noble truth. Things such as a chair or a bottle of water, for example, can display the characteristic of *dukkha*. We cannot rely on a chair or a bottle, or any other thing to last because their nature is impermanent. This sense of unreliability is *dukkha.* To put it another way, impermanent things are *dukkha* because they cannot be reliable sources of enduring happiness. The third characteristic of existence, *anatta,* is yet another perspective on the nature of things. In Pali, *atta* refers to self and *anatta* refers to not-self. Here, self refers to the incorrect view that things are independently self-arising. This view means that phenomena arise independent from causes and conditions, which is, of course, contrary to the way things actually are. As a characteristic of existence, *anatta* describes that changing phenomena are interdependent. That is, individual things depend on other things for their existence. The term emptiness is sometimes used to describe *anatta* in that things, including you and me and my chair and bottle, are empty of inherent self-existence.

Insight has many levels. At an ennobling level, insight about the three characteristics of existence has a generalizing effect with clinical implications. Seeing the impermanence *(annica)* and interdependence *(anatta)* of something external such as melting snow turning into a flowing stream can be generalized to something internal such as painful thoughts and emotions, and seeing that they too are changing, dependent on other things for their arising and passing and need not be taken personally. One of the aims of MBCT (Segal et al. 2002) is the development of meta-cognitive insight. Meta-cognitive insight refers to "experiencing thoughts as thoughts (that is as events in the mind rather than direct readouts on reality" (Teasdale et al. 2002, p. 286). By developing meta-cognitive insight, MBCT participants resist feeding into ruminative thoughts, thereby short circuiting a process that previously bound them to relapse with depression. Meta-cognitive insight can develop by shifting the focus of attention from the contents of thoughts to the relationship with thoughts as well as seeing the general unreliability or *dukkha* of these events.

3.8 Right Intention

Right intentions are also sometimes called right thought. Here, thought has a resolute or purposeful nature. At a macro level, intentions can steer us through the bigger picture of our whole life. When we are clear about what causes suffering and what leads away from suffering, it is easier to make important decisions about the direction we wish our lives to take. At a micro level, intentions are involved in the moment-to-moment actions of our everyday life. At the micro level we may have thousands of intentions every day. If we want to short circuit reactive patterns of *dukkha,* it helps to be mindful of skillful and unskillful intentions. Skillful intentions are those intentions that lead to happiness for our self and other beings in the long run. Unskillful intentions are those intentions that lead us to act in a manner that may complicate our lives or harm our self or others. The Buddha explained that unwholesome intentions are those directed by craving, ill will, and ignorance and eventually lead to harm. In direct opposition to this, right intentions are those based on wisdom, letting go, and good will that do not result in harm.

The first type of right intention is renunciation. Renunciation involves letting go of craving, grasping at, and clinging to views, concepts, and experiences. Intentions of good will are the second type of right intentions. Unwholesome intentions driven by ill will are major obstacles to meditation and the cause of much suffering. The direct opposite and remedy for ill will is loving-kindness or *metta. Metta* is the cultivation of unconditional care, goodwill, and warm friendliness towards self, other beings, and experience in general. The third type of skillful intention is harmlessness. Compassion is a human response to suffering and is the wish for beings (including ourselves) to be free from suffering. The aspiration to avoid harm and foster compassion are examples of the third types of right intentions.

3.9 Ethical Training

Intentional actions that do not cause harm could be considered as ethical actions. Moreover, compassion and kindness could be considered as universal ethics. In Pali, the word for ethical training is *sila* which is often translated as morality or virtue. In traditional Buddhist meditation, ethical behaviors provide a level of life stability that is necessary for the cultivation of the mind. Ethical behavior provides us with enough mental composure and a lightness of conscience that enables us to concentrate and be mindful at levels that are conducive to meditation. In the traditions, ethical behaviors are considered a prerequisite for training in meditation because they are the foundation upon which the practice is built. In a Buddhist framework, the risks and dangers of meditation, such as when we arrive at stages of insight where *dukkha* becomes lucidly evident, are well known (Nanamoli 1956; Nyanaponika 1994). Having an ethical foundation and lifestyle is considered an important protective factor to help manage possible difficult negative side effects of meditation practice.

Acting with ethical integrity includes making the choice to be harmless in our actions. When we are not intentionally harming ourselves or others, it is likely that our minds will not be plagued with hatred, guilt, or fear. When we avoid harmful speech, actions, and occupations, our conscience is more likely to be clear and our minds more easily able to focus on the immediate experience of life.

3.10 Right Speech

Many of us communicate with others a lot of the time and most of us talk to our selves, most of the time. As expressions of greed, ignorance, and hatred, words have the power to inflict great harm. Through our communications we can, however, also express the qualities of generosity, wisdom, and kindness which promote healing, well-being, happiness, and awakening in self and others. Right speech involves communicating with intentions that further our journey along a path of healing and awakening. Right speech includes words that are encouraging, constructive, helpful, kind, and supportive. Right speech involves *sampajanya* or the clear comprehension of what should be spoken, when, and how, in accordance with purpose, timeliness, and appropriateness. Right speech usually involves being honest. If however, being frank is not helpful then right speech may involve telling a white lie. If it is not appropriate or timely to speak then being silent is also considered to be right speech.

3.11 Right Action

Right actions involve behaving in ways that are consistent with wholesome and wise directions. Wrong actions involve going against valued directions, resulting in unhappiness and a general increase of *dukkha*. Actions that are consistent with the eightfold path vary from one individual to the next, but the general principle is to avoid intentional harm and participate instead in actions based on generosity, kindness, compassion, and wisdom. The five Buddhist precepts reflect the themes of right action and, though they can be considered as proactively engaging in helpful behaviors (Hanh 1993), they are most often described as training to avoid behaviors that will in some form or other be harmful. The first three of the five precepts are avoid unnecessary killing, avoid taking what is not freely offered (i.e., theft) and avoid sensual misconduct, which usually means sexual contact where someone is hurt or harmed. The last two of the five precepts include avoiding false and harsh (wrong) speech and avoiding having the mind clouded by unwise use of intoxicants or drugs.

3.12 Right Livelihood

The next factor on the path is right livelihood, which refers to making a living that is consistent with liberating life directions. It refers to how we provide for the needs and desires of our self and our dependents. Most of us spend a large percentage of our time in the workplace. Our work can be can be a source of meaningfulness, excitement, joy, and fulfillment or a source of drudgery, frustration, misery, and feeling trapped. If what we do for a living is criminal, then it is for the most part harmful to someone in the long run and therefore wrong livelihood, because it produces *dukkha*. If our work involves doing something that for us is meaningless or is going in the opposite direction to what we value then, even if it is not criminal, it could be wrong livelihood for us because we increase our vulnerability to becoming unmotivated, frustrated, feeling trapped, and generally unhappy. Right livelihood is an essential component of the path and if it is ignored it negatively impacts the ability to train our mind with meditation.

3.13 Meditation Training: Serenity and Insight

In Buddhism, meditation is an integral part of the eightfold path. The Pali term for meditation is *bhavana,* which translates as bringing into being, causing to be, developing, or cultivating (Nanamoli and Bodhi 1995; Olendzki 2009). In Theravada Buddhism, meditation is sometimes called *citta bhavana. Citta* generally refers to mind. However, a more accurate English translation of *citta* is "heart–mind" because the functions of *citta* align closely with what in the West we would call the heart as well as the mind. *Citta bhavana* refers to training the heart–mind, with concentration, mindfulness, and energy in order to develop serenity and insight.

Serenity and insight are two aspects of Buddhist meditation conducive to wisdom and awakening. Meditation practitioners may focus specifically on developing the serenity aspect of meditation or they may focus on developing insight. The intentional cultivation of serenity emphasizes concentration while insight emphasizes mindfulness. Serenity meditation practices lead to unified, quiet, still, and calm states of the heart–mind. Hence, they are also commonly called tranquility, stillness, and calm meditation practices. At the other end of the meditation spectrum, insight meditation practices cultivate insight or knowing and understanding about oneself and the world. Regardless of how we meditate, or whether we incline towards serenity or insight, meditation always involves some form of effort, mindfulness, and concentration. The serenity and insight aspects of meditation could be considered as the two ends of a stick. When someone picks up one end of the stick, the other end follows. Serenity and insight are inseparable as opposite ends of the meditation spectrum.

Some meditation practices are at the extreme end of serenity-emphasizing concentration, some practices are at the extreme end of insight-emphasizing mindfulness, and some practices are in between. Within any one meditation session, an individual's attention may also go back and forward along the spectrum varying the concentration–mindfulness ratio. The two aspects of meditation work together. The serenity aspect provides sufficient calm, stillness, precision, power, and mental clarity to enable us to see what is happening and how it happens, developing insight. The insight aspect of meditation provides the discernment to not be distracted by superficial attraction or aversion and to focus attention in the most helpful way. By balancing the serenity and insight sides of meditation, it is possible to generate the wisdom and compassionate intent needed for awakening. Right effort, is the first factor in the meditation component of the path.

3.14 Right Effort

Right effort involves the decision to train the heart–mind in ways that are in accordance with our understanding and best intentions. The effort required for meditation should not be confused with the strain or struggle that sometimes might be associated with achieving a goal. Just as tuning a guitar, the string cannot be too tight or too loose, the effort for meditation is a balanced degree of energy. The type of effort required in meditation can involve rousing enthusiasm, energy, and commitment to persist. Meditation teachers, for example, sometimes describe right effort as courageous and "enduring patience in the face of suffering and difficulty" (Pandita 1992, p. 264). The opposite is also true when right effort involves knowing that there may be too much energy and enthusiasm with our meditation practice and rather than trying harder, we respond by letting go, letting be, and going with the flow of life's changes.

Balanced effort involves the diligence and zeal to cultivate healthy states of heart–mind as well as having the grace to accept and submit to what cannot be changed and let go of what is unhealthy or unhelpful. Balanced effort is often the result of wise recollection, resolve, and commitment. On a daily basis, right effort may involve wisely remembering the relationships between physical activities, events, situations, thoughts and emotions, and doing what is helpful as well as avoiding what is unhelpful. In the context of a regular meditation practice, right effort can involve wisely remembering what has worked in the past to strengthen mindfulness and concentration, then skillfully inclining towards doing what is beneficial. Meditative, courageous effort, concentration, and mindfulness are inseparable as factors of heart–mind training or *citta bhavana.*

3.15 Right Concentration *(Samma Samadhi)*

Concentration is the collection of intensification, focus, and one-pointedness of attention. Concentration is how attention remains centered on its object. The concentration that is involved in unwholesome activities such as murder, theft, or other harm is not the sort of concentration that is found on the eightfold path. This type of concentration is called wrong concentration. Right concentration, on the other hand, involves the gathering of attention in relationship to activities that are ethically wholesome. According to Bodhi (2000a), right concentration is defined as the wholesome unification of the mind.

When attention is collected and settles onto one activity or object, there is a reduction of unnecessary mental functions. Concentration decreases the tendency for attention to be dispersed, scattered, or to go from one thing to another. When our attention becomes more focused, we may also feel absorbed in what we are doing. The experience of flow, as described in contemporary psychology (e.g., Csiksenzentmihalyi 1988), is one example of a function of concentration. Flow is an optimal state of being that can occur when individuals are so engaged and absorbed in whatever they are doing that everything else fades away as insignificant.

Becoming concentrated can alter the way we experience our self and the world around us. Right concentration usually co-arises with relaxation and a sense of physical and emotional ease. As relaxation becomes deeper, physical health concerns may begin to heal, concerns fade away and problems that may have seemed entrenched, resolved. As long as we are concentrating on neutral and pleasing objects, in a way that is not harmful, concentrated attention generally leads to well-being.

Wallace (2006) noted that relaxation is the first step on the path to developing highly refined meditative concentration. The second step is stability of attention, so that attention stays where it is placed, and the third step is vividness of perception, so that whatever is perceived becomes sharp in focus and lucid. In the Theravada Buddhist traditions, meditative concentration is called *samadhi,* and *samatha bhavana* refers to serenity meditation. According to Pali scholars, the term *samadhi* is derived from *sam-a-dha* where the root *dha* means "to put or place," *a* indicates "towards," and *sam* refers to "together" (Kearney 2009). Therefore, *samadhi* literally means to collect attention together and place it on an object. The Buddhist Pali literature uses the term *samadhi* to refer to: one-pointedness as a particular mental factor; very high states of concentration called *jhāna*s along with the stages leading up to them; and a method of practice which is used to attain serenity, tranquility, or calm (Kearney 2009).

Serenity meditation *(samatha bhavana)* practices provide a systematic way of cultivating *samadhi* and a vehicle to travel along the path of awakening. As long as it is ethically wholesome, almost any object can be used to cultivate serenity. However, Theravada texts such as the *Visuddhimagga* describe up to 40 classic serenity meditation practices (Nanamoli 1956). The classic objects include the breath, colors, the elements such as earth (solidity) and wind (movement) as well as qualities of mind such as loving-kindness and compassion. Wallace (2006) explained that the primary purpose of developing highly concentrated states is to stabilize and refine vividness of attention so that enquiry into the nature of reality is enhanced.

In the process of the eightfold path, insight is the liberator and *samadhi* is the tool that makes insight possible. Like looking at the moon with a telescope, *samadhi* is the instrument that makes the vision powerful and lucid. Ultimately, *samadhi* gives muscle to insight (Wallace 2008).

Right concentration can be purposefully cultivated as part of the path of serenity meditation or it can result as a by-product on the path of insight meditation (Bodhi 2000a). While serenity meditation is mostly associated with the development of right concentration, insight meditation is related to the development of right mindfulness.

3.16 Right Mindfulness *(Samma Sati)*

In Buddhism, the type of mindfulness that leads to wisdom and awakening is called right mindfulness. Wrong or unskillful mindfulness, on the other hand, may involve remembering to be attentive in a way that does not lead to wisdom and may be harmful (Thanissaro 2006). A burglar or a sniper, as two examples again, must remember to be attentive to achieve their goals. However, this type of mindfulness does not lead to understanding. In Buddhism, right mindfulness has an ethical quality that discerns what is useful to follow and what is not. Right mindfulness grounds the practitioner in the present moment and it facilitates both serenity and insight.

The function of mindfulness in serenity meditation is slightly different than the function of mindfulness in insight meditation (Bodhi 2000a). In the context of serenity meditation practices, "*mindfulness* refers to attending continuously to a familiar object, without forgetfulness or distraction" (Wallace 2006, p. 13). According to Bodhi (2000a), the function of mindfulness in serenity meditation is to monitor concentration. In this role, it ensures that focused attention does not slip off and become lost in thought or other distractions. In serenity meditation, mindfulness serves to remember to bring attention back to the object of attention, whatever it may be. Mindfulness or insight meditation, which will be described as *satipatthana vipassana* also requires right mindfulness to be effective. The primary task of right mindfulness in mindfulness meditation is to observe, note, and discern phenomena precisely so that cause–effect relationships are understood and the three characteristics of existence (impermanence, emptiness, and unreliability) are seen clearly.

3.17 Mindfulness Meditation

What is called mindfulness meditation or insight meditation in contemporary psychology is called *satipatthana vipassana* in the Theravada traditions. *Satipatthana* is a compound Pali word derived from *sati* and *patthana* or *sati* and *upatthana* (Thanissaro 1996). *Patthana* means keeping present and foundation or source (Thanissaro 1996). The *patthanna* of *satipatthana* refers to remembering where attention is directed (Kearney 2000; Nyanaponika 1962). *Upattana* is a variation of the term and refers to establishing near or setting up near or station, with the idea that attention is stationed or established and an object is kept closely in mind (Thanissaro 1996). Thus, *satipatthana* means the foundations of mindfulness and refers to remembering to deliberately place close attention or turn the mind to what is happening. The term *vipassana* means insight, and *satipatthana vipassana* literally refers to practicing the foundations of mindfulness for the development of insight. One of the Buddha's discourses *(suttas)* called the *Satipatthana Sutta* describes the practice in detail, and a basic overview of this *sutta* follows.

The four foundations of mindfulness are:

1. Body *(kaya)*
2. Feelings *(vedana)*
3. Consciousness or heart–mind *(citta)*
4. Phenomena (*dharmas*—Sanskrit)

Each of these foundations contains sub-domains, which are different aspects of the foundation they are within. Scholars have also referred to these foundations as applications (e.g., Wallace 2011), domains, and/or frames of reference (Thanissaro 1996). The names of the different foundations also include the Pali compound word *anupassana,* which is derived from *anu,* which translates as along, and *passana,* which is seeing. *Anupassana* is usually referred to as contemplation and Pali scholars also translate this term as "to repeatedly look at" or "to closely observe" (Analayo 2003, p. 32) or "to seeing along with" or "to track" (Kearney 2014). When we closely observe and track changing conditions of body and heart–mind we begin to understand ourselves.

Analogous to walking along a path in a mysterious forest, journeying through life with mindfulness and clear comprehension *(sampajanya),* we pay attention to the present moment realities yet also keep in mind our direction and remember significant markers on the way. In this way, our wisdom grows and we become familiar with the environment of our body–heart–mind so we do not get lost.

The four foundations of mindfulness are at the heart of Buddhist meditation (Nyanaponika 1962) and they encompass the full range of all possible human experiences. They also cover the range of processes needed for the development of insight and therefore liberation from cycles of *dukkha.* Though the *Satipatthana Sutta* was directed to monks in ancient India, the instructions given are as relevant today in contemporary culture, as they were when they were originally taught 2560 years ago.

As a meditation practice, meditators can choose to establish their attention on one foundation or a sub-domain of a foundation as is appropriate. Just like changing gears on a motor vehicle to adapt to the road and the terrain, meditators can make different foundations or sub-domains central in their awareness as required and needed. Practitioners usually begin with mindfulness of body practices and progress to more refined foundations of mindfulness as their skills develop. Mindfulness of body practices are, however, often foundation practices that meditators use as an anchor to come back to when needed.

The instructions in the *sutta* are given in such a way that they lead to the cultivation of the helpful/wholesome and the abandonment of the unhelpful/unwholesome. These instructions are geared towards reducing and uprooting the causes of *dukkha* (clinging/craving, hostility/aversion, and ignorance/delusion) and cultivating insight. Regardless of which foundation or sub-domain a meditator chooses to make central, they all ultimately lead to being free from habits and patterns that cause *dukkha.* Ultimately, however, it is the realization of the four noble truths, which is key to being free from *dukkha*. As an indication of the progressive nature of the four foundations, contemplation of the four noble truths is listed as the last sub-domain in the fourth foundation.

The discourse outlines the basics of *satipatthana* by firstly establishing four mental qualities:

1. Being ardent or with diligence and energy
2. Being alert or clearly knowing and comprehending
3. Mindfulness
4. Being able to put aside greed and distress with reference to the world or detachment (Huxter 2007, p. 51)

According to Thanissaro (1996), the discourse also describes three stages in the development of satipatthana:

1. Noticing the object in and of itself, both internally (within oneself) and externally (outside of oneself), and both internally and externally (the interaction between internal and external) in the immediate time frame (the present moment).
2. Noticing how the object changes by being attentive to either its arising, its passing, or its arising and passing.
3. Having equanimity about the object, without doing anything with it, and being present with an object as it is.

3.18 Contemplation of Body: *Kayanupassana Satipatthana*

The first foundation involves contemplating the body in all possible ways and circumstances. This foundation has six sub-domains, which are as follows:

1. Mindfulness of breathing
2. Mindfulness of physical postures
3. Clear comprehension of actions (physical)
4. Mindfulness centered on the components of the body
5. Contemplation on the natural qualities or elements of body
6. Mindfulness on the nine cemetery meditations

Mindfulness of the breath is possibly one of the most common meditation practices and it can be a serenity or an insight meditation practice. For many meditation practitioners, beginner or advanced, mindfulness of breath is a popular anchor practice which is used as a regular meditation practice. While we are alive, we breathe; thus, the breath is always there as an object of attention and a way to track immediate experience.

Mindfulness of physical postures refers to being attentive to all postures whether reclining, sitting, walking, and so on. It is understandable that this sub-domain is second on the list because after breathing it is something that is always available. No matter where we are, we are in a posture.

Clear comprehension of actions (physical) refers to being aware of actions and doing them with clear understanding *(sampajanya)*. Clear comprehension of actions is more refined than merely being aware of postures as it includes awareness of the greater context of our experience. For example, regardless of whether we are sitting, walking, eating, or talking, we can be aware with clarity of the purpose, suitability, and timeliness of our actions.

Mindfulness centered on the components of the body involves being aware of the separate component of the body such as hair, skin, bones, teeth, as if visualizing these parts of the body, laid out in front of oneself. The description of this sub-domain of mindfulness may not be consistent with most popular perspectives of mindfulness. Nonetheless, when we can reflect on and be mindful of the components of the body, our conceptualization about our bodies goes deeper than our superficial perceptions. In Theravada Buddhist traditions, contemplation of parts of the body is a part of the ordination process for monks and nuns. Contemplating hair as hair, bones as bones, teeth as teeth and skin as skin, as examples, helps to break down the tendency to identify with a body.

Contemplation on the elements of the body refers to being aware of the qualities of temperature (fire), the qualities of hardness and softness (earth), the qualities of movement (air), and the quality of fluidity (water). Formal meditation practices are often steered towards mindfulness of the elements. For example, being aware of the sensations associated with how the abdomen stretches with the breath can be mindfulness of air element (movement). Being aware of all the changing experiences at the base of the foot when walking may involve tracking the experience of hardness and softness (earth element). Sometimes the elements are not directly experienced and the practitioner visualizes the parts of the body that represent these qualities. For example, feeling and visualizing the teeth and bones can represent hardness (earth element) and saliva and blood represent fluidity (water element).

Mindfulness on the nine cemetery meditations involves either visualizing or observing actual corpses at various stages of decay and being aware that one day we shall also die. Like contemplating the parts of the body above, contemplating corpses at various stages of decay is not a mindfulness practice that is commonly taught in Western settings. In most cases, it would not be appropriate. Traditionally, skilled meditation teachers prescribed this practice to students with particular temperaments. Nonetheless, being able to observe a dead body, if it is not traumatizing, can have a powerfully sobering and insightful effect. Seeing a body without life can impact dramatically on our understanding of what is means to be alive and embodied. Being able to realize that one's own body will also age, decay, and die can also transform the tendency to identify with a body as an unchanging entity.

3.19 Contemplating Feelings: *Vedananupassana Satipatthana*

The Pali term *vedana* comes from the root term *vedeti,* which means to feel and to know (Analayo 2003). *Vedana* is usually translated as feelings and it refers to the emotional flavor or the affective tones of pleasantness, unpleasantness, or neither.

Other dimensions of feelings include whether they give rise to unhelpful reactive patterns or not. Feelings are not emotions as they are considered in our everyday language, nor are they physical sensations. *Vedana* is often translated as sensations. This translation can, however, be confusing, because as described in the first domain of mindfulness sensations can refer to physical qualities such as pressure, heat, movement, and so on.

Feelings move us to act. Often our feelings about something can move us to act in ways that are wholesome and helpful in life. Feelings can also move us to act in ways that perpetuate being bound on cycles of *dukkha.* In these reactive cycles, craving to either push away or pull in, arise dependent on feelings. We cannot control our feelings about experiences because they arise as conditioned responses. We can choose, however, how we act based on our feelings. Contemplating feelings as feelings can short circuit unnecessary over reactions to experiences that come our way. As one example, contemplating feeling can help to regulate emotions and reduce cravings, thereby helping to work with addictions. Contemplating feelings also develops equanimity (resilience and peace) and can therefore be helpful for pain management.

3.20 Contemplation of *Citta* or Heart–Mind: *Cittanupassana Satipatthana*

The object of mindfulness within this domain is the heart–mind or *citta.* In Theravada Buddhism, the heart–mind thinks, feels, knows, and experiences via feelings *(vedana),* perceptions, mental fabrications/cognitions, and consciousness. It is not an enduring entity, but a sequence of momentary mental acts, each discrete, distinct and changing (Bodhi 2000a). The knowing aspect of heart–mind is awareness, and the heart–mind is both cognizant and illuminating.

It is easy to confuse the aware aspect of heart–mind with the thoughts, emotions, moods, impulses, feelings, and other events that arise within it. One of the functions of this foundation of mindfulness is to distinguish between the events that arise and pass within the heart–mind and awareness itself.

There are up to 15 sub-domains in this foundation, which include emotions, moods, thoughts, and states of mind ranging from the gross to the subtle, deluded, and awakened. The sub-domains of this foundation involve being attentive to the presence of these heart–mind events and the degree to which they represent one of the root causes of *dukkha* (greed, hatred, or ignorance) or their absence. Contemplating the heart–mind helps with emotional regulation as well as reducing the tendency to identify with transient emotional and mental events. For example, mindfully tracking the changing nature of painful emotions helps to short circuit reactive patterns often associated with these experiences. Attending to aggressive emotions and possibly labeling them, as another example, can help to provide choice with these drives rather than feeling controlled by them.

Contemplating heart–mind also includes being attentive to and tracking very subtle and refined states of heart–mind such as those associated with high levels of concentration and insight. Practicing awareness of awareness (Wallace 2005), which is a meditation practice taught in some traditions, is an example of practicing this contemplation at more refined levels.

As the objects of contemplation include reference to an unsurpassable heart–mind and a heart–mind free from unwholesome tendencies, this indicates that this foundation of mindfulness includes awareness of an awakened heart–mind.

3.21 Contemplating Phenomena: *Dhammanupassana Satipatthana*

This foundation involves contemplating *dhammas* or dharmas (Sanskrit). The word dharma most commonly refers to the truths that the Buddha and other awakened beings knew directly and taught. The term dharma or *dhamma* can also mean a range of other things. According to one Pali dictionary, its meaning includes:

> Nature, condition, quality, property, characteristic; function; object, thing, idea, phenomena; doctrine; justice; the law. (Childers 2005, p. 118)

In order to more completely understand the fourth foundation, it is also worthwhile considering how the Buddha may have explained experience and *dhammas*. For the Buddha, the world is our experience of the world, which comprises both the subjective experiencing and the object being experienced. It is evident in the discourses that the Buddha also taught that the world was not an independently existing thing, but an interdependent co-arising experience, where the self and its world were a series of experiences. In Theravada Buddhism, the units of experience are called *dhammas* and are often translated as phenomena. A *dhamma* is not an objective thing, but a thing as experienced or the experience of a thing. A *dhamma* has two essential aspects: experiencing and what is experienced (Kearney 2007).

Thanissaro (1996) noted that *dhammanupassana* (contemplating *dhammas*) includes any experience that is not included in the other foundations. Analayo (2003) stated that this foundation is more concerned with a range of specific mental qualities and patterns pertaining to the teaching of the Buddha. This foundation can also include the way thought, emotions, moods, and behaviors interact. The fourth foundation is different from the other three in that there is more active engagement and intelligent discernment about experience and less nonevaluative observation. With the first three foundations, it is enough to simply focus on an object with diligence, notice how the object changes, and be present with equanimity. With the fourth foundation, however, more emphasis is placed on following the principles involved with reducing and abandoning *dukkha,* and cultivating the factors that produce wisdom and lead to awakening. The five sub-domains of the fourth foundation are:

1. Contemplation of the five hindrances or obstacles to meditation and living a valued life
2. Contemplation of the five aggregates of experience that together we call a self
3. Contemplation of the six sense bases
4. Contemplation of seven factors of awakening
5. Contemplation of the four noble truths

3.22 Contemplation of the Five Hindrances

This sub-domain refers to contemplating five hindrances that block the path of freedom and obscure awareness of an awakened heart–mind. They are:

1. Obsessive and unnecessary sensual desire or craving
2. Hostility, ill will, or unhelpful aversion
3. Lethargy, mental stiffness, and dullness
4. Agitation, worry, rumination, and restlessness
5. Paralyzing uncertainty and doubt

3.23 Contemplation of the Five *Kanda* or the Aggregates of Clinging

In Buddhism, the "self" consists of five groups or aggregates of experience. When there is clinging to the groups as an independent and permanent self, there is *dukkha*. The five groups of clinging include form, feelings, perceptions, mental formations, and consciousness. The instructions in the *Satipatthana Sutta* are to merely note the arising and passing of these conditions. When impermanence is perceived and insight develops, the tendency to reify and cling to the aggregates as a solid lasting independent self, is released. In Buddhist insight meditation practices, there is a general enquiry about what it is to be human. Sometimes this is verbalized internally as "what or who am I?" Within this particular sub-domain, the focus of the contemplation is completely on the nature of self and insight arises about the self. The aim of this sub-domain of mindfulness is to wake up to ourselves and in doing so we release the grip on who and what we think we are. To release clinging to changing body–heart–mind experiences as a self is to also realize complete awakening.

3.24 Contemplation of the Six Sense Spheres

The six senses spheres are sight, sound, smell, touch, taste, and mental experience. In Buddhism, the heart–mind is considered a sense preceptor and it perceives mental objects. The instructions in the *sutta* are to notice the sense organ and the sense object. Further to this, the meditator is instructed to notice either the presence or absence of craving and clinging dependent on the sense perception. Attention is also brought to knowing how clinging has arisen, how it can be discarded once arisen and also how the tendency to cling can be kept at bay. Thus, hearing sounds, as one example, we can note impermanence of the sounds, and know how to let go of the tendency to cling to pleasant sounds or reject and condemn unpleasant sounds.

3.25 Contemplation of the Seven Factors of Awakening

The seven factors of awakening are seven positive cognitive, affective, and behavioral qualities that help lead to awakening. In Buddhist psychology, they are considered as sequential in that one positive factor leads on to the next. In order they are: mindfulness, investigation/interest, energy/enthusiasm, rapture/joy, tranquility/calm, concentration/unification, and peacefulness/being centered or equanimity. In the teachings of the Buddha, the factors have both refined noble and basic ennobling levels. The instructions in the *sutta* are to simply observe whether one or more of the factors are present or not, then to apply strategies to cultivate, nourish, nurture, and maintain them. Developing the seven awakening factors has an opposite outcome to the effects of being bound up in the five hindrances because they lead to awakening and not away from it. At an ennobling level, the cultivation of the factors is therapeutic. For example, developing skills and qualities such as awareness, enquiry, motivation, relaxation, joy, concentration, peacefulness, etc., are often basic components of many psychotherapeutic approaches.

3.26 Contemplation of the Four Noble Truths

The description of the contemplation of the four noble truths is inseparable from describing reflections and contemplations of the whole of the Buddha's teaching. This is because the four noble truths are the essence of what the Buddha taught and to realize the four noble truths is to realize the teaching of the Buddha. Mindfulness in this sub-domain refers to remembering to be attentive to these realizations and track them.

The final messages at the end of the *sutta* are predictions about the results of practicing the four foundations of mindfulness. According to the Buddha, the results of practicing mindfulness are not only the reduction of *dukkha* but also its complete release through awakening. These predictions point to how causes have effects.

That is, when mindfulness is practiced in a right, complete, or skillful way, it has the result of leading to insight, timely realizations, and ultimately full and complete awakening.

3.27 Conclusion

In the past 30 years, mindfulness has gained popularity in the contemporary world. The trend began with psychotherapeutic programs and interventions and now it is a mainstream and marketable interest. However, mindfulness is often taught in a way that is separate from the context of its Buddhist roots. The aim of this chapter was to illuminate the foundations of mindfulness in the context of the Buddha's noble eightfold path. Mindfulness was explained by referring to the original Pali term *sati,* which literally means memory. The traditional description of mindfulness and the contemporary description differ in that the Buddhist approach emphasizes wise discernment while contemporary mindfulness-based programs most often emphasize bare attention. Taking into account both the traditional and contemporary approaches to mindfulness Bhikkhu Bodhi, described mindfulness as: "to remember to pay attention to what is occurring in one's immediate experience with care and discernment" (Shapiro 2009, p. 556). From a Buddhist perspective, right mindfulness cannot be separated from the context of seven other factors, each supporting the other in the direction of awakening.

The eightfold path comprises three components: the wisdom component (right view and right intention), the ethics component (right speech, action, and livelihood), and the meditation component (right effort, mindfulness, and concentration). The Buddha's ennobling eightfold path empowers individuals to change what causes them suffering and experience the results of healing and increased well-being. The Buddha's noble eightfold path leads to radical transformations in consciousness, impeccable behaviors, and complete freedom from suffering and its causes. The meditation component of the path has two aspects: serenity where concentration is emphasized and insight where mindfulness is emphasized. These two sides of Buddhist meditation mutually support each other with serenity, providing the functions of focus, stillness, and calm to facilitate insight, while insight enables discernment to steer focused attention in the right direction. Insight meditation is represented by the four foundations of mindfulness, the practice of which has been explained in a comprehensive and detailed way in the *Satipatthana Sutta.* These foundations are contemplations of body, feelings, heart–mind, and phenomena.

The Buddha's approach to mindfulness is a timeless, sophisticated, and refined practice that can be adopted by any individual and any culture. Mindfulness is key in developing the understanding that motivates us to release what is not helpful and cultivate instead what is wholesome and liberating. When there is no cause for suffering, there is no suffering. Thus, it is one way to address and reduce psychological distress in whatever way it manifests. Moreover, the practice of mindfulness is a way to awakening and thus a powerful factor to realize complete psychological freedom. It is worthwhile to pay homage to the historical Buddha, the one who taught the foundations of mindfulness and the profound way of the noble eightfold path to awakening.

References

Allen, N. B., Chambers, R., Knight, W., Blashki, G., Ciechomski, L., Hassed, C., Gullone, E., McNab, C., & Meadows, G. (2006). Mindfulness-based psychotherapies: A review of conceptual foundations, empirical evidence and practical considerations. *Australian and New Zealand Journal of Psychiatry, 40,* 285–294.

Analayo. (2003). *Satipatthana: The direct path to realization.* Birmingham: Windhorse.

Beck, A. T. (1976). *Cognitive therapy and the emotional disorders.* New York: New American Library.

Baer, R. A. (2003). Mindfulness training as a clinical intervention: A conceptual and empirical review. *Clinical Psychology: Science and Practice, 10*(2), 125–143.

Bodhi, B. (2000a). *The noble eightfold way: Way to the end of suffering.* Onalaska: BPS Pariyatti Editions.

Bodhi, B. (Ed.) (2000b). *A comprehensive manual of Abhidhamma: Pali text, translation & explanatory guide.* Onalaska: BPS Pariyatti Editions.

Brown, D. P. (1986). The stages of meditation. In K. Wilber, J. Engler, & D.P. Brown (Eds.), *Transformations of consciousness: Conventional and contemplative perspectives on development.* Boston: Shambala.

Carroll, M. (2011). *The mindful leader: Awakening your natural management skills through mindful meditation.* Boston: Trumpeter.

Childers, R. C. (2005). *A dictionary of the Pali language.* Delhi: Munshiram Manoharlal Publishers Pvt Ltd.

Csiksenzentmihalyi, M. (1988). The flow experience and human psychology. In M. Csiksenzentmihalyi & I. S. Csiksenzentmihalyi (Eds.), *Optimal experience: Psychological studies of flow in consciousness.* Cambridge: Cambridge University Press.

Davidson, R. J., Kabat-Zinn, J., Schumacher, J., Rosenkranz, M., Muller, D., Santorelli, S. F., Urbanowski, F., Harrington, A., Bonus, K., & Sheridan, J. F. (2003). Alterations in brain and immune function produced by mindfulness meditation. *Psychosomatic Medicine, 65,* 564–570.

Dawson, G., & Turnbull, E. (2006). Is mindfulness the new opiate of the masses? Critical reflections from a Buddhist perspective. *Psychotherapy in Australia, 12*(4), 2–6.

Didonna, F. (2009). *Clinical handbook of mindfulness.* New York: Springer.

Goleman, D. (1988). *The meditative mind.* London: Thorsons.

Hanh, T. N. (1975). *The miracle of mindfulness: A manual on meditation.* Boston: Beacon.

Hanh, T. N. (1993). *For a future to be possible.* Berkeley: Parallax.

Hanh, T. N. (1998). *The heart of the Buddha's teachings.* Berkeley: Parallax.

Hayes, S. C., Strosahl, K. D., & Wilson, K. G. (1999). *Acceptance and commitment therapy.* New York: Guilford.

Huxter, M. J. (2007). Mindfulness as therapy from a Buddhist perspective. In D.A. Einstein (Ed.), *Innovations and advances in cognitive behaviour therapy.* Bowen Hills: Australian Academic Press.

Huxter, M. J. (2009). The Buddha's psychology of awakening: A personal spiritual practice and framework for therapy. *Inpsych, 31*(4), 12–13.

Huxter, M. J. (2013). Buddhist mindfulness: A paradox of harmony and incompatibility. Paper presented at the First International Conference on Mindfulness, Rome, Italy.

Kabat-Zinn, J. (1990). *Full catastrophe living. Using the wisdom of your body and mind to face stress, pain, and illness.* New York: Guilford.

Kabat-Zinn, J. (2003). Mindfulness based interventions in context: Past present and future. *Clinical Psychology: Science and Practice, 10*, 144–156.
Kabat-Zinn, J. (2009). Forward to: Clinical handbook of mindfulness. In F. Didonna (Ed.), Clinical handbook of mindfulness. (pp. xxv–xxxiii). New York: Springer.
Kearney, P. (1995). Developing awareness. *Sakyamuni News*. Sakyamuni Buddhist Centre. Lynehan, Australia.
Kearney, P. (2000). *Introduction to Satipatthana*. A talk given at the Kuan Yin Centre in Lismore, NSW, Australia.
Kearney, P. (2007). *Introducing dependent arising*. Notes from the Dharma salon workshops at the Dharma Gathering. Yarrahappini, NSW, Australia.
Kearney, P. (2009). *Cultivating the heart-mind with mindfulness: A workshop for therapists*. A workshop conducted with Malcolm Huxter at the Ballina Beach Resort, Ballina, NSW, Australia.
Kearney, P. (2014). *Mindfulness and vipassana meditation practice*. Talks provided at The Blue Mountains Insight Meditation Centre on a month long silent retreat. Medlow Bath, NSW, Australia.
Linehan, M. M. (1993). *Cognitive-behavioral treatment of borderline personality disorder*. New York: Guilford.
Nanamoli, B. (1956). *The path of purification (Visuddhimagga) by Bhadantacariya Buddhaghosa*. Singapore: Singapore Buddhist Meditation Centre.
Nanamoli, B., & Bodhi B. (1995). *The middle length discourses of the Buddha: A new translation of the Majjhima Nikaya*. Boston: Wisdom.
Narada, M. T. (1956). *A Manual of Abhidhamma*. Kuala Lumpur: The Buddhist Missionary Society.
Nyanaponika, T. (1962). *The heart of Buddhist meditation: A handbook of mental training based on the Buddha's way of mindfulness*. Kandy: Buddhist Publication Society.
Nyanaponika, T. (1994). The progress of insight (Visuddhinana-katha): A modern treatise on Buddhist Satipatthana meditation by Venerable Mahasi Sayadaw. Downloaded from http//www.accesstoinsight.com. Accessed Sept 2014.
Olendzki, A. (2009). Mindfulness and meditation. In F. Didonna (Ed.), *Clinical handbook of mindfulness* (pp. 37–44). New York: Springer.
Pandita, S. U. (1992). *In this very life: The liberation teaching of the Buddha*. Boston: Wisdom.
Segal, Z. V., Williams, J. M. G., & Teasdale, J. D. (2002) *Mindfulness-based cognitive therapy for depression*. New York: The Guilford.
Shapiro, S. L. (2009) The integration of mindfulness and psychology. *Journal of Clinical Psychology, 65*(6), 555–560.
Singh, N. N., Lancioni, G. E., Wahler, R. G., Winton, A. S. W., & Singh, J. (2008). Mindfulness approaches in Cognitive Behavior Therapy. *Behavioural and Cognitive Psychotherapy, 36*, 659–666.
Stone, M. (2014). Abusing the Buddha: How the U.S. Army and Google co-opt mindfulness. *Salon*. http://www.salon.com/2014/03/17/abusing_the_buddha_how_the_u_s_army_and_google_co_opt_mindfulness/. Accessed Sept 2014.
Teasdale, J. D., Moore. R. G., Hayhurst, H., Pope, M., Williams, S., & Segal, Z. (2002). Metacognitive awareness and prevention of relapse in depression: Empirical evidence. *Journal of Consulting and Clinical Psychology, 70*(2), 275–287.
Thanissaro, B. (1996). *The wings to awakening*. Barre: Dhamma Dana.
Thanissaro, B. (2006). The integrity of emptiness. http://www.accesstoinsight.org/lib/authors/thanissaro. Accessed Sept 2014.
Walsh, R. (1980). The consciousness disciplines and the behavioral sciences: Questions of comparison and assessment. *American Journal of Psychiatry, 137*(6), 663–673.
Wallace, B. A. (2005). *Genuine happiness: Meditation as the path to fulfillment*. New Jersey: Wiley.
Wallace, B. A. (2006). *The attention revolution: Unlocking the power of the focused mind*. Somerville: Wisdom.

Wallace, B. A. (2008). A mindful balance. *Tricycle, 17*(3), 60–63.
Wallace, B. A. (2011). *Minding closely: The four applications of mindfulness*. New York: Snow Lion.
Wallace, B. A., & Shapiro, S. L. (2006). Mental balance and well-being: Building bridges between Buddhism and western psychology. *American Psychologist, 61*(7), 690–701.
Williams, J. M. G, & Kabat-Zinn, J. (2013). *Mindfulness: Diverse perspectives on meanings, origins and multiple applications at the intersection of science and dharma*. Oxon: Routledge.
Wilson, J. (2014). From monastery to marketplace. *Tricycle*. http://www.tricycle.com/blog/monastery-marketplace. Accessed Sept 2014.

Malcolm Huxter has had confidence in the teachings of the Buddha since 1975. He was a Buddhist monk in Thailand for 2 years in the late 1970s and has attended intensive retreats in Burma, Thailand, Australia, and the USA. Mal is a registered clinical psychologist in both Australia and the UK. A psychologist since 1991, he has worked in a variety of settings including inpatient and community mental health, detention centers for asylum seekers, and private practice. He has been using mindfulness-related strategies in clinical settings for over 20 years and has written and conducted mindfulness-based programs for different clinical populations including those with panic, bipolar disorder, and generalized anxiety disorder. Mal has conducted workshops, seminars, and retreats for therapists since 2001.

Chapter 4
Understanding and Practicing the *Ānāpānasati-sutta*

Bhikkhu Anālayo

4.1 Introduction

Mindfulness of breathing is a frequently practiced form of meditation in different Buddhist traditions. The *Ānāpānasati-sutta,* the "Discourse on Mindfulness of Breathing," offers a detailed exposition on how this form of meditation can be undertaken.

The *Ānāpānasati-sutta* is part of the collection of middle length discourses, the *Majjhima-nikāya,* of the Pāli canon preserved by the *Theravāda* tradition. The discourses now found in the Pāli canon are the final result of centuries of oral transmission of the texts believed to have been spoken originally by the Buddha and his disciples. These orally transmitted discourses eventually reached Sri Lanka and were then committed to writing. According to the traditional report in the Ceylonese chronicles, this happened shortly before the beginning of the Common Era. By then, at least four centuries had passed since the time when the Buddha would have lived.

The Pāli canon transmitted by the *Theravāda* tradition is not the only product of the oral transmission of the early Buddhist discourses. Other Buddhist schools in India also preserved their records of the Buddha's teachings, and it seems fairly probable that, at about the time of the writing down of the Pāli canon in Sri Lanka or soon after, these other transmission lineages also came to be written down.

Due to the climatic conditions in Sri Lanka and most of the Indian subcontinent, written records of the teachings made on a material like palm leaves are in constant need of being redone. With the eventual disappearance of Buddhism from India, the process of copying manuscripts came to an end and much of the material committed to writing has been lost. Fortunately, by that time, collections of discourses from

Bh. Anālayo (✉)
Numata Center for Buddhist Studies, University of Hamburg, Alsterterrasse 1,
20354 Hamburg, Germany

E. Shonin et al. (eds.), *Buddhist Foundations of Mindfulness,*
Mindfulness in Behavioral Health, DOI 10.1007/978-3-319-18591-0_4

different Buddhist schools had been brought to China and translated into Chinese. As far as we know, the discourse collections had also reached Tibet, but, during the persecution of Buddhism under the King Glang dar ma in the ninth century, these appear to have been lost. Therefore, the present-day Buddhist canon preserved in Tibetan translation does not have counterparts to the four Pāli discourse collections, the *Nikāyas,* but only some selected discourses preserved on their own or as citations in other works. Another source of early Buddhist discourse material can be found in manuscripts that mostly come from Central Asia. Due to the dry climatic conditions in Central Asia, texts written on a material like birch bark endure much longer than manuscripts in Sri Lanka or South India, and, even in recent days, substantial manuscript finds from Central Asia have made headlines.

The Chinese canon contains counterparts to each of the four Pāli discourse collections in the form of the *Āgamas,* although these belong to different schools. In the case of the *Ānāpānasati-sutta*, thanks to the existence of these Chinese *Āgamas,* we have access to a parallel version from a collection of discourses connected by topic, a *Saṃyukta-āgama*. This *Saṃyukta-āgama* was translated into Chinese in the early fifth century of the present era, apparently based on a text that the Chinese pilgrim Faxian had brought with him from his travels in India and Sri Lanka. This *Saṃyukta-āgama* collection appears to have been transmitted within a Buddhist school known as *Mūlasarvāstivāda,* corresponding to the monastic tradition still nowadays followed in Tibetan Buddhism.

Besides this *Saṃyukta-āgama,* parallels to the *Ānāpānasati-sutta*, or more precisely to its instructions on mindfulness of breathing, are extant in canonical texts on monastic discipline. These are the Vinayas of the *Mahāsāṅghika*, *Mūlasarvāstivāda*, and *Sarvāstivāda* schools, which are also extant in Chinese translations. The relevant part from the three Vinayas presents only a description of the 16 steps of mindfulness of breathing. The three Vinayas are therefore only a parallel to the actual instruction, whereas for the remainder of the *Ānāpānasati-sutta*, which is concerned with relating the 16 steps to progress to liberation, only the *Saṃyukta-āgama* parallel provides material for comparison.

These extant versions—the *Ānāpānasati-sutta* of the *Theravāda Majjhima-nikāya,* its parallel in the *Mūlasarvāstivāda Saṃyukta-āgama,* and the relevant portions in the *Mahāsāṅghika*, *Mūlasarvāstivāda* and *Sarvāstivāda* Vinayas—can in principle lay an equal claim to being authentic records of the early Buddhist teachings on meditation. They each stem similarly from one of the various oral transmission lineages that attempted to preserve the teaching of the Buddha and each of these became part of the canonical textual collection of one of the Buddhist schools, once these had come into being. In the case of the parallel versions preserved in Chinese, there is of course the problem of translation errors. Rendering an Indic text into Chinese involves two languages that are substantially different, making it a rather demanding task to transform a text from one language to the other without a change or even loss of the meaning.

Comparing different versions of a particular teaching takes us beyond the confines of any particular school and helps to access the earliest level of Buddhist teaching that we are able to reach through the medium of the texts that have been preserved. The vision of early Buddhist teachings that emerges from such comparative study can at times be different from the doctrinal position of the *Theravāda* tradition, for example, which developed since the transmission of Buddhism to Sri Lanka during the reign of King Asoka. Early Buddhism, in contrast, stands for the period from the time of the Buddha until King Asoka.

Now, when comparing the instructions given in the four extant versions for the 16 steps of mindfulness of breathing, a close degree of similarity emerges. In principle, close correspondence between parallel versions transmitted by different schools points to a common early core (Anālayo 2012). In the present case, it therefore seems safe to conclude that the basic instructions for the 16 steps of mindfulness of breathing can be considered an integral part of early Buddhist meditation theory. From an academic perspective, there would be little ground for assuming that these 16 steps are the result of later elaborations.

In what follows, I take up these 16 steps in 4 groups of fours—four tetrads—beginning with the instructions given in the *Ānāpānasati-sutta*. Whenever opportune, I bring in the comparative perspective based on examining the parallels. In line with the title of this chapter, my main aim is to develop an understanding of the significance of the discourse for the actual practice of mindfulness of breathing; a comparative study of the *Ānāpānasati-sutta* and its *Saṃyukta-āgama* parallel meant for the more academically interested reader can be found in *Anālayo* (2011, pp. 664–673).

4.2 The First Tetrad

The instructions for the 16 steps of practice in the *Ānāpānasati-sutta* and its parallels are preceded by an indication that the meditator should retire to a secluded spot to sit down for actual meditation practice. This indication is noteworthy insofar as it gives the impression that, in early Buddhist thought, mindfulness of breathing was considered a form of meditation best cultivated in a setting free from outer disturbances, instead of being a practice one undertakes alongside everyday activities. There does in fact not seem to be an explicit reference in the early discourses to undertaking mindfulness of breathing while one is engaged in some form of activity, such as having a conversation, going somewhere, doing some kind of manual work, etc. Even in the case of descriptions of walking meditation, the instructions are to keep the mind free from defilements, not to watch the breath while one is walking.

Of course, it will always be beneficial to keep the breath in mind, in whatever situation one may be in. Nevertheless, a problem can arise at least for some practitioners when trying to maintain mindfulness of breathing while, at the same time, having to engage in various daily activities and conversations. The fact that the breath is a relatively subtle object naturally requires some degree of mental focus, in order to be kept in mind. The stronger one's mind focuses on anything, however, the less it will be able to attend to a range of other things that may be happening at the same time. At least in situations where one is actively engaged in a particular task, it can at times be preferable to use a less subtle object to sustain continuity of mindfulness.

An alternative to the breath would be, for example, mindfulness of the whole body. The entire body is a comparatively less subtle and more easily discerned support for mindfulness, making it less of a challenge to be kept in mind while engaging in various activities.

The actual instructions in the *Ānāpānasati-sutta* for being aware of the breath, once one has sat down in a secluded place, begin by directing mindfulness to the phenomenon of the breath as such, reading: "Mindful one breathes in, mindful one breathes out" (MN III 82; translated in Ñāṇamoli 1995, p. 943). The basic distinction between inhalation and exhalation introduced in this way sets a pattern that continues throughout the entire scheme of practice. The distinction between the breath that comes in and the breath that moves out inculcates a continuous awareness of the impermanent nature of the breath, which keeps changing all the time. This already points to the insight potential inherent in mindfulness of breathing, something that becomes particularly prominent with the last tetrad in the 16-step progression. Before coming to that, however, I first survey the preceding tetrads.

The instructions for the first tetrad direct mindfulness to the following aspects while being aware of breathing in and out:

1. Know breaths to be long
2. Know breaths to be short
3. Experience the whole body
4. Calm the bodily formation

In practical terms, this means that, after having become mindful of the breath moving in and out, the meditator next becomes aware of the length of these breaths. These could be either long or short. Here, it is noteworthy that in the Pāli version, the instructions for steps (1) and (2) are worded as alternatives, evident in the use of the disjunctive particle *vā,* which means "or." In other words, the point at stake is not that one should be having first long breaths and then short breaths, but rather that one is aware of either long or short breaths.

A distinct characteristic of the early Buddhist approach to meditation on the breath is in fact an emphasis on mere observation, instead of attempting to control the breath in the way this would be the case for someone engaging in a type of practice that involves an intentional controlling of the breathing process. Elsewhere, the early discourses report that, during the period of his quest for awakening, the Buddha-to-be did engage in breath control, yet he found that this did not lead him to liberation (MN I 243; translated in Ñāṇamoli 1995, p. 337 f.).

In principle, the breath is an aspect of the body that happens naturally, but which can also be influenced through one's intentions. Breathing happens even when no attention is being paid to it, yet one can freely decide to take a deep and long breath, for example.

Instead of attempting to control the breath, however, implementing the instructions in the *Ānāpānasati-sutta* would simply require being aware of the length of the breath as it naturally occurs in the present moment. This length should then be distinguished into two types: belonging to either the category of long breaths or the category of short breaths.

The next step then requires experiencing the whole body. Here, the instructions in the *Ānāpānasati-sutta* show a shift of terminology, as the discourse proceeds from referring to an act of "knowing," employed for the first two steps, to using the expression "training," a term used throughout the remainder of the 16 steps. In the *Ānāpānasati-sutta,* then, with step (3) concerned with experiencing the whole body, a form of training begins, one trains oneself to experience the whole body while breathing in or breathing out.

The parallel versions differ, as the *Saṃyukta-āgama* speaks of "training" in the case of each of the 16 steps (T II 206a), including the first two, whereas the three Vinayas do not mention the need for any "training" at all (T XXII 254c, T XXIV 32c, and T XXIII 8a).

The notion of engaging in a form of training in relation to mindfulness of breathing, even though this clearly does not imply an attempt to control or even suppress the breath, does point to some degree of intentional monitoring of a natural process that for the most part unfolds on its own.

The impression that actual practice involves some degree of intentional monitoring finds further support in the instructions given for the 16 steps. Had there not been a need for some degree of intentional effort or directing of the mind, there would have been little reason for detailed instructions on how to proceed through the 16 steps. So some extent of "training" is indeed required, inasmuch as the practitioner does incline the mind in such a way that the ensuing step can take place. Yet, at the same time, such "training" is not a forceful matter that involves a strong degree of control, but is probably best understood as a soft kind of nudging of the mind in the proper direction.

The proper direction to be taken for this third step requires some degree of discussion, as the Pāli commentarial tradition takes the expression "body" in the instruction "to experience the whole body" as intending the body of the breath (Vism 273; translated in Ñāṇamoli 1956/1991, p. 266). That is, the practitioner should become aware of the full length of the breath, being able to distinguish between its beginning, middle, and final parts.

This interpretation is not entirely straightforward, as awareness of the breath in its full length has already been the task of the preceding steps (1 and 2). Unless one has been aware of the whole breath, from its beginning all the way to its final parts, it would not be possible to know if this breath should be reckoned "long" or "short." So on the explanation suggested by the Pāli commentarial tradition, the third step would not be introducing something distinctly new to the progression of practice, but would just amount to a repetition, or perhaps better a refinement, of awareness of the whole breath.

Here, the parallel versions in the three Vinayas provide a helpful indication, as they formulate the third step in terms of "pervading the body." Such pervading would indeed present a distinctly new element for the progression of practice, in that from having become aware of the breath in its entire length, the meditator now moves on to becoming aware of the whole body in the sitting posture. This would be a natural progression when turning attention inward, where the breath as an easily noticeable bodily process would then lead on to noticing other and more subtle bodily sensations occurring elsewhere in the body. On this understanding, the third step in the progression would involve a conscious broadening of the field of awareness from the breath alone to the breath experienced within an awareness of the whole body.

The final step in the first tetrad then requires a calming of the bodily formation. Here, the term formation, *saṅkhāra,* can be understood to mean in particular the breath itself. In addition, the same term could also be taken to stand for any other bodily activity. On this understanding, the instruction would then entail a relaxing of the body in the sitting posture until it becomes naturally still and stable, as well as a calming of whatever other bodily activity may be going on within the body, to the extent that one is able to calm these down. These two interpretations are mutually supportive insofar as a calming of the breath will naturally lead to an increased general tranquility of the body, and tranquility of the body in turn will enhance the calmness of the breathing process. So it seems safe to conclude that step (4) requires calming the breath and the body.

In sum, then, a way of practically implementing the first tetrad of mindfulness of breathing could proceed from becoming aware of the breath to recognizing its length (in terms of either long or short breath), followed by broadening the field of one's awareness from the breath to the whole body in the sitting posture and then relaxing breath and body, allowing them to become calm. Chief themes of actual practice would then be a firm establishing of mindfulness on the breath and the body together with a gradual calming of both.

4.3 The Second Tetrad

The instructions for the second tetrad in the 16-step practice model delineated in the *Ānāpānasati-sutta* describe the progression of practice to be undertaken while remaining aware of breathing in and out as follows:

5. Experience joy
6. Experience happiness
7. Experience mental formation
8. Calm mental formation

The instructions for steps (6) and (7) refer to joy *(pīti),* often alternatively translated as "rapture," and to happiness *(sukha)*. Joy and happiness are qualities characteristic of the first and second absorption *(jhāna)*. Although this clearly draws attention to the potential of mindfulness of breathing to lead to deep concentration and the attainment of absorption, mental conditions of joy and happiness can already manifest at stages of practice that fall short of being full absorption attainment.

A perusal of the early discourses in general gives the impression that the attainment of absorption represents a deeply concentrated mental condition in which the mind is quite literally absorbed in its object and has become thoroughly unified (Anālayo 2003, 75 and the following pages). On adopting such an understanding of the nature of absorption attainment, the instructions in this part of the *Ānāpānasati-sutta* and its parallels would then appear to refer to lesser levels of concentration, in the sense that the mind would be unified and collected only up to such a degree that one can still be distinctly aware of the difference between inhalation and exhalation. Already during such lesser levels of concentration, wholesome forms of joy and happiness can be experienced that will become more intense when the mind proceeds to deeper levels of concentration. Whatever understanding of the nature of absorption one may advocate, it seems fair to conclude that steps (5) and (6) need not be seen as confined to actual attainment of a form of mental absorption during which one is no longer able to sense distinctly inhalations and exhalations.

From a practical perspective, then, the basic degree of bodily and mental calm established through the preceding four steps leads at the present juncture to the arising of a wholesome form of joy (step 5). Practitioners might even consciously encourage the arising of joy by reviewing the pleasant condition of tranquility that one is experiencing after having proceeded through the first tetrad. Joy, which at times can be quite exuberant and rapturous, eventually leads over to the calmer experience of happiness (step 6) in the sense of a pleasantly contented condition of body and mind. With step (7), awareness of joy and happiness leads on to becoming aware of any other mental formation or activity present in the mind. This and the next step in this tetrad are similar to the last two steps in the preceding tetrad, inasmuch as in each case meditation proceeds from awareness of bodily or mental formations to their calming (step 8).

The description of these four steps in the parallel versions is closely similar, a minor but noteworthy difference is that step (8) in the *Mahāsāṅghika* and *Sarvāstivāda* Vinayas require "letting go" of mental formations, an expression these two versions also used in relation to step (4). This in a way could be seen as a complementary description of the calming enjoined in the *Ānāpānasati-sutta*. It is precisely when one has a mental attitude of being willing to let go bodily and mental formations that these become calm. In the present context, this would involve, in particular, the willingness to let go of joy and happiness; however, powerfully attractive these may be in actual experience, in order to be able to proceed further in the practice.

Understood in this way, steps (5) and (6) clearly show that wholesome joy and happiness have a central part to play in the practice and should be encouraged, a topic that comes to the fore again in relation to the awakening factors, to which I will turn later. At the same time, however, steps (7) and (8) show that joy and happiness should be experienced with an attitude that is willing to let go of them, allowing them to subside naturally once the time for that has come.

A way of practically implementing the second tetrad of mindfulness of breathing would then be to proceed from the joy that comes from the calming down of bodily processes to the calmer experience of happiness, which via becoming aware of any other mental activity that might be taking place at that time then leads over to a calming of these mental activities. Chief themes of such practice would then be giving proper place to joy and happiness as integral parts of the practice, combined with aiming at a calming down of mental processes.

4.4 The Third Tetrad

The practice of the 16 steps of mindfulness of breathing described in the *Ānāpānasati-sutta* proceeds to a third tetrad, which relates awareness of breathing in and out to the following steps:

9. Experience the mind
10. Gladden the mind
11. Concentrate the mind
12. Free the mind

The parallel versions agree closely on these four steps. Meditation at the present juncture moves from being aware of the contents of the mind to becoming aware of the mind itself. So far, the progress of practice involved a shift from awareness of the body (or of aspects of the body) with the first tetrad to the experience of mental activities or qualities (like joy and happiness) with the second tetrad. Progression to the third tetrad involves a further degree of refinement. The ability to know that one is breathing in or breathing out does not require much meditative expertise, and even to know if one is joyful or happy can still be reckoned part of average experience. Of course, in both cases, through intentional directing of mindfulness one learns to notice these more clearly than one would have done earlier. At the present juncture, however, to become aware of the mind as such, in the sense of recognizing that which is aware of the breath or aware of joy and happiness, clearly requires some degree of meditative expertise and familiarity with introspection. The present step does continue along the same trajectory taken earlier, but this continuity requires some degree of meditative expertise for a practitioner to be able to navigate the transition from awareness of what is experienced to awareness of experience itself.

In practical terms, successfully navigating this shift from step (8) to step (9) can take place through a turning back of awareness, or a turning inside of awareness, so to say. From being mindful of the breath, one turns back awareness to that which knows the breath. From being mindful of the experience of joy and happiness, one turns awareness inside to that which knows the experience of happiness. Thanks to the calming of mental formations experienced in the preceding step (8), it becomes easier to recognize the mind itself, to experience that which knows experience.

Awareness of the mind itself then leads naturally to the arising of gladness, because such turning back or inward of awareness results in a much more subtle and calm type of experience. The type of gladness that arises at this stage of practice is one that easily leads to concentration, to the mind becoming collected and unified (step 11). In this way, the mind comes to be increasingly freer from any obstruction or mental hindrance. Having become naturally concentrated, at the present juncture, the mind is also free from any interference on the side of the meditator, however subtle it may be. Instead of interfering, the mind is simply allowed to rest in calm composure. The freedom of this calm composure is what the practitioner is aware of (step 12), alongside the constantly changing rhythm of inhalation and exhalation.

So one way of practically implementing the third tetrad of mindfulness of breathing would be to turn awareness back to that which knows, and then proceed from the naturally arisen gladness that results from such turning back to collecting the mind and liberating it. Chief themes of practice undertaken in this way would be to know the mind as such and to allow it to become free from any distraction or interference.

4.5 The Fourth Tetrad

The final tetrad in the 16 steps of practice in the *Ānāpānasati-sutta* proceeds by combining awareness of breathing in and out with the following insight-related themes:

13. Contemplate impermanence
14. Contemplate fading away/dispassion
15. Contemplate cessation
16. Contemplate letting go

With the first of these steps, the fact of impermanence, which anyway was present at the background of the practice throughout the preceding steps by way of remaining aware of the breath coming in and going out, now moves to the center stage of attention. With step (13), not only the impermanent nature of the breath, but also the impermanent nature of all aspects of experience becomes the object of contemplation. This includes the impermanent nature of any joy and happiness experienced as well as the impermanent nature of that which knows—the mind. Even though the ability to know is a constant given in all experiences, the very fact that one is able to know different things makes it clear that the mind must also be changing itself. Were it permanent, then it would be forever frozen in the condition of knowing only a single thing. According to early Buddhist thought, the entire gamut of body and mind is nothing but a changing process, without any exception all of it is subject to the law of impermanence.

From a full appreciation of impermanence, the practice then moves on to *virāga,* which could be translated as "fading away" or else as "dispassion" (step 14). Both translations bring out related nuances of what in actual experience are closely interrelated aspects in the progress of insight. Seeing that everything changes and is bound to fade away arouses dispassion, one naturally becomes disenchanted and disillusioned with what anyway is impermanent. In this way one's passion will inevitably diminish and fade away. Such dispassion through seeing the fading away of impermanent phenomena in a way brings out the characteristic of *dukkha,* making it unmistakably clear that impermanent phenomena are incapable of yielding lasting satisfaction. All conditioned phenomena are indeed "unsatisfactory," and this insight brings about increasing degrees of dispassion and inner freedom through detachment.

From dispassion, the instructions in the *Ānāpānasati-sutta* proceed to cessation *(nirodha)*. This could be understood in the sense of attending to the disappearance aspect of whatever is experienced. Be this the breath or joy, or whatever else one knows in the present moment, it all is bound to cease, bound to disappear, giving room to the arising of something else. Contemplating cessation in this way sharpens insight into impermanence, bringing to the fore of attention the aspect of impermanence that is the most threatening one: Things are bound to cease and vanish. Another and complementary aspect of the practice at the present juncture would be that dispassion (step14) leads by degrees to the cessation of *dukkha*. While the final cessation of *dukkha* requires full awakening in early Buddhist thought, minor cessations of craving and clinging can be experienced already much earlier, as long as dispassion is being cultivated.

The more the practitioner comes to be at peace with cessation (step 15), learning to allow things to end, the easier it becomes to let go (step 16). Letting go or relinquishing here refers to letting go of any form of attachment, most importantly perhaps to letting go of all sense of identification and appropriation of any aspect of experience in terms of "I" or "mine." Such letting go points directly to the final goal of liberation.

Some parallel versions differ from the presentation in the *Ānāpānasati-sutta* regarding steps (14) to (16). In their presentation, practice continues from contemplating impermanence to contemplating eradication (step 14), dispassion (step 15), and cessation (step 16). Following this mode of presentation, contemplation of impermanence would then lead to eradicating, which could be understood to intend the gradual eradication of clinging and attachment. This would naturally lead on to dispassion and then cessation.

A way of practically implementing the fourth tetrad of mindfulness of breathing as described in the *Ānāpānasati-sutta* would be to proceed from the apperception of the changing nature of the breath to awareness of the impermanent nature of all aspects of experience. Clear awareness of impermanence would then be the foundation for arousing dispassion, proceeding to cessation in the sense of allowing things to end, and finally letting go in the most comprehensive manner possible. Alternatively, on following the parallel versions preserved in Chinese translation, based on insight into impermanence, one could turn to the eradication of attachment and then move on to dispassion and cessation. The chief theme of implementing the instructions for the last tetrad of mindfulness of breathing, whichever mode one may prefer, is clearly the cultivation of insight based on awareness of impermanence.

4.6 The Four Establishments of Mindfulness

After delineating the above 16 steps of mindfulness of breathing, the *Ānāpānasati-sutta* continues by relating them to the four establishments of mindfulness, *satipaṭṭhāna*. The early discourses recurrently refer to these four *satipaṭṭhāna*s in short, which require directing awareness to the following four aspects of experience:

- The body
- Feelings
- Mental states
- Dharmas

A detailed exposition of how the four *satipaṭṭhānas* can be practically undertaken is found in the *Satipaṭṭhāna-sutta,* a discussion of which forms a separate chapter in this book (see Chap. 5).

For the present purpose of exploring the practice of mindfulness of breathing, it is particularly remarkable that, whereas the *Satipaṭṭhāna-sutta* moves through different exercises in order to cover the four establishments of mindfulness, the *Ānāpānasati-sutta* accomplishes the same based on a single exercise: mindfulness of breathing. In this way, what taken on its own is an aspect of the body, namely the breath, can according to the *Ānāpānasati-sutta* be used as the basis for moving from contemplation of the body to contemplation of feelings, mental states, and dharmas. This shows a rather flexible approach to meditation, where the fact that the object used for contemplation is a bodily phenomenon does not automatically imply that actual practice needs to be confined to observation of the body. This well reflects what cultivation of mindfulness is about, namely a broadening of perspective.

The *Saṃyukta-āgama* parallel agrees with the *Ānāpānasati-sutta* on correlating the four tetrads of mindfulness of breathing with the four establishments of mindfulness, although the two versions show some minor differences in the rationale they provide for this correlation (Anālayo 2007). As mentioned above, the three Vinayas only cover the 16 steps of practice, so that for the present correlation and what follows in the *Ānāpānasati-sutta,* only the *Saṃyukta-āgama* provides material for comparative study.

Regarding the first tetrad, when being aware of long breath, short breath, the whole body, and calming the bodily formation, one is operating within the field of contemplation of the body, the first establishment of mindfulness, *satipaṭṭhāna.*

With the second tetrad, one becomes aware of joy and happiness, followed by attending to mental formations and their calming. In terms of *satipaṭṭhāna* meditation, this corresponds to the second establishment of mindfulness, contemplation of feelings.

The third tetrad involves invariably the mind: experiencing it, gladdening it, concentrating it, and freeing it. Clearly, this corresponds to contemplation of the mind or of mental states, the third *satipaṭṭhāna.*

Progressing through insight-related perspectives that build on impermanence—such as dispassion, cessation, and letting go (or else eradication, dispassion, cessation)—fulfills contemplation of dharmas, the fourth establishment of mindfulness. The relationship between the fourth tetrad of mindfulness of breathing and the fourth *satipaṭṭhāna* becomes particularly evident when one takes into consideration an exercise found in all of the three discourse versions of the *Satipaṭṭhāna-sutta,* namely the awakening factors. These are the qualities that need to be established in the mind in order to be able to break through to awakening. In fact, the *Ānāpānasati-sutta* and its *Saṃyukta-āgama* parallel continue their exposition by showing how mindfulness of breathing can lead to the cultivation of the awakening factors. Similar to the main purpose of these awakening factors, the themes delineated in the fourth tetrad of mindfulness of breathing prepare the mind for the breakthrough to awakening. Understood in this way, a thrust towards awakening is what emerges as a common theme of the fourth tetrad in the 16-step scheme of mindfulness of breathing and contemplation of the awakening factors as one of the exercises belonging to the fourth *satipaṭṭhāna*.

4.7 The Awakening Factors

Based on having established the relationship between the four tetrads of mindfulness of breathing and the four establishments of mindfulness, the *Ānāpānasati-sutta* and its *Saṃyukta-āgama* parallel continue by indicating that, with practice undertaken in this way, the seven factors of awakening *(bojjhaṅga)* can be cultivated. As their name indicates, the factors of awakening are those mental factors or qualities that according to early Buddhist meditation theory need to be cultivated in order for the mind to awaken. The seven awakening factors are as follows:

- Mindfulness
- Investigation of dharmas
- Energy
- Joy
- Tranquility
- Concentration
- Equipoise

The *Ānāpānasati-sutta* and its *Saṃyukta-āgama* parallel show in closely similar ways that through mindfulness of breathing one can establish the first and foundational of these awakening factors, which is mindfulness itself. Based on having established mindfulness, one then investigates and examines one's experience in the present moment. This results in the cultivation of the second awakening factor, investigation of dharmas. One also needs to make an effort to some degree while investigating, in order to avoid distraction, and the very activity of investigation in turn yields a momentum that arouses further energy. In combination, this then results in the third awakening factor of energy becoming established.

The form of energized investigation undertaken in this way is one that sooner or later will lead to the arising of wholesome forms of joy, which is the next awakening factor. For this to happen, it is important that investigation and energy do not result in the arising of tension and agitation, which can happen when practice becomes too pushy. Instead, investigation and energy are at their best when only taken up to the point of a continuous and sustained interest in the present moment's experience. Out of this, joy can arise, and this joy in turn is of a type that results in calmness of body and mind. The calmness of body and mind that pervades meditation at the present juncture can then turn into manifestations of the awakening factor of tranquility. Out of bodily and mental tranquility, the next awakening factors arise: concentration in the sense of a collected mind that is aloof from distraction. When the mind has become concentrated in this way, it becomes very finely balanced and reaches equipoise *(upekkhā)*, and the seventh of the awakening factors has come into being.

In this way, the task is to cultivate and maintain these seven mental qualities, from mindfulness to equipoise, alongside one's actual practice of mindfulness of breathing. Executing this task adds another dimension to the practice of the 16 steps described above. Somewhat comparable to the shift from knowing something to becoming aware of that which knows at the transition point from the second tetrad to the third tetrad of mindfulness of breathing, engaging in the cultivation of the awakening factors requires a similar act of turning inward. Through such turning inward, by monitoring one's own mental state of affairs, one learns to be aware of the actual condition of one's mind and cultivate it in such a way that the awakening factors arise and become established.

In order to bring into being the trajectory of the awakening factors from mindfulness to equipoise, the early discourses provide additional information on the dynamics underlying the awakening factors. These fall into three distinct groups (Anālayo 2013, p. 202 ff.). Here, mindfulness forms a group of its own, as it were, since mindfulness as the foundational factor of awakening is required in any situation or circumstance. The remaining six fall into two groups. One group comprises investigation, energy, and joy as awakening factors that energize. The other group contains tranquility, concentration, and equipoise as awakening factors that calm and tranquilize.

In actual practice, then, if while monitoring with awareness one's practice of mindfulness of breathing one notices that the mind has become a little sluggish, one could give emphasis to investigation, energy, and joy in order to energize the practice. If instead one notices that the mind has become slightly agitated, emphasis could instead be given to the qualities of tranquility, concentration, and equipoise. By navigating in this way through whatever fluctuations occur during actual practice, the seven factors of awakening can become increasingly well established in the mind.

4.8 Knowledge and Liberation

The *Ānāpānasati-sutta* and its *Saṃyukta-āgama* parallel continue by explaining how, once the seven awakening factors have been established with the help of mindfulness of breathing, progress to awakening can take place. This requires combining one's meditative practice of mindfulness of breathing, undertaken by cultivating the factors of awakening, with four insight-related themes. According to these four themes, the factors of awakening should be cultivated as follows:

- In dependence on seclusion
- In dependence on dispassion
- In dependence on cessation
- Culminating in letting go

Several of the themes mentioned here are familiar from the last tetrad of mindfulness of breathing, which in the *Ānāpānasati-sutta* similarly involves the progression towards dispassion, cessation, and letting go. The first term mentioned in the above set of four themes is seclusion, which in the present context could be taken to refer in particular to seclusion from anything detrimental in the mind. Based on such a mental condition of seclusion, it will be possible for the awakening factors to become fully established and lead to supreme seclusion, when through full awakening all defilements will forever be eradicated from the mind. Progress in this direction takes place through dispassion, cessation, and letting go, whose implications are as described above in relation to the fourth tetrad of mindfulness of breathing. A minor but noteworthy difference in presentation here is that the first three—seclusion, dispassion, cessation—are what one depends on in order to progress to the culmination point of letting go.

In a way, each of these three already involves some form of letting go. With the coming into being of seclusion any unwholesome mental condition is being let go off, as well as anything else that may stand in contrast to one's secluded mental condition. Dispassion is the letting go of passion and attachment, and cessation requires letting go of the wish for things to exist and last, for them to be always new and fresh, instead of passing away and disappearing. All these forms of letting go eventually can culminate in the supreme letting go that takes place with the attainment of awakening.

Awakening is in fact the main purpose of mindfulness of breathing in early Buddhist thought, where its function is clearly to become a vehicle for progress to full liberation. Whatever other benefits the practice of mindfulness of breathing may have, from an early Buddhist viewpoint these are only secondary compared to the central purpose of such meditation practice in leading to total freedom.

With full liberation attained, according to early Buddhist doctrine a practitioner has forever eradicated mental defilements from the mind. Anger and ill will, sensual desire and greed, depression and anxiety, and a whole host of other detrimental mental conditions no longer have a scope to arise in one's mind, which has become thoroughly liberated from their influence. The mind of one who has taken the practice of mindfulness of breathing in 16 steps up to its final culmination point is thus freed in all these respects. Such a one has fully realized the human potential and thereby reached the acme of mental health recognized in early Buddhism.

In this way, the exposition in the *Ānāpānasati-sutta* and its *Saṃyukta-āgama* parallel of mindfulness of breathing in 16 steps as a way of cultivating the four establishments of mindfulness and bringing into being the seven factors of awakening well exemplifies the general thrust of mindfulness meditation in early Buddhist thought: The predominant function of mindfulness meditation in its original historical context is clearly to lead to the goal of Nirvāṇa.

Abbreviations

MN	*Majjhima-nikāya*
T	*Taishō* edition
Vism	*Visuddhimagga*

References

Anālayo, Bh. (2003). *Satipaṭṭhāna, the direct path to realization*. Birmingham: Windhorse.
Anālayo, Bh. (2007). Mindfulness of breathing in the Saṃyukta-āgama. *Buddhist Studies Review, 24*(2), 137–150.
Anālayo, Bh. (2011). *A comparative study of the Majjhima-nikāya*. Taipei: Dharma Drum.
Anālayo, Bh. (2012). The historical value of the Pāli Discourses. *Indo-Iranian Journal, 55*, 223–253.
Anālayo, Bh. (2013). *Perspectives on Satipaṭṭhāna*. Cambridge: Windhorse.
Ñāṇamoli, Bh. (1956/1991). *The path of purification (Visuddhimagga) by Bhadantācariya Buddhaghosa*. Kandy: Buddhist Publication Society.
Ñāṇamoli, Bh. (1995). *The middle length discourses of the Buddha, A translation of the Majjhima Nikāya*. Boston: Wisdom.

Bhikkhu Anālayo is a professor of Buddhist studies at the Numata Center for Buddhist Studies of the University of Hamburg, and a researcher at the Dharma Drum Institute of Liberal Arts in Taiwan. He earned his doctoral degree with a study of the *Satipaṭṭhāna-sutta* at the University of Peradeniya in Sri Lanka, and his habilitation with a comparative study of the *Majjhima-nikāya* at the University of Marburg. His primary research interests are the Chinese *Āgamas*, meditation, and women in Buddhism. With over 250 publications, he is a leading scholar in research on early Buddhism.

Abbreviations

Chapter 5
Understanding and Practicing the *Satipaṭṭhāna-sutta*

Bhikkhu Anālayo

5.1 Introduction

The *Satipaṭṭhāna-sutta*, the "Discourse on the Establishments of Mindfulness," provides detailed instructions on how mindfulness can be cultivated so as to lead to the realization of Nirvāṇa. In line with the title of this chapter, my main aim in what follows is to develop an understanding of the significance of the discourse for the actual practice of mindfulness; a comparative study of the *Satipaṭṭhāna-sutta* meant for the more academically interested reader can be found in Anālayo (2011a, pp. 73–97).

The *Satipaṭṭhāna-sutta* is the tenth discourse in the collection of middle-length discourses, the *Majjhima-nikāya*, found in the Pāli canon preserved by the Theravāda tradition. A discourse, that for the most part is closely similar, occurs under the title *Mahāsatipaṭṭhāna-sutta* as the 22nd text in the collection of long discourses, *Dīgha-nikāya*, of the same Theravāda tradition.

The instructions in the *Satipaṭṭhāna-sutta* are addressed to "monks," in line with a recurrent usage in the early discourses of directly addressing only those in a particular congregation that, according to ancient Indian standards, were considered its more eminent members. This does not mean that mindfulness instructions and its practice were only meant for male monastics, in fact, elsewhere the discourses refer to nuns as well as lay disciples who are proficient in *satipaṭṭhāna* meditation (Anālayo 2003, pp. 275 f.).

The *Satipaṭṭhāna-sutta* has two discourse parallels that are part of the textual transmission of different Buddhist schools (on the significance of comparing parallels versions from different schools, see the first part of the chapter on the *Ānāpānasati-sutta*). One of these parallels is a discourse in the *Madhyama-āgama*, a collection of middle-length discourses probably transmitted by Sarvāstivāda reciters. The other parallel is a discourse in the *Ekottarika-āgama*, a collection of

---

Bh. Anālayo (✉)
Numata Center for Buddhist Studies, University of Hamburg, Alsterterrasse 1, 20354 Hamburg, Germany

E. Shonin et al. (eds.), *Buddhist Foundations of Mindfulness*, Mindfulness in Behavioral Health, DOI 10.1007/978-3-319-18591-0_5 numerical discourses whose reciters might have been members of the Mahāsāṅghika school. The school affiliation of this collection is a matter of continued discussion among academics, so that at present it is probably best to consider it as uncertain.

The practical instructions in the *Satipaṭṭhāna-sutta* follow a basic division of *satipaṭṭhāna* meditation into four main areas of contemplation, which are concerned with:

- The body
- Feelings
- Mental states
- Dharmas

Elsewhere, the early Buddhist discourses recurrently refer to these four areas for establishing mindfulness, without, however, providing a detailed account comparable to the *Satipaṭṭhāna-sutta* and the *Mahāsatipaṭṭhāna-sutta* regarding how each of these four can be put into practice. Contrary to the case of the *Ānāpānasati-sutta,* where the parallel versions show fairly close agreement, the *Satipaṭṭhāna-sutta* and its parallels exhibit considerable variations. These manifest in particular in relation to the first and fourth areas of contemplation, concerned with the body and with dharmas.

5.2 Contemplation of the Body

The *Satipaṭṭhāna-sutta* describes six distinct modes of contemplating the body, this being the first of the four *satipaṭṭhāna*s. These six modes involve directing mindfulness to the following:

- The breath
- Bodily postures
- Bodily activities
- The anatomical constitution of the body
- The material elements that make up the body
- A corpse in successive stages of decay

5.3 Contemplation of the Body: The Breath

The instructions for contemplation of the body in the *Satipaṭṭhāna-sutta* begin with the breath (MN I 56, translated in Ñāṇamoli 1995, p. 145). Having retired to a secluded spot and become aware of the breath, one progresses through the four steps of mindfulness of breathing that make up the first tetrad of practice in the *Ānāpānasati-sutta* (see Chap. 4 on this discourse for a more detailed discussion of the practical implications of this tetrad). The four steps are:

- Know breaths to be long
- Know breaths to be short
- Experience the whole body
- Calm the bodily formation

The *Satipaṭṭhāna-sutta* illustrates the first two steps of practice with the example of a turner who makes a long or a short turn on his lathe. The simile is not found in the parallel versions, in fact, the *Ekottarika-āgama* parallel does not mention mindfulness of breathing at all (T II 568a, translated in Anālayo 2013, pp. 286–295).

5.4 Contemplation of the Body: Bodily Postures and Activities

The next two exercises listed in the *Satipaṭṭhāna-sutta* are also absent from its *Ekottarika-āgama* parallel. The first of these concerns awareness of one's bodily posture, covering:

- Walking
- Standing
- Sitting
- Lying down

In addition to these four main postures, any other posture of the body could also become the basis for establishing mindfulness. The main task in this exercise is to be as continually as possible aware of one's bodily posture. This establishes a grounding in an embodied form of mindfulness that facilitates continuity of awareness in situations outside of formal meditation practice. The whole body in any posture offers a readily available support for establishing mindfulness in daily life situations, which can become a stabilizing factor for remaining aware of whatever else takes place in the present moment.

The second exercise, concerned with clearly knowing bodily activities, is also closely related to having built a foundation in embodied mindfulness. Such embodied presence of awareness then leads to a way of undertaking one's daily activities that is endowed with the presence of clear knowing or clear comprehension. According to the *Satipaṭṭhāna-sutta,* such clear knowing can be practiced when one walks or looks here and there, when one moves one's limbs, when one dresses, when one eats and drinks, when one falls asleep and wakes up, and even when one responds to the calls of nature. The main point of this exercise seems to be to use any bodily activity as an arena for the cultivation of mindfulness and clear knowing. Their presence will invest such activities with an inner centeredness and result in acting with a dignified and graceful manner, because of the very fact of being carried out with full awareness. Taken together, awareness of one's bodily posture and clear knowing of various bodily activities establish a grounding of mindfulness in bodily experience.

5.5 Contemplation of the Body: Anatomical Parts and Elements

The *Satipaṭṭhāna-sutta* continues with two analytical forms of contemplation. These are found in all of the three discourse versions. The first of these two exercises directs mindfulness to an examination of the anatomical constitution of the body. The practitioner reviews his or her own body as made up of various anatomical parts, such as hair, nails, teeth, skin, flesh, bones, various organs, and bodily liquids.

What is particularly noteworthy about such reviewing of the anatomical constitution of the body is that this form of mindfulness practice is explicitly accompanied by an element of evaluation. One should review the body as being "unclean," *asuci,* which could alternatively even be translated as "impure." Another qualification found in other contexts for this same exercise encourages seeing the body as "not beautiful," *asubha.* There can be little doubt that the present form of meditation encourages, even requires, a form of evaluation aimed at the deconstruction of the notion of bodily beauty. The point at stake here is not a deconstruction of the general notion of beauty as such, but in particular of bodily beauty as something that is sensually attractive and sexually alluring. This deconstruction has its foundation in the early Buddhist assessment of sensual attraction as being based on an erroneous mode of perception. In order to free the mind from such erroneous modes of perception and their negative consequences, contemplation of the anatomical parts aims at arousing a sense of detachment towards bodily beauty.

Here, the point of the exercise is not to arouse an attitude of negativity towards the body. Becoming disgusted with the body would simply be a way of succumbing to another unhealthy attitude towards the body. The aim of the exercise is to lead to a form of mental balance instead. This can be seen from a simile that comes with this exercise in the *Satipaṭṭhāna-sutta* and in its *Madhyama-āgama* parallel (T I 583b, translated in Anālayo 2013, pp. 269–286). According to this simile, the contemplation of the anatomical parts should be undertaken in a way comparable to looking at various grains in a type of utensil apparently employed in ancient India for sowing. Needless to say, looking at various grains will not stimulate sensual desire, but it will also not lead to aversion and disgust. Similar to the relatively neutral attitude that would result from looking at various grains, one should look at one's own body, and eventually also at the bodies of others.

The theme of detachment in relation to the body continues with the next exercise, which requires reviewing the material elements that according to ancient Indian thought are the raw material out of which a human body and any other manifestation of matter are made. The *Satipaṭṭhāna-sutta* lists four primary elements for this purpose. These are earth, water, fire, and wind. The four elements stand for basic properties of matter, namely solidity, wetness, temperature, and motion. By enjoining a mental dissecting of one's own body into these basic constituents of matter, the present exercise aims at undermining the solid sense of an embodied self that usually accompanies an unawakened experience. What easily is taken to be "my" body, on closer inspection turns out to be just a combination of material qualities that in themselves are not different from manifestations of matter outside in nature. The main thrust of this exercise, thus, would be the arousing of insight into the not-self nature of the body, leading to a lessening of identification with and appropriation of the assemblage of four material elements that makes up this body. At the same time, undertaking this exercise can foster a sense of connectedness to the nature outside of one's own body and to the environment as a whole, based on the growing understanding that this body and any other manifestation of matter outside of it are of the same nature.

The *Satipaṭṭhāna-sutta* and its parallels illustrate this form of contemplation with the example of a cow that has been slaughtered and cut up into pieces. A butcher selling these pieces no longer thinks in terms of "a cow," but rather in terms of its various pieces. In this way, his earlier perception of the cow as a compact unit has disappeared. Similarly, for a practitioner of this form of mindfulness practice, the perception of his or her own body as a compact unit gradually begins to dissolve, to be replaced by an apperception of basic material qualities that are found inside the body as well as outside of it. In this way, the de-identification strategy of this form of practice, in combination with a strengthening of one's sense of relatedness to the wider environment, results in undermining one's sense of separateness and uniqueness, of one's own body being somehow special in terms of race, gender, beauty, or whatever else it may be. Instead, the body is simply a conglomeration of hardness, wetness, temperature, and motion, with little in it to justify the creation of a sense of ego in relation to it.

5.6 Contemplation of the Body: Cemetery Contemplations

The *Satipaṭṭhāna-sutta* and its parallels depict in closely similar ways successive stages of decay of a corpse that has been left out in the open to rot away. The description proceeds from such a corpse becoming bloated and being devoured by various animals to its gradual falling apart, when at first the skeleton becomes visible, then all flesh disappears while the skeleton is still held together by tendons, and once these rot away the skeleton disintegrates into various bones scattered here and there, which eventually turn into dust.

A central purpose of this form of contemplation is to throw into relief the mortality of the human body and make it unmistakably clear that one's own body is bound to fall apart and disintegrate; it is definitely not exempt from that fate. Death is the inescapable destiny of all human bodies.

The formulation used in the *Satipaṭṭhāna-sutta* to introduce the stages of decay of a corpse gives the impression as if the actual practice were to involve some degree of imaginative reflection, perhaps even visualization, reading, "just as though one were to see a corpse thrown aside in a charnel ground." In the same way, one should reflect that one's own body "is of the same nature, it will be like that, it is not exempt from that fate."

This is remarkable in so far as it extends the range of mindfulness practice to forms of reflection and even to what seems to border on some degree of visualization. When considered in conjunction with the fact that contemplation of the anatomical parts requires an element of evaluation, it becomes clear that the form of practice envisaged in these body contemplations in the *Satipaṭṭhāna-sutta* and its parallels, arguably the earliest records of Buddhist conceptions of mindfulness, cannot be adequately understood as standing for an invariably nonconceptual and nonevaluative form of awareness.

Certainly, the absence of concepts and freedom from evaluative judgments is an important aspect in the cultivation of mindfulness as a tool for progress on the path to liberation. But the early Buddhist conception of mindfulness practice is clearly not confined to such modes of meditation. Now central task of mindfulness is certainly to emerge out of habitual patterns of judgmental evaluation. Nevertheless whenever opportune for the sake of progress to awakening, evaluations, reflections, and perhaps even visualizations have their place. They do have their place in as much as—and only as long as—they are able to contribute to the overarching aim of liberating the mind from defilements.

5.7 Contemplation of the Body: Summary

Practice of contemplation of the body undertaken according to the *Satipaṭṭhāna-sutta* proceeds from mindfulness of the breath to becoming aware of the body in various postures and activities as a grounding in an embodied form of mindfulness. This builds a foundation for analytical contemplations of the body through examining its anatomical constitution and the elements that make up its material aspects. Undertaking these two exercises has the purpose of deconstructing the sexual attraction of bodily beauty and undermining the tendency to appropriate the body as something special that is one's personal possession. The final exercise in this first of the four *satipaṭṭhāna*s quite vividly brings home the mortality of the body and its nature of being unavoidably destined to fall apart.

The last three exercises—concerned with the anatomical parts, the elements, and a corpse in decay—are similarly found in the two discourse parallels to the *Satipaṭṭhāna-sutta,* giving the impression that these three exercises reflect an early and common core of the conception of contemplation of the body in early Buddhist thought. This in turn suggests that contemplation of the body is not so much about using the body to establish mindfulness. Of course, this is an important aspect in the cultivation of mindfulness, referred to recurrently elsewhere in other discourses as "mindfulness of the body," *kāyagatā sati*. But the main thrust of contemplation of the body as a *satipaṭṭhāna* meditation practice evident in these three exercises appears to be to cultivate mindfulness so as to understand the true nature of the body. In short, the body is neither truly beautiful nor truly one's own, and invariably bound to disintegrate and fall apart. Such insights point directly at the main aim of *satipaṭṭhāna* meditation as a whole: progress towards liberation.

5.8 Contemplation of the Body: The Refrain

The *Satipaṭṭhāna-sutta* gives additional room to this overall thrust towards liberation in a paragraph that comes like a refrain after the description of each of the individual exercises for each of the four *satipaṭṭhānas*, from contemplation of the body to contemplation of dharmas. This refrain stipulates several alternative modes of practicing, as indicated by the disjunctive particle *vā*, which means "or." These alternative modes are followed by one final statement that is relevant to all forms of mindfulness practice, as can be seen from the fact that this statement is introduced with the conjunctive particle *ca*, which means "and." According to this final statement, the practitioner should dwell independently, without clinging to anything in the world. This, in short, is the gist of the whole practice of *satipaṭṭhāna*.

The alternative modes of practicing, introduced by the disjunctive particle *vā* in the *Satipaṭṭhāna-sutta*, are:

- Internal, external, both
- Arising, passing away, both
- Bare awareness

The first of these modes directs attention to what is internal and what is external. As far as other early discourses allow us to judge, the point here is to proceed from contemplation concerned with oneself to contemplating others (Anālayo 2013, pp. 17–19). So the main import of this instruction appears to be that mindfulness should not only be aimed at oneself—internally—but also at others—externally—so as to lead to a comprehensive understanding of what one is contemplating. In the case of the three body contemplations that are found in the *Satipaṭṭhāna-sutta* as well as in its two parallels—anatomical parts, elements, and corpse in decay—this understanding would seem to yield a feasible form of meditative cultivation. In actual practice, this then means being aware of the fact that not only one's own body but also the bodies of others are not inherently beautiful, simply a combination of elements, and bound to die and fall apart.

The second of the alternative modes of practicing is concerned with impermanence. Whatever one is mindful of should be recognized as being of a changing nature, by contemplating its arising, its passing away, and its arising and passing away.

The third aspect then involves a bare form of awareness, where one is just mindful of there being the body, merely for the sake of knowing and mindfulness. This counterbalances the more directed and, in a way, informed modes of mindfulness described earlier and shows that bare receptive awareness has its place within the *satipaṭṭhāna* scheme. Whichever of these three modes one may decide to practice, the central requirement remains the same: dwelling independently, without clinging to anything.

5.9 Contemplation of Feelings

The need to avoid clinging receives a further spotlight with the second of the four *satipaṭṭhāna*s. According to the standard exposition of dependent arising *(paṭicca samuppāda),* the conditioned genesis of *dukkha* can be traced back to clinging, which in turn arises because of craving. Craving then arises in relation to feeling. Whereas feeling is an integral part of the daily experience of anyone, from the average person who does not even meditate up to one who has reached full awakening, the same does not hold for craving and clinging. According to early Buddhist meditation theory, craving and clinging can and in fact should be removed and overcome. This inevitably puts feelings into the limelight as the place where craving and clinging can, but do not have to, come into being.

The term "feeling" translates to *vedanā,* which does not stand for emotions. An emotion is a complex phenomenon in Buddhist thought that has its closest equivalent in certain states of mind, *citta*. States of mind are the object of the third *satipaṭṭhāna*. The second *satipaṭṭhāna,* contemplation of feelings, is instead concerned with the basic affective condition of present moment's experience. This could be:

- Pleasant
- Unpleasant
- Neutral

The task of contemplation of feelings is to inculcate a clear recognition of these three basic affective tones of being pleasant, unpleasant, and neutral. Based on these three affective tones, subsequent reactions take place only too easily: desiring the pleasant to last and increase, wanting the unpleasant to diminish and disappear, and wishing for something more attractive and entertaining than the neutral, which is often experienced as boring and dull.

Building on the successful cultivation of the ability to recognize these three affective tones, contemplation of feeling then moves on to a further distinction. This distinction divides each of these three feelings into worldly and unworldly types. The distinction between worldly and unworldly feelings, found similarly in the *Satipaṭṭhāna-sutta* and its parallels, appears to be aimed at inculcating an awareness of an ethical dimension in the experience of feelings. The underlying rationale for such an ethical dimension comes from the early Buddhist assessment that some forms of pleasure and pain are better avoided, but others can become vehicles for the path to liberation. While worldly feelings of sensual pleasure, for example, are an obstruction to the gaining of mental freedom, unworldly feelings of non-sensual pleasure are an important aid for progress on the path. The distinction of each feeling tone into worldly and unworldly types intends to equip the practitioner of *satipaṭṭhāna* with a clear understanding of this crucial distinction.

In sum, then, contemplation of feelings trains one in clear recognition of the affective tone of present moment's experience as pleasant, unpleasant, or neutral, and moreover inculcates sensitivity to the ethical dimension of each of these feelings, in as much as their experience may further or counter progress to awakening.

5.10 Contemplation of Mental States

From having become aware of the affective tone of experience as that which conditions mental reactions, the *Satipaṭṭhāna-sutta* and its parallels continue by directing awareness to the condition of the mind. They do so by listing several possible mental states. In the *Satipaṭṭhāna-sutta,* this listing begins with the presence of lust and its absence, followed by the presence of anger and its absence, and the presence of delusion and its absence. A fourth set lists distraction and its absence, followed by several mental states that appear to be related to more advanced stages of meditation practice, when mindfulness has the function to monitor practice by recognizing if the mind has become great, unsurpassable, concentrated, or liberated, listed together with their opposites.

The fact that these mental states invariably come in pairs has a noteworthy practical implication. In the case of experiencing sensual lust or anger, for example, the task is not only to recognize when these are present in the mind. This is, in a way, only half of what the meditator is expected to do. The other half of the task is that one should recognize as well when the mind is free from lust and anger. Recognition of the positive quality of a mental condition that is at least temporarily free from defilement is an important aid for successful practice, providing an immediately accessible and self-evident source for encouragement and inspiration that will fortify the practitioner against the challenges that inevitably manifest during the progress of practice.

Self-inspection is anyway a key aspect of *satipaṭṭhāna* meditation, but its potential becomes particularly evident with the third *satipaṭṭhāna* and its emphasis on identifying one's own mental condition, be this a mood in the present moment or a recurrently manifesting character trait. The importance of honest recognition finds a highlight in another discourse, which shows the crucial importance of accurately discerning one's own mental condition. Being in a defiled condition, one needs first of all to become aware of that. Only upon honest recognition will it be possible to make an effort to emerge from the defiled condition. Similarly, it is also important to know when one is in an undefiled mental condition, otherwise one will not make an effort to protect and nurture such a mental condition (MN I 24, translated in Ñāṇamoli 1995, p. 108).

The instructions in the *Satipaṭṭhāna-sutta* and its parallels for the third *satipaṭṭhāna* are aimed at equipping the practitioner with the skills required for such recognition. The actual task here is to look beyond or through any particular train of thoughts and associations that may arise in the mind and clearly apperceive the underlying current, the basic mental condition that informs the stream of mental ideas and thoughts. Instead of giving in to various self-rationalizations and projections, one honestly acknowledges what is really going on in one's own mind.

In sum, contemplation of mental states trains the practitioner in clear and honest recognition of one's own mental condition, inculcating a mindful monitoring of the present moment's experience that ranges from moments of sensual lust and anger to awareness of the development of the mind during more advanced stages of meditation practice.

5.11 Contemplation of Feeling and Mental States: The Refrain

In accordance with the stipulation given in the "refrain" part of the discourse, the second and third *satipaṭṭhāna*s can be undertaken internally as well as externally. External practice here would refer to recognizing from the facial expression or tone of voice of another if something that has just happened has led to pleasant or painful feelings, or even to mental reactions of lust or anger, etc. Such externally directed awareness can be of considerable help for skillfully navigating even difficult situations and challenging interpersonal relations in everyday life.

According to the same "refrain" part, feelings and mental states are also to be seen as impermanent phenomena. In the case of feelings, awareness of their changing nature can go a long way in divesting them of their apparent importance. Pleasure and pain will have considerably less leverage in the mind once the fact that they are anyway bound to change is clearly held in awareness. In the case of the mind itself, from the viewpoint of early Buddhist thought any mental state, be it a particular mental condition of being defiled or undefiled, bare awareness, or a profoundly deep condition of mental absorption, is subject to the law of impermanence. In other words, that which knows experience, that which is aware of phenomena, is itself also a changing phenomenon. The fact that this knowing quality forms a constant given in experience can easily lead to the assumption that there must be something permanent that is beyond change. Sustained practice of mindfulness, undertaken in accordance with early Buddhist meditation theory, will uncover that even that apparently constant quality of knowing is merely a succession of moments of being conscious, a stream of awareness that is as impermanent as the phenomena it cognizes. Being impermanent, such awareness is also a conditioned phenomenon, it is also a dependently arisen state.

5.12 Contemplation of Dharmas: The Hindrances

Conditionality is a theme that comes more explicitly to the foreground with the next of the contemplations in the *Satipaṭṭhāna-sutta,* which takes up the five hindrances, the first exercise in the fourth *satipaṭṭhāna* concerned with contemplation of dharmas. The mental states and conditions assembled under the heading of being "hindrances" are what early Buddhist meditation theory considers to be particularly obstructive for attempts to use the mind to its fullest potential. The five hindrances are:

- Sensual desire
- Anger
- Sloth and torpor
- Restlessness and worry
- Doubt

The actual listing covers seven distinct mental states, where sloth and torpor are grouped together due to their similar effect on the mind. The same holds for restlessness and worry.

The theme of conditionality underlies the instructions given in the *Satipaṭṭhāna-sutta* for contemplation of these hindrances. One should not only know if one of these hindrances is present in the mind or else absent, but one should also recognize the conditions that have led to the arising of a hindrance and the conditions that will lead to its removal and prevent its subsequent re-arising. Such direct drawing of attention to conditionality acquires its rationale from the overall thrust of the present exercise, which of course is to overcome the hindrances. Nevertheless, the actual overcoming of the hindrances is the task of another factor in the conception of the path to liberation in early Buddhist thought, which comes under the header of being an eightfold path. Here, right mindfulness in the form *satipaṭṭhāna* meditation is only one of eight factors required for progress to liberation. Another factor is right effort, which involves precisely the effort to overcome defilements in the mind.

As particularly evident in the preceding contemplation of the mind, a central task of *satipaṭṭhāna* is receptive recognition. Neither contemplation of the mind nor contemplation of the hindrances describes the taking of active measures to emerge from a defiled mental condition. This is noteworthy, since it brings out a central characteristic of mindfulness meditation in the form of receptive awareness. As the various exercises found under contemplation of the body show, such receptive awareness can at times come with an element of purposeful evaluation and reflection, as long as this fosters the overall soteriological orientation of the practice. Nevertheless, mindfulness itself remains a mental quality of receptive awareness.

Such receptive awareness functions as a crucially important stage in the overall attempt to emerge from a defiled mental condition. Instead of immediately reacting and perhaps in a combative attitude trying to force the defilement out of the mind, the procedure is rather to become, first of all, just aware of what is happening. Full awareness of the defiled condition of one's own mind, how it happened, and also how it negatively affects one's present well-being, lay the proper foundation for then being able to take efficient action. At times, bare recognition may in fact suffice for a particular defilement or hindrance to go into abeyance. Should this not suffice, then the time has come to bring in the path factor of right effort in order to emerge from a hindrance or defilement. By then one has fully explored the situation with receptive mindfulness and is well equipped for handling the situation as effectively as possible.

The chief aim of contemplation of the five hindrances is thus to enable clear recognition of their presence or absence and insight into the conditions whose understanding can help in emerging from the hindrances.

5.13 Contemplation of Dharmas: The Aggregates

The *Satipaṭṭhāna-sutta* continues next with contemplation of the aggregates, an exercise not found in its two parallels in the *Madhyama-āgama* and the *Ekottarika-āgama*. The five aggregates serve as an overview of central aspects of personal experience that could be identified with and appropriated as one's own. These are:

- The body
- Feelings
- Perceptions
- Volitional formations
- Consciousness

Here the body stands for what is material, whereas the remaining four cover the mental side of experience. Feelings to some extent stand in a middle position, since even though they are mental phenomena, feelings often affect the body and are the part of the mind that directly senses the body. Perception stands for the mind's ability to recognize what is experienced with the help of concepts and labels that are the result of previous learning and acquaintance. Volitional formations stand for the intentional aspect of the mind, the tendency, or at least the potential, to react and take decisions. Consciousness is the part of the mind which cognizes experience.

The meditative task in this case is to recognize each of these five facets of personal experience or existence and then become aware of their impermanent nature. The instructions in the *Satipaṭṭhāna-sutta* indicate that, for example, in the case of consciousness, one should know that "this is consciousness, this is its arising, this is its passing away." In this way, the theme of impermanence, which anyway is taken up in the refrain after each individual exercise, acquires such prominence here that it is built into the actual instructions.

The chief target of contemplation of the five aggregates is insight into the impermanent and therefore not-self nature of all aspects of personal experience.

5.14 Contemplation of Dharmas: The Sense-Spheres

The next exercise in the *Satipaṭṭhāna-sutta* directs mindfulness to the sense-spheres, an exercise also found in the *Madhyama-āgama* parallel. Contemplation of the six sense-spheres in a way complements contemplation of the five aggregates, in as much as the sense-spheres also serve as an analysis of personal experience. These sense-spheres cover the material senses as well as the mind, resulting in the following listing:

- The eye and forms
- The ear and sounds
- The nose and odors
- The tongue and flavors
- The body and tangibles
- The mind and mental objects

It is remarkable that in this way early Buddhist thought places the mind on a par with other physical sense-doors. While the mind is what makes sense out of the information received from the other senses, the conceptual information derived in this way is considered as not necessarily superior to bare sense-door experience of forms, sounds, odors, flavors, and tangibles.

Behind this stands a clear awareness of the potentially deceptive nature of concepts and their tendency to lure the mind into reactions, opinions, and even dogmatic views. Nevertheless, early Buddhist thought does not consider concepts to be problematic as such, but rather attempts to use them wisely as stepping stones for progress on the path. In fact, *satipaṭṭhāna* meditation clearly takes place in reliance on concepts, even in the case of the second and third *satipaṭṭhāna,* which prominently feature a receptive form of awareness. Actual practice requires the use of concepts or even labels of the type "pleasant feeling" or "unpleasant feeling," as well as "mind with anger" or "mind without anger," etc. The instructions in the *Satipaṭṭhāna-sutta* for these categories are explicitly worded in such a way that these labels come as direct speech, making it unmistakably clear that some form of mental verbalization is involved, however subtle it may be.

The actual contemplation of the sense-spheres in the *Satipaṭṭhāna-sutta* then requires recognizing the six senses and their objects, as well as the mental fetter that might arise in dependence on them. As in the case of the hindrances, here again conditionality is brought into play, in as much as, alongside recognizing the fetter, one should also know how this fetter arose, how it can be overcome, and how its re-arising can be prevented. As before, the task of mindfulness is the full exploration of these conditions with receptive awareness, the taking of actual measures to overcome a fetter belongs to the domain of right effort.

The main target of contemplation of the sense-spheres is to draw attention to the fettering force of all forms of experience, in order to learn to withstand and overcome this tendency to mental bondage.

5.15 Contemplation of Dharmas: The Awakening Factors

From the two analyses of experience, by way of the aggregates and the sense-spheres, the *Satipaṭṭhāna-sutta* proceeds to the awakening factors. Notably, this is the only exercise that is also found in the two parallel versions, the *Madhyama-āgama* and the *Ekottarika-āgama*. The seven awakening factors are as follows:

- Mindfulness
- Investigation of dharmas

- Energy
- Joy
- Tranquility
- Concentration
- Equipoise

In the context of *satipaṭṭhāna* meditation, the task is to know whether these seven mental qualities are present in the mind or else absent. In line with the emphasis on the conditionality of mental events already evident with the hindrances and the sense-spheres, in the present context the practitioner should also be aware of how the awakening factors can come to arise and how they can become fully established.

In early Buddhist meditation theory, the seven awakening factors occupy a central position as the mental qualities whose presence in the mind makes awakening possible (see in more detail the discussion of the awakening factors in Chap. 4). The central aim of the present exercise is the development of the ability to recognize the awakening factors and to know how they arise and can be nourished so that they come to be fully established.

5.16 Contemplation of Dharmas: The Four Truths

The last exercise in the *Satipaṭṭhāna-sutta* also stands in a close relationship to awakening; in fact, the scheme of the four truths is on record as the foundational teaching given by the recently awakened Buddha to his first disciples. The four truths take up the following topics:

- *Dukkha*
- Its arising
- Its cessation
- The path to its cessation

Proper appreciation of the implications of this central doctrine in early Buddhist thought requires a careful handling of the term *dukkha*. The standard rendering of this term as "suffering" is prone to lead to misunderstandings, and a better rendering of *dukkha* would be "unsatisfactory" (Anālayo 2003, p. 244 f.).

The need for care when translating this term can be exemplified with the case of feelings. All feelings fall under the sway of *dukkha,* yet not all feelings are "suffering." Some feelings are painful, but others are pleasant. Even the changing nature of these feelings is not "suffering." While one may suffer when a pleasant feeling changes and disappears, when a painful feeling changes and disappears this will not be experienced as suffering. All feelings are clearly not suffering. But all feelings are unsatisfactory, as due to their impermanent nature none of them is able to offer truly lasting satisfaction.

So the first truth does not involve a proclamation that the whole world is suffering. Instead, it highlights that whatever one experiences, even the most sublime pleasure, cannot yield lasting satisfaction, because it is inevitably bound to change.

The dissatisfaction experienced when things change is, according to the early Buddhist analysis, a direct reflection of the degree to which one is attached to them; in other words, the degree to which one has craving. This is the theme of the second truth, which shows that one's own craving is a central conditioning factor for whatever dissatisfaction, frustration, or mental pain one might experience. Conditions in the outer world are often enough beyond one's control and direct influence, but how one reacts to them does fall within the sphere of what one can control and influence. The second truth thus reveals the need to take responsibility for the part that one contributes oneself to any dilemma or problem experienced.

The complement to this revelation then comes with the third truth, which asserts that it is possible to be completely free from craving. With the cessation of craving and ignorance, the whole chain of the dependent arising of *dukkha* ceases, and the supreme peace of Nirvāṇa is realized.

The fourth truth then delineates the actual path to be undertaken to reach Nirvāṇa, which is the eightfold path, consisting of:

- Right view
- Right intention
- Right speech
- Right action
- Right livelihood
- Right effort
- Right mindfulness
- Right concentration

Based on a preliminary acquaintance with the four truths as one's right view, one rectifies any mental, verbal, and physical activities (including livelihood) in accordance with this right view. Through mental training that proceeds based on the framework of the four truths, one arouses the effort to emerge from defilements and remain free from them, cultivates mindfulness in the form of *satipaṭṭhāna,* and develops concentration in the form of absorption attainment.

The scheme of the four truths appears to be based on an ancient Indian medical diagnostic scheme. While there is no firm evidence for the existence of such a scheme in non-Buddhist literature of that time, it seems fairly probable that some such scheme was in existence at a popular medical level (Anālayo 2011b). The basic pattern underlying this scheme, as applied to the four truths, is as follows:

- Disease
- Pathogen
- Health
- Cure

The use of a medical scheme of analysis conveys an eminently pragmatic orientation of early Buddhist thought, which approaches the problem of *dukkha* from what is a predominantly psychological perspective.

The instructions for working through this scheme in the *Satipaṭṭhāna-sutta* are fairly brief. The practitioner should simply recognize *dukkha* as it really is, its arising, its cessation, and the path leading to its cessation.

As mentioned earlier, the collection of long discourses, the *Dīgha-nikāya,* has a discourse under the title *Mahāsatipaṭṭhāna-sutta,* the "Great Discourse on the Establishment of Mindfulness." The main difference between the *Satipaṭṭhāna-sutta* and the *Mahāsatipaṭṭhāna-sutta* manifests in relation to the present exercise. The *Mahāsatipaṭṭhāna-sutta* goes into considerably more detail in relation to contemplation of the four truths by delineating various aspects of each (DN II 304, translated in Walshe 1987, p. 344 ff.). The parallels to the *Satipaṭṭhāna-sutta* in the *Madhyama-āgama* and the *Ekottarika-āgama,* however, do not take up the four truths at all.

5.17 Contemplation of the Dharmas: The Refrain

According to the stipulation made in the refrain, each of the various contemplations of dharmas surveyed so far should be applied to oneself as well as to others. Moreover, the impermanent nature of each should be clearly recognized. Alternatively, one can simply be aware of them. The final point in each case is invariably that one should dwell independently, without clinging to anything.

5.18 Contemplation of the Dharmas: Summary

Undertaking the whole set of the contemplations of dharmas according to the instructions given in the *Satipaṭṭhāna-sutta* could begin by examining the mind for the presence of any of the hindrances. Next, the practitioner could continue by analyzing present moment's experience with the help of the five-aggregate scheme and attending to it from the viewpoint of the six sense-spheres and their potential to result in a mental fetter. The next step would be establishing the awakening factors, leading to insight into the four truths.

When considered from a comparative perspective, it is remarkable that only the awakening factors are common to the expositions of contemplation of dharmas in the *Satipaṭṭhāna-sutta* and its two parallels in the *Madhyama-āgama* and the *Ekottarika-āgama*. The hindrances are also part of contemplation of dharmas in the *Madhyama-āgama* discourse, whereas in the *Ekottarika-āgama* version they are just mentioned in an earlier part of the discourse.

Similar to the case of body contemplation, this brings out an essential aspect of contemplation of dharmas as a *satipaṭṭhāna* practice. The main thrust of such contemplation does not appear to be on contemplating various aspects of the Dharma, the teaching of the Buddha, but much rather about monitoring progress on the path to awakening. This requires in particular the cultivation of the awakening factors (which needs to be based on successfully emerging from the hindrances).

This perspective makes it more easily understandable why the last tetrad of mindfulness of breathing in the 16-step scheme described in the *Ānāpānasati-sutta* should be reckoned a mode of contemplating dharmas. This last tetrad requires progress through four insight-related perspectives: impermanence, dispassion, cessation, and letting go. Just as the awakening factors are mental qualities aimed at the breakthrough to awakening, in the same way these four themes directly aim at the breakthrough to awakening. Understood in this way, a thrust towards awakening is what emerges as a common theme of the fourth and last section in the 16-step scheme of mindfulness of breathing and what is common in the fourth and last *satipaṭṭhāna* described in the *Satipaṭṭhāna-sutta* and its parallels.

5.19 Purpose of *Satipaṭṭhāna*

The final part of the *Satipaṭṭhāna-sutta* turns to the purpose of properly undertaken practice, indicating that within a time period that could vary from 7 years to 7 days the attainment of non-return or full awakening would be possible. A similar prediction can be found in the *Madhyama-āgama* parallel, which even envisages such a possibility for a single day and night of proper practice. The use of such numbers is to some extent symbolic, simply serving to indicate that progress is certain, but the time it takes can vary.

In early Buddhist thought, the attainment of non-return or full awakening corresponds to the higher two of four levels of awakening, the other two being stream-entry and once return. What distinguishes these two higher levels is the definite, complete, and irreversible removal of any form of sensual desire and anger from the mind. In this way, the *Satipaṭṭhāna-sutta* and its *Madhyama-āgama* parallel present the practice of mindfulness they describe as capable of leading to a mental condition in which neither sensual desire nor anger will have any more scope to manifest.

The strong soteriological orientation that emerges in this way is already evident right at the outset of the *Satipaṭṭhāna-sutta,* which introduces the practice of *satipaṭṭhāna* as the way to overcoming all *dukkha* and to realizing Nirvāṇa. The same is also a continuous theme throughout. According to a stipulation given in the *Satipaṭṭhāna-sutta,* contemplation of the body, feelings, mental states, and dharmas requires combining diligent energy with mindfulness and clear knowing in such a way that one stays free from desire and discontent in regard to the world. The same theme is also the recurrent finale of the "refrain" that comes after each exercise, which instructs that contemplation should lead to dwelling independently and without clinging to anything in the world.

The achievement of a state of complete mental health through the lasting removal of clinging is the central aim and purpose of mindfulness practice in early Buddhist thought. Although early Buddhist thought clearly recognizes the potential of mindfulness to lead to physical health and psychological well-being (Anālayo 2015), *satipaṭṭhāna* has its predominant function as the direct path to the realization of Nirvāṇa.

Abbreviations

DN *Dīgha-nikāya*
MN *Majjhima-nikāya*
T Taishō edition

References

Anālayo, Bh. (2003). *Satipaṭṭhāna, the direct path to realization*. Birmingham: Windhorse.
Anālayo, Bh. (2011a). *A comparative study of the Majjhima-nikāya*. Taipei: Dharma Drum Publishing Corporation.
Anālayo, Bh. (2011b). Right view and the scheme of the Four Truths in Early Buddhism. The Saṃyukta-āgama parallel to the Sammādiṭṭhi-sutta and the simile of the four skills of a physician. *Canadian Journal of Buddhist Studies, 7,* 11–44.
Anālayo, Bh. (2013). *Perspectives on Satipaṭṭhāna*. Cambridge: Windhorse.
Anālayo, Bh. (2015). *Healing in Early Buddhism*. Buddhist Studies Review (forthcoming).
Ñāṇamoli, Bh. (1995). *The middle length discourses of the Buddha: A translation of the Majjhima Nikāya*. Boston: Wisdom Publications.
Walshe, M. (1987). *Thus have I heard: The long discourses of the Buddha*. London: Wisdom Publications.

Bhikkhu Anālayo is a professor of Buddhist studies at the Numata Center for Buddhist Studies of the University of Hamburg and a researcher at the Dharma Drum Institute of Liberal Arts in Taiwan. He earned his doctoral degree with a study of the *Satipaṭṭhāna-sutta* at the University of Peradeniya in Sri Lanka and his habilitation with a comparative study of the *Majjhima-nikāya* at the University of Marburg. His primary research interests are the Chinese *Āgamas*, meditation, and women in Buddhism. With over 250 publications, he is a leading scholar in research on early Buddhism.

Chapter 6
Sīla and *Sati:* An Exploration of Ethics and Mindfulness in Pāli Buddhism and Their Implications for Secular Mindfulness-Based Applications

Steven Stanley

6.1 Introduction

The growth of the mindfulness movement seems to be at its zenith. In clinical medicine and clinical psychology, standardised evidence-based mindfulness courses such as mindfulness-based stress reduction (MBSR; Kabat-Zinn 1990; Stahl and Goldstein 2010) and mindfulness-based cognitive therapy (MBCT; Segal et al. 2013) are becoming increasingly recognised as interventions for people suffering from stress, anxiety, depression and other mental health difficulties. Third-wave acceptance-based cognitive behavioural therapies, dialectical behaviour therapy (DBT) and acceptance and commitment therapy have been developed which teach mindfulness skills to clients (see Baer 2006; Didonna 2009). Eclectic and nonstandardised applications of mindfulness in counselling and psychotherapy have also emerged (Barker 2013). Looking further afield, and outside of clinical contexts, we now find mindfulness-based applications in diverse fields such as education, sport and business (see Bush 2011; Weare 2014; Chaskalson 2011; for an overview, see Ie et al. (2014)).

From the perspective of research, the multidisciplinary field of mindfulness studies appears to be growing rapidly, such that it is arguably impossible for any one individual researcher to keep up with research trends and publications on the topic. *Mindfulness Monthly* is an Internet publication which aims to document and summarise mostly clinical research articles about mindfulness published each month (American Mindfulness Research Association 2014). Indeed, interest in mindfulness has become so pronounced—with mindfulness turning up in perhaps unexpected places such as American and British politics (Ryan 2012; The Mindfulness Initiative

S. Stanley (✉)
School of Social Sciences, Cardiff University, Glamorgan Building, King Edward VII Avenue, CF10 3WT Cardiff, Wales, UK
e-mail: StanleyS1@Cardiff.ac.uk

E. Shonin et al. (eds.), *Buddhist Foundations of Mindfulness*,
Mindfulness in Behavioral Health, DOI 10.1007/978-3-319-18591-0_6

2014), transnational corporations (Tan 2012) and even the US military (Stanley 2014)—that it has recently been described as a "movement" in American society (Wilson 2014). This burgeoning interest and popularity have led to a backlash in some quarters, with commentators arguing that mindfulness is being oversold (Brazier 2013). The majority of critiques seem to be made by Buddhist commentators, whose central concern seems to be that mindfulness meditation, as a practice with roots in ancient and modern Buddhist traditions, might have become denatured, or cut off from its Buddhist roots, with undesirable consequences (e.g. Titmuss 2013). It is now recognised by some of the founders of the most well-known mindfulness-based applications that it is time to pause and reflect on the mindfulness movement: to be mindful about mindfulness (e.g. Williams and Kabat-Zinn 2011). This chapter follows this trend by exploring the Buddhist roots of mindfulness, specifically the relation between mindfulness and ethics in early Buddhism, and their implications for secular mindfulness-based applications.

6.2 Mindfulness, Ethics and Buddhism

The topic arguably given the most attention in critical discussions of secular mindfulness courses, as taught outside of Buddhist contexts, is ethics or morality (for a discussion of various "'gains" and "losses" of mindfulness as a medical and therapeutic tool, see Clower and Peng (2014)). Arguably, one of the most common concerns expressed by Buddhist commentators who reflect upon the modern mindfulness movement is that secular adaptations, when presented as equivalent to Buddhist mindfulness, seem to lack the grounding in ethical reflection and morality which is central to some (but not all) Buddhist traditions (see Purser and Milillo 2014; Wallace and Bodhi 2006). In being made modern and secular, they argue that mindfulness risks losing its moorings in Buddhist ethics, the Buddhist path to liberation and what it means to live a good life. When looking at the mindfulness movement from this angle, it could be said that in being taken out of its Buddhist contexts, secular mindfulness might be a demoralised version of Buddhism: appropriated as a therapeutic or self-help tool, but without the liberative and soteriological potentials of *dharma* practice (on the wider demoralisation of Western culture, see Fevre (2000)). Buddhist teachers and scholars have been the most overtly critical of the apparent lack of a clear ethical framework and grounding for secular mindfulness teaching in contrast to the teaching of mindfulness in Buddhist contexts. Most notably, applications of mindfulness meditation in transnational corporations such as Google's *Search Inside Yourself* program (Tan 2012) and in the US military application *Mindfulness-Based Mind Fitness Training* (MMFT®; Stanley 2014) have been subject to the most critical attention (e.g. Titmuss 2013).

Leaving aside for a moment corporate and military applications of mindfulness, in a general sense, it is rare for patients, students or clients who are taught mindfulness skills or mindfulness meditation in clinical, educational or business contexts to be instructed to adhere to explicit ethical codes of conduct, as they might in a

Buddhist context. Whilst mindfulness teachers themselves are likely to explicitly follow professional ethical codes of conduct (e.g. an ethical duty of non-harming), their students will not necessarily be bound by such codes, or necessarily frame their practice of mindfulness ethically or morally. Instead, it is perhaps more likely that students of mindfulness will frame their understandings psychologically or therapeutically, that is, without giving explicit and special attention to ethical and moral matters (however, this is a hypothesis which has yet to be the subject of empirical research). Indeed, when it is approached in a modern context, mindfulness is most commonly interpreted as a psychological therapy. Recent collections framing mindfulness as a style of clinical psychology intervention or way of enhancing wellbeing attest to this orientation by containing very little, if any, discussion of ethics or morality (see, for example, Didonna 2009; Ie et al. 2014). According to McCown (2013), the mindfulness teaching community in America shows "little interest in engaging the ethical" (p. 17). He writes that the ethical is an "under explored realm" (p. 33) in secular mindfulness teaching. This is particularly noteworthy given the apparent Buddhist influence upon mindfulness-based applications on the one hand and the crucial importance of ethical and moral investigation and purification in the early Buddhist teachings, on the other.

Some critics have argued that secular definitions of the concept of mindfulness have become de-ethicised, making ethically questionable applications possible, and that there is a need to re-ethicise our conceptual understanding of mindfulness by engaging with Buddhist thought, especially Pāli Buddhism (e.g. Bodhi 2012; Kang and Whittingham 2010; Purser and Milillo 2014; Stanley 2013). The Pāli canon contains some of the earliest documented teachings of the historical Buddha and is therefore a crucial resource for scholars seeking to understand the ancient roots of mindfulness as a style of meditation, especially its ethical and moral moorings. The Pāli canon was committed to writing in Sri Lanka around the middle of the first century BC (Keown 1996). This collection of discourses comprises one of the core sources for one of the earliest documented schools of Buddhism, the Theravadā School, which means "Abiding Teaching" or "Original Teaching" (ibid.; for a detailed discussion of Pāli, see Gombrich (1994)).

However, other commentators have argued that rather than secular mindfulness demoralising Buddhism, it might be more accurate to speak of the remoralising of mindfulness as a result of it being recontextualised for Western audiences (Williams and Kabat-Zinn 2011). It has been argued that notions of the good life, goodness and rightness (i.e. morality) are inherent to both Buddhism and the secular mindfulness movement. Wilson (2014) argues that proponents of the mindfulness movement make a moral distinction between the mindful (good) and the mindless (bad) and propose mindfulness as a solution to the problem of a "mindless" society at the level of individual psychology. Social change is envisaged as beginning with the individual: One mindful individual at a time. Mindfulness is not only understood as giving immediate practical benefits and short-term solutions to individual psychological and emotional problems—such as eating disorders, attention deficit or sexual difficulties—but it is also often combined with a broader social vision and project of social emancipation and change, even freedom and revolution (i.e. practising mindfulness to make the world a better place, such as achieving world peace, e.g., Tan (2012)). In Wilson's (2014) view, the boundaries between the religious and the secular are not as clear-cut as might be implied when we talk about a "secular" mindfulness movement.

> No matter how much effort is expended to remove the religious nature of mindfulness, it still continues to have the capacity to operate in a religious manner. We might call this a secular religion, one devoid of the supernatural and the afterlife yet operating as a deep well of values, life orientation, and utopian vision. (p. 185)

Whilst in this chapter I present mindfulness-based applications as secular and, therefore as distinct from religion, it is important to address the ambiguity of the religious status of the mindfulness movement. Kabat-Zinn (2011) described the work of MBSR as "sacred as well as secular" (p. 301) in part due to it arguably containing a "universal dharma" which is taught in secular settings. Williams and Kabat-Zinn (2011) similarly described mindfulness-based interventions such as MBSR and MBCT as "Dharma-based portals" (p. 12). In response to such claims, Shonin et al. (2013) discussed the ambiguity of mindfulness-based interventions vis-à-vis religion and spirituality, the ethics and credibility of such claims, and the potential "identity crisis" of MBSR. By contrast, in relation to MBCT in the UK, Gilpin (2008, p. 228) distinguished a Theravāda spiritual perspective—grounded in monastic religious contexts—and the secular perspective of MBCT, grounded in an evidence-based clinical psychology.

Despite this ambiguity between the secular and religious (spiritual or sacred) meanings of mindfulness, I still want to preserve a distinction between the ancient Buddhist and the secular contexts of mindfulness. Modern secular mindfulness courses are arguably quite different to most Buddhist contexts in which mindfulness is taught, including the ancient contexts, not least because mindfulness-based teachers often disclaim the Buddhist status of their ideas and practices (e.g. Kabat-Zinn 1990). In addition, in many Buddhist contexts, there is often explicit attention given to investigation and purification of the moral dimensions of intention as a foundation for meditation practice—in both lay and monastic settings. Indeed, Olendzki (2014) suggested that in the early Buddhist teachings, "moral integrity is a precondition for the efficacy of meditation…the mind is simply unable to become concentrated if it is permeated with such unwholesome states as sensual desire, ill-will, restlessness, sluggishness, or doubt" (p. 63). He goes on to highlight the "fundamental role of ethics in early Buddhist mental training" (p. 72). Indeed, Thomas William Rhys Davids (1890), the first scholar to translate the Pāli canon into a European language (in collaboration with his wife Caroline), described early Buddhist teachings as comprising an "ethical psychology" (p. 58). By returning to the ancient sources of Buddhism, we can arguably engage more directly with the ethical and moral basis of the psychology of mindfulness, and potentially better understand and evaluate the social and political meanings and functions of mindfulness-based applications in modern day society.

When ethics and morality are discussed in relation to mindfulness-based applications, this is often in relation to the *teaching* of mindfulness rather than its practice by students (e.g. Kabat-Zinn 2011; McCown 2013; but see Cullen 2011; Kang and Whittingham 2010). In his investigation of the ethics of mindfulness-based pedagogy, which involves a reflection on his own experience as a mindfulness teacher, McCown (2013) argued that exploration of the ethical space in mindfulness-based interventions is overdue and that such investigation might make an important contribution to attempts to define mindfulness and ensure the integrity of mindfulness-based teaching. McCown suggested that there is already an implicit theory of the ethical space in mindfulness-based pedagogy, which needs to be made explicit (e.g. the cultivation of *mettā* or loving-kindness in some MBIs involves an "inherent ethical stance", p. 48; Kabat-Zinn (2011) makes a similar argument). A mindfulness course is a cocreation between the teacher and students. It is a shared ethical space. McCown suggested that individualistic discourses dominate the clinical and research perspectives towards mindfulness and that instead a relational view is needed which is in fact already present within the conduct of the pedagogy of mindfulness-based applications themselves. McCown suggested that whilst it is a temptation to look to Buddhist thought for an ethical psychology to ground or supplement our mindfulness teaching, for a number of reasons this is undesirable and inappropriate. Considering that the ethical dimension is arguably already implicitly present in mindfulness courses, it is better to instead articulate and understand what is already present within the pedagogy of secular courses. Whereas Kabat-Zinn (2011) suggested MBSR contains a "universal dharma" primarily derived from Buddhist thought and practice, McCown (2013) disagreed that the ethical space of MBSR is, or should necessarily be, Buddhist, not least because mindfulness courses need to present themselves with a secular face in most contexts (for a related discussion, see Shonin et al. (2013)). Cullen (2011) made a similar argument and suggested ethics is a "formality" in Buddhist traditions and that it is "equally possible to integrate a foundation of ethical behavior into the practice of mindfulness itself" through personal experience of the relationship between "skilful behavior and personal flourishing" (p. 189). Cullen suggested ethical sensitivity would arise naturally from the practice of mindfulness, which in itself is inherently wholesome. I will return to this argument below.

In this chapter, I take a different path to McCown (2013) and Cullen (2011), by investigating ethics and mindfulness in the ancient Pāli Buddhist discourses and considering their potential relevance for modern secular understanding and practice of mindfulness. I suggest that we can learn something from these early discourses that might help us to develop our application of secular mindfulness in ethically sensitive ways. The chapter does not offer an overview of ethics and mindfulness in early Buddhism in the abstract, but rather integrates into the discussion comparisons to claims made about mindfulness in modern secular applications of mindfulness in psychosomatic medicine and clinical psychology. The chapter aims to integrate ancient and modern accounts of the relations between mindfulness and ethics. My basic argument is that we can learn from the ethical psychology of early Buddhism and this encounter may enrich secular mindfulness teaching.

6.3 Modern Mindfulness and Ancient *Sati*

Peacock (2014) suggested there is a clash between the ancient traditions of Buddhism and modern mindfulness-based approaches in mental health care. This is evident in a divide between clinical empirically based scientific approaches to mindfulness and Buddhist religious approaches to *sati*. He suggested there is a "mutual suspicion that has arisen amongst practitioners on both sides of the 'divide'" (p. 2). Whilst clinicians and scientists may suggest the Buddhist background to mindfulness is unnecessary or irrelevant, Buddhist practitioners tend to characterise mindfulness-based approaches as "somehow 'dharma' light" (p. 2). Peacock suggests that such suspicions on the part of clinicians and scientists are largely based on misunderstandings of the teachings of the historical Buddha found in the Pāli canon. If clinicians better understood these ancient teachings on mindfulness, then there is a chance that the mutual suspicion on both sides of the divide will be lessened.

Let us start with a brief consideration of the ways in which mindfulness tends to be understood in professional clinical and research circles. When we use the word mindfulness, it is easy to assume that we are speaking about the same thing. But there is actually a range of meanings given to mindfulness in secular contexts. I find it helpful to map these meanings on a continuum according to their relative dependence upon Buddhist traditions of meditation, starting with the least dependent.

First, and at one end of the continuum, is mindfulness as a form of information processing distinct from "mindlessness". Langer's (1989) social cognitive understanding of mindfulness comprises: (i) the creation of novel conceptual distinctions and categories; (ii) openness to new information; (iii) awareness of more than one perspective. It is contrasted with "mindlessness". This definition is rooted in a Western (American) social cognitive tradition of experimental social psychology and does not take influence from Asian religious or meditative traditions. It is beyond the scope of this chapter to consider Langer's definition much more than this. For more information on Langer's definition and tradition of research and how it compares with Buddhist-influenced concepts of mindfulness, see Ie et al. (2014).

Second, in the middle of the continuum, is mindfulness as a technique or skill. Acceptance and commitment therapy (ACT), which is considered a third-wave cognitive behavioural therapy, uses "mindfulness techniques" or "mindfulness skills" as part of its therapeutic approach in order to teach clients to watch their minds and observe their thoughts mindfully (Hayes et al. 2012; Varra et al. 2009). These skills are not based upon meditation practice on the part of the therapist or client. Although it is not based on Buddhist ideas, but rooted in scientific cognitive behaviour therapy, there are parallels with Buddhism (Hayes 2002). Notably this perspective engages with clients' values. Similarly, DBT, a psychotherapy developed for individuals who are chronically suicidal and diagnosed with borderline personality disorder, also approaches mindfulness as a skill (Swales and Heard 2009). Tailored to the specific needs of its client group, DBT teaches seven short "mindfulness skills" taken from Zen Buddhism: wise mind, three "what" skills or practices (observing, describing, participating), and three "how" skills (nonjudgementally, one-mindfully, effectively). As in ACT, mindfulness is not dependent upon meditation practice, and mindfulness skills are taught didactically to clients in a one-on-one setting.

Third, and at the end of the continuum, are mindfulness-based approaches, applications and interventions that are based on an understanding of mindfulness as being dependent upon mindfulness meditation practice. Chiesa and Malinowski (2011) showed that even "mindfulness-based approaches" are not all the same and do not conceptualise or practice mindfulness in the same way. There is disagreement about how to categorise secular mindfulness-based courses: as mindfulness meditation, mindfulness-based interventions (perhaps in clinical contexts) or mindfulness-based applications (perhaps in nonclinical contexts). It gets even more complex once we introduce distinctions between mindfulness-influenced and mindfulness-informed counselling and psychotherapy (see Barker 2013). Nevertheless, there seems to be a consensus in mindfulness-based circles that mindfulness can be characterised following Kabat-Zinn's (2003) operational definition of mindfulness, which is influenced by specific Buddhist traditions. For Kabat-Zinn (1994, p. 4), mindfulness is an awareness which emerges when we pay attention in a particular way: intentionally, in the present moment, and nonjudgementally to experience from moment to moment. In both MBSR and MBCT, mindfulness is an awareness which is cultivated through mindfulness meditation and which reorients or decenters consciousness, allowing the practitioner to alternate between "being" and "doing" modes of mind (Segal et al. 2013). In mindfulness-based applications, mindfulness is dependent upon meditation practice and much more likely to be seen broadly and expansively as a way of living or being, that is, rather than as a delimited technique or skill. It is taught in a psycho-educational group-based format to diverse clinical and nonclinical populations.

I have focussed upon arguably the three most well known and relatively distinct uses of mindfulness in the literature on mindfulness. A commonality of all of these definitions is that they tend to approach mindfulness from a psychological perspective and assume that it is a mental entity existing within the mind of the individual person, that is, rather than a relational practice existing between people (for a critique of this orientation and articulation of a relational view, see Stanley (2012b)). This continuum of secular perspectives on mindfulness misses out research debates in psychometrics about the measurement of mindfulness as a trait using self-report scales, of which currently there are around a dozen (for a review, see Baer (2011); for a critique, see Grossman and Van Dam (2011)), as well as discussions in cognitive neuroscience about mindfulness' mechanisms of action, that is, how it produces its effects (e.g. Hölzel et al. 2011). Nevertheless, these discussions are similarly psychological and tend to define mindfulness as a psychological construct. This broadly psychological orientation goes partly towards explaining the lack of discussion of ethics and morality in mindfulness-based approaches.

Later in this chapter, I distinguish between mindfulness and *sati*. I use the English word mindfulness to denote the third end of the continuum described above: modern mindfulness-based applications, that is, mindfulness meditation as it is employed as a therapeutic tool in clinical and nonclinical settings for stress reduction, anxiety reduction or depression relapse prevention. This captures the modern Buddhist-influenced psychological understandings of mindfulness as employed in standardised and manualised mindfulness-based applications such as MBSR and MBCT. These are applications that understand mindfulness as dependent upon meditation practice. However, to better distinguish the ancient and the modern, where possible I will use *sati* to denote the ancient understanding of mindfulness employed in the Pāli discourses. (Where Pāli scholars use the word mindfulness for *sati* I will preserve their use of mindfulness.) *Sati* concerns the ancient use of the word *sati* and especially *satipaṭṭhāna* (ways of establishing mindfulness) practice as it is described in the Pāli canon and related discourses. A later section of the chapter is devoted to understanding the ethical orientation of *sati* in early Buddhist discourse. This is done in order to better contrast the ancient with the modern secular application of mindfulness.

There is a common misunderstanding, or at least an absence of understanding, which exists amongst mindfulness researchers and mindfulness teachers about the origins of contemporary mindfulness-based applications. The Buddhist-influenced practices which inform secular mindfulness courses (e.g. MBSR and MBCT), such as mindfulness of breathing or body scanning, had already been subject to modernising and psychologising (and other) influences prior to their uptake as relatively standardised and manualised therapeutic or self-help programs (McMahan 2008; Samuel 2014; Wilson 2014). For example, contemporary mindfulness-based interventions in the USA were most immediately influenced by modern American Buddhist traditions (e.g. West and East Coast Insight Meditation; see Glieg (2011, 2012)), which are in turn influenced by modernising Southeast Asian Buddhist ("Neo-*vipassanā*") reform movements of the late nineteenth and early twentieth centuries, especially in Sri Lanka, Burma and Thailand. These reformed versions of Buddhism have been called Modern Buddhism or Protestant Buddhism and need to be understood against the backdrop of British colonialism in parts of Southeast Asia (other contextual influences are important too, see Gombrich (1988) and McMahan (2008)). Scholarship in Buddhist studies helps us to understand that the origins of secular mindfulness-based approaches are much more recent than we might otherwise assume. For example, the "meditation centre" is a very recent modern phenomena, its roots lying in the lay meditation movements of Southeast Asia in the early to mid-twentieth century, rather than being an age-old ancient practice originating 2500 years ago (on Sri Lanka, see Gombrich (1983); on the commodification of meditation in Thailand, see Schedneck (2014)). When we look to the Pāli canon, we do not find meditation centres, and even more interestingly and relevant for present purposes, nor do we find a definition of mindfulness as *solely* denoting a present-centred and nonjudgemental way of paying attention, or "bare attention" (Wallace and Bodhi 2006). Therefore, it is worth distinguishing the ancient from the modern Buddhist understandings of mindfulness. When we do this, we can appreciate that it is misleading to suggest, as many researchers and teachers of mindfulness do, that mindfulness is an ancient style of meditation that has been carried out uninterrupted and unchanged for 2500 years (for a development of this argument, see Sharf (1995, 2000)).

6.4 Mindfulness as a Translation of *Sati*

We often use the word mindful to mean remembering to do something, being careful, heedful or cautious, intending, being conscious or aware, attentive or thoughtful. This meaning has been part of the English language at least since the fourteenth century (OED 2014). Around the sixteenth century, the noun mindfulness came to be used to denote attention, memory or intention. However, it seems that the first use of the English word mindfulness as meaning a style of meditation informed by Indian and Southeast Asian Buddhist traditions is in the late nineteenth century (for a historical discourse analysis, see Sun (2014)). Mindfulness is the English word used by the Buddhist scholar Thomas William Rhys Davids (1843–1922) to translate the ancient Pāli language word *sati*. As a young man, Rhys Davids worked as a civil servant in Ceylon, now Sri Lanka, then under British colonial rule. One of his early duties was as a magistrate. He was asked to preside over a case concerning the occupation of a village monastery. A document was produced before the court as evidence in a language no one could understand. The language was Pāli. Rhys Davids, who was already well versed in Latin and Sanskrit, became a student of the Sinhalese scholar monk Yātrāmullē Unnānsē and learnt how to translate the document. This was the beginning of a lifelong scholarly and personal commitment to the translation and study of early Buddhism (for further biographical detail on Rhys Davids, see Carpenter (1923), Chalmers (2004) and Wickremeratne (1985)).

Rhys Davids' abiding legacy for the contemporary mindfulness movement is clear: He established mindfulness as the accepted translation of *sati*. He wrote that *sati* is "one of the most difficult words…in the whole Buddhist system of ethical psychology to translate" (Rhys Davids 1890, p. 58). Its etymological meaning is memory, and indeed in his first book Rhys Davids (1877) translated *sati* as memory or recollection. One of the meanings of *sati* is memory, the verb *sarati* meaning to remember. However, Rhys Davids argued that the Buddha of the Pāli canon more commonly gave *sati* an ethical meaning: "that activity of mind, constant presence of mind, wakefulness of heart, which is the foe of carelessness, inadvertence, self-forgetfulness…it is a very constant theme of the Buddhist moralist" (Rhys Davids 1890, p. 58; see also "the active, watchful mind", Rhys Davids (1881, pp. 144–145)). Rhys Davids said he sometimes rendered *sati* as self-possession, but in modern times his translation of *sati* as mindfulness has endured. Rhys Davids and his wife Caroline influenced modern Western understandings of Buddhism in other important ways (see Snodgrass 2007; on the "intercultural mimesis" between Europe and "the Orient" in the nineteenth century, exhibited in the work of Rhys Davids, see Hallisey (1995)). But for the purposes of this chapter, it is Rhys Davids' translation of *sati* as mindfulness which is the most important influence.

In a recent chapter exploring the meaning of *sati* as memory, Peacock (2014) rendered *sati* as "present moment recollection" (p. 6) rather than mindfulness. He said that *sati* "'recollects' or 'remembers' what activity one is engaged in, in the present moment. This…is different from historical recollection or remembrance, as this is a 're-collecting' or 're-membering' of the mind from states of fragmentation and into some degree of wholeness—no matter how fleeting this may be" (p. 6; for an alternative reading of the relation of *sati* to memory, see Anālayo (2003, 2013)). Peacock (2014) also emphasised the ethical intoning of *sati*. "Close attention was to be paid, in particular, to one's ethical life because morally dubious and unethical behavior hardened into character, what the Buddha referred to as 'the shape of one's life'" (p. 7). Morality is a prerequisite for meditation in this early tradition.

6.5 Ethics, Morality and Virtue

This chapter concerns the domains of life covered by the related words ethics, morality and virtue. Although Buddhism has not developed an ethics or science of morality to the same degree as Western philosophy, there is still a significant recent literature exploring Buddhist ethics, either doing so relatively independently (Saddhatissa 1970; Tichibana 1926) or in relation to Western ethical systems (Harvey 2000; Keown 1992; Keown and Prebish 2013). Outside of the world of academic philosophy, the words ethics and morality tend to be used interchangeably. Indeed, this tends to be the case in Buddhist studies literature. Most texts tend to pass over explaining the specific meanings of ethics and morality and use them interchangeably. However, we might usefully make a simple distinction between ethics, morality and virtues, which will be used later in distinguishing the ancient and modern perspectives on mindfulness.

One understanding of ethics is as a science of morality often involving the philosophical study and systematising of moral principles. The *Oxford English Dictionary* (2014) defined ethics as "moral principles, or a system of these". Ethics includes the "codes of conduct or moral principles recognized in a particular profession, sphere of activity, relationship, or other context". The Greek *ethos* concerns the character or customs of a social group. An example in the context of academic psychology, which is relevant to mindfulness research, is the *British Psychological Society* Code of Ethics and Conduct (2009) and its ethical principles of respect, competence, responsibility, integrity, along with indicative ethical values and standards. Such ethical codes of conduct help to guide academic psychologists to make informed ethical choices and decisions in their relationships with clients and research participants. For example, such codes of conduct often contain an ethical injunction to refrain from harming the participants of psychological research.

One understanding of morality is knowledge and judgement of rightness and wrongness (or goodness and badness) of actions in everyday life (i.e. moral conduct or practical morality). Morality is "ethical wisdom, knowledge of moral science" (OED 2014) as it is enacted in the "workaday world" (McCown 2013). Morality includes the "branch of knowledge concerned with right and wrong conduct, duty, responsibility" (OED 2014). Latin *mos* (plural *mores*) refers to the manners and customs of everyday life. Morals concern specific "points of ethics; moral principles or rules"; they are "a particular moral system or outlook; moral thought or conduct in relation to a particular form of activity". We might understand morality as the lived reality and enactment (or otherwise) of ethical codes.

Virtue concerns moral qualities (especially religious ones), which are considered good or desirable in a person (OED 2014). We will see later that Buddhism emphasises the cultivation of specific virtues in the person. If we momentarily turn to MBSR, the seven attitudinal foundations of mindfulness listed by Kabat-Zinn (1990), which capture something of the secular orientation of mindfulness practice and meditation, might be seen as modern virtues of mindfulness practitioners: acceptance, patience, trust, nonjudging, non-striving, letting-go, beginner's mind. These can be compared to core virtues of early Buddhism: generosity, loving-kindness, empathetic joy and compassion.

A consideration of ethics, morality and values in a discussion of mindfulness places emphasis upon our relationships with others and how we treat others, which concerns our outward social actions, along with the interior life of the mind (Anālayo 2003; Kuan 2008; McCown 2013). At the same time, whilst ethical codes of conduct tend to concern the professionals' protection of *others* from harm (e.g. clients or participants of research), as we shall see in the discussion of the early Buddhist tradition, mindfulness might also function to protect or guard *professionals* from harming themselves (i.e. if they practice *sati* or *satipaṭṭhāna*). Buddhist ethical precepts encourage us to *investigate* relationships of harm in our personal and professional lives. In this sense, they are not commandments or rules. A consideration of the ethics of mindfulness might help us to extend ethical guidelines to include professionals' relationships to themselves as well as to others. "Psychologists have a responsibility to be mindful of any potential risks to themselves" (BPS 2009, p. 18).

We will consider below how the definition of mindfulness embedded in MBSR and MBCT might relate to the understanding of *sati* in the Pāli canon, which in turn will allow us to discern more clearly the ethical (or otherwise) understanding of mindfulness in MBSR and MBCT along with the ethics of their various applications. Before considering the ethical role and functions of *sati* in the early discourses, it is important to contextualise *sati* in relation to important ethical teachings of the historical Buddha.

6.6 Ethical Dimensions of Early Buddhism

The Pāli word *sīla* is translated variously as ethics, morality and virtue. There are a number of images used to depict the multiple functions of *sīla* in the Buddhist spiritual life (Keown 1992): basis or foundation (especially organic metaphors of seeds, earth and branches), protection (e.g. a coat, shelter, cave, umbrella, refuge, friend), motion or ascent (e.g. feet), purification (e.g. water, wind) and precious object (e.g. perfume). *Sīla* is given a central role in early Buddhist thought and practice. It is "the necessary foundation for the entire spiritual project envisaged by Buddhism" (Keown 1992). Indeed, in common understanding Buddhism is widely respected as "one of the world's most ethical religions" (Keown 1996, p. 9). An important overall guiding ethic in Buddhism is the principle of non-harming *(ahiṃsā)* towards all living creatures, a principle which might have been derived from Jainism, an ancient Indian religion contemporaneous with Buddhism, which also comprises renunciation (Gombrich 2009).

Keown (1992) suggested Buddhist ethics rest upon "the cultivation of personal virtue in the expectation that as spiritual capacity expands towards the goal of enlightenment ethical choices will become clear and unproblematic" (p. 2). In this sense, according to Keown, Buddhist ethics arguably parallel Aristotle's "virtue ethics" and Kantian intuitionism, rather than utilitarianism or situational ethics. However, at the same time, there are also ethical precepts in early Buddhism, which frame the conduct of good Buddhist practitioners. In the following sections, I will outline some of the important threads to contextualise the use of *sati* in Buddhist ethical psychology.

6.6.1 Precepts and Virtues

We can understand *sīla* as combining both moral duties and virtues. Keown (1996) paralleled Buddhist morality to a coin: on one side are the precepts, and on the other are the virtues. The precepts are duties of the good Buddhist and are phrased as ethical training rules or guidelines, that is, as practices of investigation as much as items of moral duty. In their everyday life, lay Buddhist practitioners take five precepts *(pañcasīla)* to undertake an ethical rule of training to refrain from taking life *(pānātipāta),* taking what has not been given *(adinnādāna),* sexual misconduct *(kāmesu-micchācāra),* telling lies *(musāvāda)* and taking intoxicants (*surā-meraya-majja-pamādathānā;* Keown 1992). Harvey (2000) suggested that the fifth precept, sobriety, can act as an aid to right mindfulness: "when one is intoxicated, there is an attempt to mask, rather than face, the sufferings of life, there is no mental clarity or calm, and one is more likely to break all the other precepts" (p. 77; see pp. 77–79 for a summary of varying applications of the fifth precept; see also Anālayo (2003)).

Core Buddhist virtues which frame the ethico-moral intoning of intentions and actions are: nonattachment *(arāga),* benevolence *(adosa)* and understanding *(amoha)*. These are the opposites of the three roots of evil (or fires): greed *(raga),* hatred *(dosa)* and delusion (*moha;* Keown 1996). Goldstein (2013) suggests that *sati* is not only a present moment awareness but also an awareness which is without craving or thirst, grasping, greed, hatred, and confusion. He articulated a holistic understanding of mindfulness as requiring the supports of virtues including equanimity, generosity, friendliness, kindness, compassion and wisdom.

6.6.2 Intention, Action and Result

In early Buddhism, intention is a crucial determinant of the moral quality of an action. "The Buddha taught that all thoughts, words and deeds derive their moral value, positive or negative, from the intention behind them…the basic criterion for morality is intention" (Gombrich 2009, p. 13). *Cetanā* is variously translated as intention, motivation or moral choice. It is the "compass-needle" (Keown 1992, p. 211) or "pivot around which virtue and vice revolve" (p. 165). Intention does not solely refer to cognition (thought) but also to emotion. In turn, mindfulness allows one to become more aware of one's mental states, especially intentions and motives (Harvey 2000). In this early Buddhist ethical psychology, emphasis is placed upon the importance of moral choice and discernment, especially concerning intention. The Buddhist practitioner discerns the morality of their intentions: neutral, good or bad. "The psychological springs of motivation are described in Buddhism as 'roots', and there are said to be three good roots and three bad roots. Actions motivated by greed, hatred and delusion are bad *(akusala)* while actions motivated by their opposites—non-attachment, benevolence and understanding are good" (*kusala*; Keown 1996).

Gombrich (2009) explained that the word commonly used by the Buddha for a morally good act is *kusala.* He noted that there is a debate amongst scholars about whether this word should be translated as "healthy, wholesome" or "skilful". Gombrich opted for skilled because for the Buddha a good moral choice was an "intelligent and informed choice" (p. 15). However, Keown (1992) noted that skilful implied Buddhist ethics are utilitarian and indeed may risk demoralising Buddhism (by turning practitioners into craftspeople rather than saints) and suggested "virtue" or "goodness" as the most natural translation for *kusala* when used in a moral context. He continued: "*kusala* is the term which *par excellence* denotes ethical goodness" (p. 124). This debate in turn relates to the Mahāyāna emphasis on skill in means *(upāya-kauśalya),* compassion *(karuna)* and the Bodhissatva path to liberation, which is outside of the scope of this chapter (see Keown 1992).

Moral choice is followed by an act—bodily, vocal, and mental. The word for action in Pāli is *kamma* (Sanskrit *karma*). In the literature of the Brahminical religion, *karma* means ritual act (Gombrich 2009). The historical Buddha was critical of the Brahminical emphasis upon the ritual performance of action and caste-bound ethics; equally, he was critical of the Jain placing of morality within actions themselves. The Buddha replaced the word ritual for the word intention: "It is intention that I call *karma*" (Buddha, cited in Kuan (2008, p. 50)). By *kamma,* the Buddha meant ethical volition or moral causality. Instead of caste-bound ritual, the Buddha recommended a focus on ethical intention. The Buddha understood social mores were man-made and not divinely created: "what brahmins believed to be ingrained in nature was nothing but convention" (Gombrich 2009, p. 26). Who you are depends upon the intentions that inform your actions, not your caste-bound performance of ritual action. "In popular usage karma is thought of simply as the good and bad things that happen to people, a little like good and bad luck. The literal meaning of the Sanskrit word karma is 'action', but karma as a religious concept is concerned not with just any actions but with actions of a particular kind. Karmic actions are moral actions, and the Buddha defined karma by reference to moral choices and the acts consequent upon them" (Keown 1996, p. 36). For Gombrish (2009, p. 35), the "whole universe is ethicized" in the Buddha's teaching: "all sentient beings throughout the universe are morally responsible and can be reborn in a higher or lower station because of the good and evil they have done". This understanding of early Buddhism requires belief in karma and rebirth as metaphysical processes. For an approach to early Buddhism without the requirement of such beliefs, see Batchelor (1997, 2010).

An implication of this teaching is that actions bring consequences for the actor. The notion of good karma in the early tradition is merit *(puñña)*. According to Keown (1992), this refers to the experiential or felt consequences of moral activity on the part of the moral actor. One of the purposes of moral action is to purify the mind and specifically the intention. *Puñña kamma* is purifying action. Morally purified action brings good fruit *(phala)*. "The metaphor is an agricultural one: performing good and bad deeds is like planting seeds that will fruit at a later date" (Keown 1996, p. 37). Sow a seed, cultivate (or grow) it—*bhāvanā* means cultivation—and then reap the harvest. "Sow an act, reap a habit; sow a habit, reap a character; sow a character, reap a destiny" (Keown 1996, p. 36).

6.6.3 Right and Wrong Mindfulness

Sammā sati (right mindfulness) is one element of the (Noble) Eightfold Path to liberation, which in turn is the fourth Noble Truth. The Eightfold Path is often grouped into three sections: *sīla* (ethics or morality or virtue) comprising right speech, right action, right livelihood; *samādhi* (meditation) comprising right effort, right mindfulness, right concentration or unification; and *paññā* (wisdom or understanding) comprising right view or understanding, right effort.

To practice *sammā sati,* one is instructed to follow the scheme of the four *satipaṭṭhānas* or ways of establishing *sati*. Anālayo (2013) noted that the four *satipaṭṭhānas* are an elaboration of the path factor of right mindfulness. "Mindfulness is a function or quality of mind, but it is often described as something to be practiced or cultivated" (Kuan 2008, p. 1). This is done through following the instructions given in the discourses on ways of establishing mindfulness in four domains or pastures: body (including breath), feelings, mind and *dhammas*. It is beyond the scope of this chapter to describe in detail the four *satipaṭṭhānas* in the various early discourses (for more information, see Chap. 5; Anālayo 2003, 2013). According to Kuan (2008), mindfulness prevents *saññā* (apperception or conception; elsewhere translated as cognition) from going astray to conceptual proliferation *(papañca)*. Mindfulness functions to direct *saññā* in "a proper way" which means not being caught up in desire and aversion. The "absence of mindfulness results in the mind being overwhelmed by sensual desire" (Anālayo 2013, p. 21). In this sense, mindfulness is the opposite of absent-mindedness *(muṭṭhassati)*.

In the Pāli discourses, *sati* is categorised as morally either right or wrong. *Sammā sati* is right mindfulness and *micchā sati* is wrong mindfulness (Rhys Davids and Stede 1925). This moral intonation of mindfulness in the Pāli discourses as right or wrong contrasts with the idea that mindfulness is an inherently right (or wholesome) mental factor whenever it is present, as suggested by the Theravādin Abhidhamma

—a later scholarly systematising of the Pāli canon—as well as in most mindfulness-based applications, which assume mindfulness is an inherent good (see the argument presented above by Cullen (2011)), or even as a *panacea* for the ills of the world (as sometimes implied in MBSR and MBCT; see Gilpin 2008). In this sense, the understanding of mindfulness in mindfulness-based applications might parallel the Theravādin Abhidhamma understanding of *sati* more than the historically prior Pāli discourses. In the later commentarial tradition, mindfulness is "a wholesome response that simply sees things as they are, without favoring or opposing, which allows for a radical nonattachment to all experience" (Olendzki 2014, p. 67). However, in the Pāli discourses, mindfulness is not always right. Wrong mindfulness is not only possible but also a constant threat to right mindfulness (on the various interpretations of mindfulness as an inherently right, universal or occasional mental factor, see (Olendzki 2011) and Anālayo (2013, pp. 178–181)).

Micchā sati concerns what is the opposite of *sammā sati,* that is, the opposite of the instructions given in the *satipaṭṭhāna* contemplations. Anālayo (2003, p. 52) stated that right mindfulness cooperates with various other mental qualities including being diligent *(ātāpī)* and clearly knowing *(sampajāna)*. This suggests that wrong mindfulness lacks diligence and clear knowledge of what is happening. Whilst right mindfulness connotes a state of mind free from desires and discontent, wrong mindfulness connotes a mind state comprising clinging and aversion. In addition to requiring the support of diligence and clear knowing, right mindfulness works in tandem with the other elements of the Noble Eightfold (or sometimes tenfold) path. Wrong mindfulness is therefore mindfulness without the support of the other path factors, or indeed a mindfulness accompanied by their opposites (i.e. the ignoble path).

Buddhism does not define what is right or appropriate *(sammā)* as independent from what is good or wholesome (*kusala*; Keown 1992). As such, *micchā sati* is described as a wrong or unwholesome path (or way or course) which is to be abandoned (or worn away, washed away or purged) through *sammā sati.* One way of discerning whether mindfulness is right or wrong is to notice the result of its conduct or practice (i.e. its consequences). "The result of wrong mindfulness is bad both in this present life and in future lives" (Buddha, cited by Bodhi (2012, p. 1501)). Wrong mindfulness leads to suffering, harm and failure, whereas right mindfulness leads to great fruit (e.g. happiness), benefit and success—for ourselves and for others.

"The numerous bad unwholesome qualities that originate with wrong mindfulness as condition: these are harmful" (Buddha, cited by Bodhi (2012, p. 1494)). Harmful forms of mindfulness are especially involved when the ethical precepts are contravened, such as the precept against taking life. This is well illustrated in a discourse which uses the metaphor of a "false path" for the wrong Eightfold path:

"Suppose, bhikkhus, that in a wooded range there was a great low-lying marsh near which a large herd of deer lived. Then a man appeared desiring their ruin, harm, and bondage, and he closed off the safe and good path to be traveled joyfully, and he opened up a false path, and he put out a decoy and set up a dummy so that the large herd of deer might later come upon calamity, disaster, and loss. But another man came desiring their good, welfare, and protection, and he reopened the safe and good path that led to their happiness, and he closed off the false path, and he removed the decoy and destroyed the dummy, so that the large herd of deer might later come to growth, increase, and fulfilment" (Buddha, cited by Ñāṇamoli and Bodhi (2005, pp. 209–210)). In this discourse, the "false path" is the wrong Eightfold path (including wrong mindfulness), which is the opposite of the "safe and good" noble Eightfold path "to be travelled joyfully". For further examples of discourses mentioning wrong mindfulness, see Anālayo (2003, p. 52, fn #31).

6.7 Functions of *Sati*

Sati is a nuanced and complex concept used throughout the Pāli canon. The word *sati* is used in multiple ways throughout the Pāli canon and its meaning varies depending upon its context of use. There is not space in this chapter to discuss all of its meanings and functions (for comprehensive analyses see Anālayo (2003, 2013) and Kuan (2008)). Instead, the focus is upon (i) its common functions which have relevance for secular mindfulness adaptations and (ii) its ethical and moral dimensions. Whilst instructions for the practice of *sati* are contained in the *satipaṭṭhāna* discourses, which describe the establishment of mindfulness in relation to four domains of experience (body, feelings, mind, *dhammas*), there are related discourses which contain remarks on the meanings, practice and functions of *sati*—not only Pāli discourses but also Chinese, Sanskrit, and Tibetan discourses (see Anālayo 2003, 2013; Kuan 2008). Analysing Pāli, Chinese and Sanskrit sources, Kuan (2008) categorised the functions of *sati* as simple awareness, protective awareness, introspective awareness and deliberately forming conceptions. We will consider each of these functions in turn along with their potential similarities and differences to modern secular understandings of the functions of mindfulness practice.

Simple Awareness Kuan (2008) suggested that psychologists often understand mindfulness as comprising a simple awareness of what is happening in experience, that is, a present moment awareness and acceptance. Kornfield (1977) offered a description of mindfulness which emphasises its so-called bare attention dimension: "The attitude of non-judgmental, directed observation allows all events to occur in a natural way. By keeping attention in the present moment, we can see more and more clearly the true characteristics of our mind and body process" (p. 13). Kuan (2008) described this function of *sati* as "the conscious registering of the presence of objects, which can be any incoming sensory data or experiences, whether in normal daily activities or during meditation" (p. 41). According to Peacock (2014), simple awareness is one of the most basic and foundational functions of *sati* that the other functions are built upon: "non-judgmental recognition and acknowledgement of what has arisen in one's psychophysical experience" (p. 8). Anālayo (2003) illustrated the bare recognition element of *sati* using the example of anger: "By simply remaining receptively aware of a state of anger, neither the physical reaction nor the mental proliferation is given scope. If, on the other hand, one abandons the balanced state of awareness and resents or condemns the arisen anger, the act of condemnation becomes just another manifestation of aversion. The vicious cycle of anger continues, albeit with a different object" (p. 191).

Another example of the simple awareness element of mindfulness practice is the Buddha's instructions to Bāhiya: "When in the seen will be only what is seen, in the heard only what is heard, in the sensed only what is sensed, in the known only what is known, you will not be by that; when you are not by that, you will not be therein; when you are not therein, you will be neither here nor there nor in between. This is the end of *dukkha* [suffering or unsatisfactoriness]" (Anālayo 2003, p. 230).

Peacock (2014) argued that whilst "simple non-judgmental observation of experience" is vital and indeed a foundation for the other functions of *sati,* practised this *alone* will ultimately change very little in one's life. Nevertheless, the simple awareness function of mindfulness is an essential foundation and prerequisite for its other functions.

Protective Awareness This is the protecting or guarding function of *sati. Sati* is intimately related to the guarding and protective restraint of the senses in order to prevent unwholesome states and unethical conduct from arising. Protective awareness "actively disengages individuals from potential unwholesome activity" (Peacock 2014, p. 9). Peacock suggested this protective function might distinguish *sati* from the mindfulness of secular mindfulness-based approaches. Kuan (2008) noted that the protective function of mindfulness is related to restraint of the senses and "requires moral judgment" (p. 42).

In the early discourses, there is an illustration of the protective or guarding function of *sati,* in which *sati* is a wise gatekeeper to a city. "It is just as if in the king's border town a chief officer has been appointed as gatekeeper, one who is sharp-witted and wise in making decisions, brave and resolute, of excellent counsel, who allows entry to the good and keeps out the bad, in order to ensure peace within and control outside enemies. In the same way, a noble disciple continuously dwells with mindfulness, achieves right mindfulness, always recalling and not forgetting what was practised or heard long ago. This is a noble disciple's gaining of mindfulness as the gatekeeper, as the chief officer, who removes what is bad and unwholesome [desire and aversion] and develops wholesome states" (Anālayo 2013, pp. 29–30).

The gatekeeper guards the six gates to the city in the same way that a Buddhist practitioner should guard the six sense doors (eye, ear, nose, tongue, body, mind). The gatekeeper keeps out strangers and admits acquaintances; similarly, the Buddhist practitioner allows wholesome sense objects to enter and disallows unwholesome sense objects from entering the mind. "Just as the presence of the gatekeeper prevents those not entitled from entering the town, so too the presence of well-established *sati* prevents the arising of unwholesome associations and reactions at the sense doors" (Anālayo 2003, p. 56).

A further example from the early discourses illustrates the application of sense restraint in relation to sexual desire experienced by a renunciate. "A foolish and ignorant person, who dwells in dependence on a village, puts on the robes in the morning, takes the alms bowl, and enters the village to beg for alms without properly guarding the body, without restraint of the sense-doors, and without the mind being collected through mindfulness. On seeing women, he arouses improper attention and, grasping the sign of their bodily form, lustful sensual desires appear in his mind. Lustful sensual desires having appeared, he is ablaze with the fire of sensual desire, which burns his body and mind" (Anālayo 2013, p. 22). Whilst this example might not seem relevant to lay secular mindfulness-based applications, Gombrich (2009) suggests that when "the Buddhist layman vows 'not to act wrongly in respect of sense desires'; this can be used in any society, no matter what its sexual mores, more it is just a promise to abide by those mores" (Gombrich 2009, p. 27). This teaching also promotes investigation of the third precept concerning the meaning of sexual misconduct in the context of one's life.

There are several other metaphors in the early discourses illustrating the protective functions of mindfulness, which are beyond the scope of this chapter to discuss: the good charioteer (Anālayo 2013, pp. 37–38), the thorny forest (Kuan 2008, p. 42), the post or pillar (Kuan 2008, p. 44) and the bowl of oil (Kuan 2008, p. 44).

"Being fully aware of what is taking place right now without reacting in unwholesome ways is central to the protective function of mindfulness" (Anālayo 2013, p. 24). The domains of *satipaṭṭhāna* practice—body, feeling, mind, *dhammas*—are considered a "safe ground that enables one to withstand the allure of sensually enticing objects" (Anālayo 2013, p. 27) and without getting caught in reactive patterns of desire and aversion. Gilpin (2008, p. 229) discussed the function of mindfulness as moral protection for self and others in the context of Theravadā and MBCT. He suggested that the decentring from ruminative thinking that produces metacognitive insight in MBCT is compatible with the attenuation of mental proliferation *(papañca)* occurring in sense-restraint and the protective function of *sati* (p. 242). However, he noted there are also notable differences. Whilst a body scan conducted in MBCT might be viewed as "useful for developing non-judgemental bodily awareness and learning how to shift one's attention, the Theravādin approach is chiefly concerned with counteracting sensual desire" (p. 244). Nevertheless, Gilpin (2008) went on to make the important point that despite the emphasis on the simple awareness aspects of mindfulness in MBCT, such as acceptance and nonjudgement, MBCT nevertheless "makes a clear judgement about the undesirability of…ruminative mental processes, and suggests skilful courses of action to counter these" (p. 245). He concludes that MBCT "does engender some degree of ethical sensibility in the meditator although, unlike Buddhism, this is not made in explicit terms, nor is it a core motivation that defines and shapes its practice" (p. 245). I would also add that the emphasis on what is skilful in mindfulness-based applications like MBCT might suggest mindfulness practice is equivalent to utilitarian ethics. The emphasis on what is skilful in terms of the consequences of an action might also risk distracting the practitioner from the moral status of their intention. Nevertheless, it does appear that when seen from the perspective of early Buddhism, there might be some minimally protective functions to mindfulness when it is applied in secular interventions.

Introspective Awareness It might be assumed that mindfulness meditation, as a way of becoming aware of and observing the inner life of the mind, is equivalent to introspection as it was used in the early history of psychology. Whilst there are similarities with introspection, mindfulness meditation has some important differences (Stanley 2012a). When it is used as a form of introspective awareness in early Buddhism, *sati* works to examine unwholesome states that have invaded the person. "Suppose…a man were wounded by an arrow thickly smeared with poison…. A surgeon would cut around the opening of the wound with a knife, then he would probe for the arrow with a probe, then he would pull out the arrow and would expel the poisonous humour without leaving a trace of it behind" (Buddha, cited by Kuan (2008, p. 51)). Kuan explained that the "wound" designates the six senses whilst the "poisonous humour" and "arrow" stand for ignorance and craving, respectively. The "probe" designates *sati.* This metaphor captures the function of *sati* to investigate the location and nature of unwholesome states that exist within the person prior to their removal. "Like the surgeon's probe, whose function is to provide information about the wound for subsequent treatment, so too the "probe" *sati* can be used to carefully gather information, thereby preparing the ground for subsequent action" (Anālayo 2003, p. 53). The introspective function of *sati* is an important illustration of its ethical discernment.

Deliberate Forming of Concepts This function of *sati* involves deliberate conceptualising which directly contradicts the idea that *sati* solely comprises a simple awareness (or bare attention). Kuan (2008) explained that *anussati* is to "deliberately conceptualize what is accounted spiritually wholesome and beneficial according to a set of credal statements or formulae" (p. 53). Certain subjects are to be remembered and called to mind by Buddhists in their meditation and daily life, such as the six recollections of the Buddha (awakened one), *Dhamma* (Buddhist teachings or truth), *Saṅgha* (community of monks and nuns), one's ethical conduct, one's liberality, and of heavenly beings (devas; Anālayo 2003, pp. 46–47). But perhaps more relevant to secular mindfulness-based applications is Peacock's (2014) discussion of the cultivation of boundless friendliness *(mettā bhāvanā)* as an example of *sati* functioning to deliberately conceptualise. "Just as a mother would protect her own son, her only son, with her life, so one should develop the immeasurable mind towards all beings and loving-kindness towards the whole world. One should develop the immeasurable mind, upwards, downwards and across, without obstruction, without hatred and hostility. Standing, walking, sitting, or lying down, as long as one is free from drowsiness, *one should practice this mindfulness*. They say, 'This is a divine dwelling in this world'" (Buddha, cited in Kuan (2008, p. 55); emphasis added). Kuan (2008) pointed out that the development of *mettā* is "unique for its altruistic aspect" which seems to be lacking in the other functions of *sati.* "The practice of mindfulness is not only concerned with oneself, but it can also be altruistic. The process of developing loving kindness (*mettā*) is a type of mindfulness that should be practiced to form one's ethical attitude towards all beings" (Kuan 2008, p. 139).

The social ethics of mindfulness and its relevance for interpersonal relationships is illustrated particularly well in the parable of the acrobat and his apprentice Medakathālikā: "Just as the apprentice Medakathālikā said to the teacher: 'I shall protect myself', monks, thus should *satipaṭṭhāna* be practiced. 'I shall protect others', thus should *satipaṭṭhāna* be practised. One who protects oneself protects others. One who protects others protects oneself. And, monks, how does one who protects oneself protect others? By practicing, developing and cultivation. Thus one who protects oneself protects others. And, monks, how does one who protects others protect oneself? By forbearance, harmlessness, loving-kindness and compassion" (Buddha, cited in Kuan (2008, p. 56)). Chappell (2003) described this as a "social mindfulness" which includes dialogue as a practice. "Moral development in Buddhism never occurs at the expense of one's own long-term good: it benefits both oneself and others" (Keown 1992, p. 231).

In sum, we can recognise that in the Pāli discourses, *sati* is not only a simple awareness of what is happening from moment to moment, being present, or being awake. These are the aspects most often emphasised in secular psychological understandings of mindfulness (i.e. simple awareness or "bare attention"). In addition to the simple awareness of what is happening in and around us, mindfulness also functions in other ways, which are ethically intoned. The practice of the four *satipaṭṭhānas* is intimately related to restraint of the senses, which is illustrated especially by the guarding or protective role played by *sati* in the metaphors used to illustrate its practice.

6.8 Conclusion

Buddhism has been interpreted in diverse and numerous ways across history and culture, in different times and places, and with different emphases: as a religion, a philosophy, a science, a psychology, a psychotherapy, a way of life and a code of ethics (see *inter alia* Gombrich 2009; Keown 1996; Lopez 2012). In this sense, there are multiple "Buddhisms" which change across time and place, rather than there being a single and monolithic "Buddhism". A currently dominant understanding of Buddhism is as a therapeutic means of alleviating suffering *(dukkha)* compatible with modern medicine, psychotherapy and scientific research. One of the possible risks of interpreting Buddhism as a psychology or psychotherapy and mindfulness as a therapeutic self-help technique or skill is that it potentially de-ethicises or demoralises the practice of mindfulness. The overly psychological orientation of much interest in mindfulness risks limiting our point of view to our psychologies only as experienced introspectively, without a focus on the ethics of our intentions, rather than also encompassing our social and relational lives with their inevitable ethical and moral dimensions (i.e. how we treat others as well as ourselves). One way to remedy the neglect of ethics and morality is to engage more deeply with the ancient Pāli canon and the close alliance made between mindfulness and moral choice (intention), action and discernment of the consequences of our actions.

Doing this allows us to make a simple distinction between the implicit morality of a secular mindfulness-based course and the explicit ethics of traditional Buddhist teaching of mindfulness (Gilpin 2008, p. 245). On the basis of this distinction, we might wonder whether a more explicit ethics is required in secular courses and, if so, how it might be expressed.

However, a focus solely on the early Buddhist discourses is potentially limiting because we risk ignoring or sidestepping contemporary ethical issues not addressed by the historical Buddha and which are global in their consequences, such as consumerism, sustainability and social and economic inequality. The Buddhist focus on non-harming, generosity, kindness, empathetic joy and compassion perhaps needs to be supplemented with attention towards and discussion of the equally important issues of justice, rights, freedom and fairness (see Harvey 2000). In addition, we still need to explore the social and political meanings of "mindful consumption" (Badiner 2002) in the context of consumer capitalist societies (see Armstrong 2012).

The chapter, being restricted to a consideration of the relation between mindfulness and ethics in the early Buddhist discourses, misses out important later traditions of Buddhism in which there are different ethico-moral emphases. The Mahāyāna (Greater Vehicle) emphasis on skill in means *(upāya-kauśalya),* compassion *(karuna)* and the Bodhissatva path have not been discussed (Harvey 2000). Skilful means might be interpreted as similar to situation ethics: a utilitarian hybrid (Keown 1992). It is arguably central to the ethico-moral orientation of MBSR (Kabat-Zinn 2011). Further investigation is required to understand and evaluate the influence of this orientation on secular mindfulness-based interventions.

Finally, there is a need to study empirically the conduct of practical morality in secular mindfulness teaching and learning, for example, in standardised 8-week mindfulness-based courses such as MBSR and MBCT. Without such empirical research, our theoretical discussions will remain overly abstract and ungrounded: entirely the opposite of the ethico-moral rootedness of mindfulness in the tradition of early Buddhism.

References

American Mindfulness Research Association. (2014). Mindfulness Research Monthly. http://goamra.org/publications/mindfulness-research-monthly/. Accessed 17 Nov 2014.

Anālayo. (2003). *Satipaṭṭhāna: The direct path to realization.* Cambridge: Windhorse.

Anālayo. (2013). *Perspectives on Satipaṭṭhāna.* Cambridge: Windhorse.

Armstrong, A. (2012). *Mindfulness and consumerism: A social psychological investigation.* Unpublished Doctoral Thesis, University of Surrey.

Badiner, A. H. (2002). *Mindfulness in the marketplace: Compassionate responses to consumerism.* Berkeley: Parallax.

Baer, R. A. (2006). *Mindfulness-based treatment approaches: Clinician's guide to evidence base and applications.* London: Academic.

Baer, R. A. (2011). Measuring mindfulness. *Contemporary Buddhism, 12*(1), 241–261.

Barker, M. (2013). *Mindful counselling and psychotherapy: Practising mindfully across approaches and issues.* London: Sage.

Batchelor, S. (1997). *Buddhism without beliefs: A contemporary guide to awakening*. London: Bloomsbury.
Batchelor, S. (2010). *Confession of a Buddhist atheist*. New York: Spiegel & Grau.
Bodhi, B. (2012). *The numerical discourses of the Buddha: A translation of the Aṅguttara Nikāya*. Boston: Wisdom.
Brazier, D. (2013). Mindfulness reconsidered. *European Journal of Psychotherapy and Counselling, 15*(2), 116–126.
BPS (The British Psychological Society). (2009). *Code of ethics and conduct: Guidance published by the Ethics Committee of the British Psychological Society*. Leicester: The British Psychological Society.
Bush, M. (2011). Mindfulness in higher education. *Contemporary Buddhism, 12*(1), 183–197.
Carpenter, J. E. (1923). The passing of the founder. *Journal of the Pāli Text Society, 1920–23*, 1–21.
Chalmers. (2004). Davids, Thomas William Rhys (1843–1922), rev. Richard F. Gombrich. Oxford Dictionary of National Biography: Oxford University Press. http://www.oxfordnb.com/view/article/32726. Accessed 9 Nov 2014.
Chappell, D. W. (2003). Buddhist social principles. In K. H. Dockett, G. R. Dudley-Grant, & C. P. Bankart (Eds.), *Psychology and Buddhism: From individual to global community* (pp. 259–286). London: Kluwer Academic.
Chaskalson, M. (2011). *The mindful workplace: Developing resilient individuals and resonant organizations with MBSR*. London: Wiley-Blackwell.
Chiesa, A., & Malinowski, P. (2011). Mindfulness-based approaches: Are they all the same? *Journal of Clinical Psychology, 67*(4), 404–424.
Clower, J., & Peng, T. (2014). From cushions to couches, shramanas to shrinks: What is lost and what is gained when mindfulness becomes a tool of medicine and psychotherapy. In A. Ie C.T. Ngnoumen, & E. J. Langer (Eds.), *The Wiley Blackwell handbook of mindfulness* (Vol. II; pp. 688–704). London: Wiley Blackwell.
Cullen, M. (2011). Mindfulness-based interventions: An emerging phenomenon. *Mindfulness, 2*, 186–193.
Didonna, F. (Ed.) (2009). *Clinical handbook of mindfulness*. New York: Springer.
Fevre, R.W. (2000). *The demoralization of western culture*. London: Continuum.
Gilpin, R. (2008). The use of Theravāda Buddhist practices and perspectives in mindfulness-based cognitive therapy. *Contemporary Buddhism, 9*(2), 227–251.
Gleig, A. L. (2011). *Enlightenment after the enlightenment: American transformations of Asian contemplative traditions*. Unpublished Doctoral Thesis, Rice University.
Gleig, A. L. (2012). Wedding the personal and impersonal in West Coast Vipassana: A dialogical encounter between Buddhism and psychotherapy. *Journal of Global Buddhism, 13*, 129–146.
Goldstein, J. (2013). *Mindfulness: A practical guide to awakening*. Boulder: Sounds True.
Gombrich, R. F. (1983). From monastery to meditation centre: Lay meditation in modern Sri Lanka. In P. Denwood & A. Piatigorsky (Eds.), *Buddhist studies: Ancient and modern* (pp. 20–34). London: Barnes & Noble.
Gombrich, R. F. (1988). *Theravāda Buddhism: A social history from ancient Benares to modern Colombo*. London: Routledge.
Gombrich, R. F. (1994). Introduction: What is Pāli? In W. Geiger (Ed.), *A Pāli grammar* (pp. xxiii–xxx). Oxford: The Pali Text Society.
Gombrich, R. F. (2009). *What the Buddha thought*. London: Equinox.
Grossman, P., & Van Dam, N. T. (2011). Mindfulness, by any other name …: Trials and tribulations of *sati* in western psychology and science. *Contemporary Buddhism, 12*(1), 219–239.
Hallisey, C. (1995). Roads taken and not taken in the study of Theravāda Buddhism. In D. S. Lopez (Ed.), *Curators of the Buddha: The study of Buddhism under colonialism* (pp. 31–62). London: University of Chicago Press.
Harvey, P. (2000). *An introduction to Buddhist ethics*. Cambridge: Cambridge University Press.
Hayes, S. C. (2002). Buddhism and acceptance and commitment therapy. *Cognitive and Behavioral Practice, 9*, 58–66.

Hayes, S. C., Strosahl, K. D., & Wilson, K. G. (2012). *Acceptance and commitment therapy: The process and practice of mindful change*. London: Guilford.

Hölzel, B. K., Lazar, S. W., Gard, T., Schuman-Olivier, Z., Vago, D. R., & Ott, U. (2011). How does mindfulness meditation work? Proposing mechanisms for action from a conceptual and neural perspective. *Perspectives on Psychological Science, 6*(6), 537–559.

Ie, A., Ngnoumen, C. T., & Langer, E. J. (2014). *The Wiley Blackwell handbook of mindfulness*. London: Wiley Blackwell.

Kabat-Zinn, J. (1990). *Full catastrophe living: Using the wisdom of your body and mind to face stress, pain, and illness*. New York: Random House.

Kabat-Zinn, J. (1994). *Wherever you go, there you are: Mindfulness meditation for everyday life*. London: Piatkus.

Kabat-Zinn, J. (2003). Mindfulness-based interventions in context: Past, present, and future. *Clinical Psychology: Science and Practice, 10*(2), 144–156.

Kabat-Zinn, J. (2011). Some reflections on the origins of MBSR, skillful means, and the trouble with maps. *Contemporary Buddhism, 12*(1), 281–306.

Kang, C., & Whittingham, K. (2010). Mindfulness: A dialogue between Buddhism and clinical psychology. *Mindfulness, 1*, 161–173.

Keown, D. (1992). *The Nature of Buddhist ethics*. London: Palgrave.

Keown, D. (1996). *Buddhism: A very short introduction*. Oxford: Oxford University Press.

Keown, D., & Prebish, C. (2013). Celebrating twenty years of the *Journal of Buddhist Ethics*. *Journal of Buddhist Ethics, 20*. http://blogs.dickinson.edu/buddhistethics/. Accessed 16 Nov 2014.

Kornfield, J. (1977). *Living buddhist masters*. Kandy: BPS.

Kuan, T-F. (2008). Mindfulness in early Buddhism: New approaches through psychology and textual analysis of Pali, Chinese and Sanskrit sources. London: Routledge.

Langer, E. J. (1989). *Mindfulness*. Reading: Addison-Wesley.

Lopez, D. S., Jr. (2012). *The scientific Buddha: His short and happy life*. London: Yale University Press.

McCown, D. A., Jr. (2013). *The ethical space of mindfulness in clinical practice*. Unpublished MA dissertation, Tilburg University.

McMahan, D. L. (2008). *The making of Buddhist modernism*. Oxford: Oxford University Press.

Ñāṇamoli, B., & Bodhi, B. (2005). *The middle length discourses of the Buddha: A translation of the Majjhima Nikāya*. Boston: Wisdom.

Olendzki, A. (2011). The construction of mindfulness. *Contemporary Buddhism, 12*(1), 55–70.

Olendzki, A. (2014). From early Buddhist traditions to western psychological science. In A. Ie, C. T. Ngnoumen & E. J. Langer (Eds.), *The Wiley Blackwell handbook of mindfulness* (vol. I, pp. 58–73). London: Wiley Blackwell.

OED (Oxford English Dictionary). (2014a). Ethics, n. OED Online. September 2014. Oxford University Press. http://www.oed.com/view/Entry/355823?redirectedFrom=ethics. Accessed 16 Nov 2014.

OED (Oxford English Dictionary). (2014b). Mindful, adj. OED Online. September 2014. Oxford University Press. http://www.oed.com/view/Entry/118740?redirectedFrom=mindful. Accessed 16 Nov 2014.

OED (Oxford English Dictionary). (2014c). Mindfulness, n. OED Online. September 2014. Oxford University Press. http://www.oed.com/view/Entry/118742?redirectedFrom=mindfulness. Accessed 16 Nov 2014.

OED (Oxford English Dictionary). (2014d). Morality, n. OED Online. September 2014. Oxford University Press. http://www.oed.com/view/Entry/122093?redirectedFrom=morality. Accessed 16 Nov 2014.

OED (Oxford English Dictionary). (2014e). Virtue, n. OED Online. September 2014. Oxford University Press. http://www.oed.com/view/Entry/223835?rskey=Y2iXeN&result=1. Accessed 16 Nov 2014.

Peacock, J. (2014). *Sati* or mindfulness? Bridging the divide. In M. Bazzano (Ed.), *After mindfulness: New perspectives on psychology and meditation* (pp. 3–22). London: Palgrave MacMillan.

Purser, R. E., & Milillo, J. (2014). Mindfulness revisited: A Buddhist-based conceptualization. *Journal of Management Inquiry*. doi:10.1177/1056492614532315.

Rhys Davids, T. W. (1877). *Buddhism: Being a sketch of the life and teachings of Gautama, the Buddha*. London: Society for Promoting Christian Knowledge.

Rhys Davids, T. W. (1881). *Buddhist Suttas translated from Pāli*. London: Clarendon.

Rhys Davids, T. W. (1890). *The questions of king Milinda*. Oxford: Oxford University Press.

Rhys Davids, T. W., & Stede, W. (1925). *The Pali text society's Pali-English dictionary*. London: The Pali Text Society.

Ryan, T. (2012). A mindful nation: How a simple practice can help us reduce stress, improve performance, and recapture the American spirit. London: Hay House.

Saddhatissa, H. (1970). *Buddhist ethics*. Somervi: Wisdom.

Samuel, G. (2014). Between Buddhism and science, between mind and body. *Religions, 5,* 560–579.

Schedneck, B. (2014). Meditation for tourists in Thailand: Commodifying a universal and national symbol. *Journal of Contemporary Religion, 29*(3), 439–456.

Segal, Z. V., Williams, J. M. G., & Teasdale, J. D. (2013). *Mindfulness-based cognitive therapy for depression* (2nd ed.). New York: Guilford.

Sharf, R. H. (1995). Buddhist modernism and the rhetoric of meditative experience. *Numen, 42*(3), 228–283.

Sharf, R. H. (2000). The rhetoric of experience and the study of religion. *Journal of Consciousness Studies, 7*(11–12), 267–287.

Shonin, E., Van Gordon, W., & Griffiths, M. D. (2013). Mindfulness-based interventions: Towards mindful clinical integration. *Frontiers in Psychology, 4,* 194.

Snodgrass, J. (2007). Defining modern Buddhism: Mr. and Mrs. Rhys Davids and the Pāli Text Society. *Comparative Studies of South Asia, Africa and the Middle East, 27*(1), 186–202.

Stahl, B., & Goldstein, E. (2010). *A mindfulness-based stress reduction workbook*. Oakland: New Harbinger.

Stanley, S. (2012a). Intimate distances: William James' introspection, Buddhist mindfulness, and experiential inquiry. *New Ideas in Psychology, 30,* 201–211.

Stanley, S. (2012b). Mindfulness: Towards a critical relational perspective. *Social and Personality Psychology Compass, 6,* 631–641.

Stanley, S. (2013). 'Things said or done long ago are recalled and remembered': The ethics of mindfulness in early Buddhism, psychotherapy and clinical psychology. *European Journal of Psychotherapy and Counselling, 15*(2), 151–162.

Stanley, E. A. (2014). Mindfulness-based mind fitness training: An approach to enhancing performance and building resilience in high-stress contexts. In A. Ie, C. T. Ngnoumen & E. J. Langer (Eds.), *The Wiley Blackwell handbook of mindfulness* (vol. II, pp. 964–985). London: Wiley Blackwell.

Sun, J. (2014). Mindfulness in context: A historical discourse analysis. *Contemporary Buddhism*. doi:10.1080/14639947.2014.978088.

Swales, M. A., & Heard, H. L. (2009). *Dialectical behaviour therapy: Distinctive features*. London: Routledge.

Tan, C-M. (2012). Search inside yourself: The unexpected path to achieving success, happiness (and world peace). London: HarperOne.

The Mindfulness Initiative. (2014). The mindfulness initiative: What does a mindful nation look like? http://www.themindfulnessinitative.org.uk/index.html. Accessed 17 Nov 2014.

Tichibana, S. (1926). *The ethics of Buddhism*. London: Curzon.

Titmuss, C. (2013). The Buddha of mindfulness: A stress destruction programme. http://christophertitmuss.org/blog/the-buddha-of-mindfulness-the-politics-of-mindfulness. Accessed 17 Nov 2014.

Varra, A. A., Drossel, C., & Hayes, S. C. (2009). The use of metaphor to establish acceptance and mindfulness. In F. Didonna (Ed.), *Clinical handbook of mindfulness* (pp. 111–123). New York: Springer.

Wallace, B. A., & Bodhi, B. (2006). The nature of mindfulness and its role in Buddhist meditation. http://shamatha.org/sites/default/files/Bhikkhu_Bodhi_Correspondence.pdf. Accessed 17 Nov 2014.

Weare, K. (2014). Mindfulness in schools: Where are we and where might we go next? In A. Ie, C. T. Ngoumen & E. J. Langer (Eds.), *The Wiley Blackwell handbook of mindfulness* (pp. 1037–1053). London: Wiley Blackwell.

Wickremeratne, A. (1985). *The genesis of an Orientalist: Thomas William Rhys Davids and Buddhism in Sri Lanka*. New Delhi: Motilal Banarsidass.

Williams, J. M. G., & Kabat-Zinn, J. (2011). Mindfulness: Diverse perspectives on its meaning, origins, and multiple applications at the intersection of science and dharma. *Contemporary Buddhism, 12*(1), 1–18.

Wilson, J. (2014). *Mindful America: The mutual transformation of Buddhist meditation and American culture*. Oxford: Oxford University Press.

Steven Stanley is a lecturer in the School of Social Sciences, Cardiff University, Wales, UK. Dr. Stanley is a social psychologist with research interests in the qualitative study of social life. He completed his Ph.D. thesis "Doctoral Dilemmas: Towards a Discursive Psychology of Postgraduate Education" in the School of Social Sciences at Loughborough University in 2005. In his current research, he explores the social, cultural and historical dimensions of mindfulness meditation, as both a topic and resource for critical social psychology.

Chapter 7
Mindfulness in Theravāda *Samatha* and *Vipassanā* Meditations, and in Secular Mindfulness

Peter Harvey

7.1 Introduction

Buddhism sees *sati* (Pali, Skt *smṛti*), or mindfulness, as a crucial aspect of the process of meditatively *calming down* and *waking up* so as to see things as they really are. Both of these are seen to help us to reduce the suffering that we inflict on ourselves and others. As the Discourse on the Applications of Mindfulness (*Satipaṭṭhāna Sutta, MN*.I. pp. 55–63) says, mindfulness is "the direct path for the purification of beings, for the overcoming of sorrow and lamentation, for the ending of pain and unhappiness, for acquiring the true method, and for experiencing Nirvana."

To be mindful starts by being clearly aware of what is experienced in the present moment, being present with, and paying careful attention to, the wondrous flow of here…now. When we stand back from and alertly take stock of what we are feeling and doing, this allows things to…naturally…calm…down…. We are then open to experiencing a dropping away of normal mental horizons and limitations, a kind of timeless presence, with feelings of happiness and ease. When we have developed more mindfulness, we tend to more easily notice simple natural events in the environment, such as a leaf gently falling to the ground, ripples on the surface of a river or pool, or a trickle of rain running down a car windscreen while one waits in traffic. Mindful observation of these can allow a natural delight to arise. There is a kind of open, playful curiosity about the fine-grained details of experience.

P. Harvey (✉)
University of Sunderland, Sunnyside, 18a Main Street, Riccall, York YO19 6PX, UK
e-mail: b.peter.harvey@gmail.com

E. Shonin et al. (eds.), *Buddhist Foundations of Mindfulness*,
Mindfulness in Behavioral Health, DOI 10.1007/978-3-319-18591-0_7

7.2 Mindfulness and Attention

The primary aspect of mindfulness, the basis of others, is a kind of disinterested watchfulness, a natural alertness, a standing back from the processes of body and mind, and calm observation of them. It is mind-full-ness, a full presence of mind, alert attention, mental clarity, being wide awake, fully with it, and vigilant. During a normal day, much of the time one is operating on autopilot involved in habitual actions and thought patterns, with no real contact with the world: like a rice pudding that has cooled and has a thick skin on it, closing it off from the air above. But when mindfulness arises, one is more alive and alert; something switches on that was previously inactive.

Mindfulness is a thorough observation which is not careless in its watchfulness: It sees things as they are, without overlooking aspects of them, or projecting things onto them. It is also disinterested and nonjudgmental, observing, without reacting for or against. It has balance and equanimity, not being pulled this way and that. It starts with an attention that simply notes and registers what is going on, a full awareness of what is happening in and to us, as it happens.

In the *Satipaṭṭhāna Sutta,* it is said: "he dwells contemplating the body (such as breathing) in regard to the body, diligent, clearly comprehending (Pali *sampajāno,* Skt *samprajāna*), and mindful, free from longing for and unhappiness with the world" (and then similarly with contemplation of feeling-tones, mind-states, and significant patterns in experience, such as the five hindrances). Kuan (2008, pp. 41–42) described this aspect as, "simple awareness…conscious registering of the presence of objects…non-judgmental observation and recognition," such as knowing one is breathing in long or short, or being aware of the passing sensations arising when lifting an arm, or the flow of changing feelings. It observes without preferences and self-interested concerns, without habitual reaction, but clearly acknowledging what is actually there in the flow of experience, noting its nature. Nyanaponika (1997) has described this as a kind of "bare attention" which sees things as if for the first time (Anālayo 2003, pp. 57–60).

What, though, is the relationship of mindfulness to attention in general? One can say that mindfulness is, or at least builds on, a certain *kind* of attention. This is not automatic and basic attention, which is involved in any state of mind. Even the "bare attention" aspect of mindfulness is beyond this, as it is an active and not an automatic state. Beyond basic, automatic attention, Buddhist texts distinguish between two kinds of attention *(manasikāra).* One is said to be *yoniso,* the other has the opposite quality, being *ayoniso. Yoniso* means something like wise, systematic, probing, not superficial, focusing on the fundamental nature of its object, skillfully noticing and tuning in to things which undermine greed, hatred, and delusion, and strengthen non-greed/generosity/renunciation, non-hatred/loving kindness, non-delusion/wisdom. *Ayoniso* means unwise, unsystematic, unprobing, attending only to obvious, surface features of things. It is said (*AN.*I. pp. 200–201):

> For one attending unwisely to (an object's) attractive aspect (*subha-nimitta*), unarisen attachment/lust (*rāga*) will arise and arisen attachment will increase and become strong…. For one attending unwisely to (an object's) irritating aspect (*paṭigha-nimitta*) unarisen hatred will arise and arisen hatred will increase and become strong…. For one attending unwisely, unarisen delusion will arise and arisen delusion will increase and become strong.

> … For one attending wisely to (an object's) unattractive aspect (*asubha-nimitta*), unarisen attachment will not arise and arisen attachment will be abandoned…. For one attending wisely to the liberation of mind by loving-kindness, unarisen hatred will not arise and arisen hatred will be abandoned…. For one attending wisely, unarisen delusion will not arise and arisen delusion will be abandoned.

It is also said that trust in a reliable guide aids wise attention and that while wise attention feeds into and sustains mindfulness and clear comprehension (Pali *sampajañña,* Skt *samprajānya*), unwise attention feeds into and sustains lack of mindfulness and clear comprehension (*AN.*V. pp. 113–116). Mindfulness and clear comprehension then feed into guarding the sense-doors, that is, avoiding habitual reactions of attachment and aversion to things one senses or thinks about, which sustains more wholesome actions and thoughts, and thence deeper mindfulness and the awakening of more wholesome and beneficial qualities.

Unwise attention undermines mindfulness, for attention is the leading edge of the mind; where it goes, other mental states follow. If one starts down the road of an unskillful thought or emotion, such as annoyance, one's view of things narrows; the more awake part of the mind shuts down, and one loses the wider sense of perspective that comes with mindfulness.

7.3 Mindfulness as Protective Awareness

Mindfulness has an aspect which Kuan (2008) called a "protective awareness." This "stands near" and so guards the mind against heedlessness and carelessness. It naturally brings restraint of unskillful reactions to sense-objects and so overcomes the superficial distractedness of desire for sense-pleasures, the first of the five hindrances to calm and wisdom. In this role, it acts as a guardian of the sense-doors (i.e., the five physical senses and the mind). In one passage (*SN.*IV. pp. 194–195), it is likened to a wise guardian of the six gates of a city (which stand for the five senses and mind), who only lets in those who are well disposed, especially two swift messengers, who stand for calm *(samatha)* and insight *(vipassanā),* which bring the message of Nirvana, having traveled along the route which is the noble eight-factored path. It is this protective aspect that helps those who have suffered from depression from lapsing back into it. It does this by helping them stand back from negative thoughts that may arise, without identifying with them and being drawn into them.

7.4 Mindfulness as Clear Memory and Introspective Awareness

As well as not losing track of what is in the immediate present, mindfulness also remembers clearly. Indeed to stay in the present, one has to keep remembering to do so! If the mind has wandered off from a selected object of contemplation, mindfulness reminds one to return to it. Mindfulness is said (*Miln.* pp. 37–38) to have the characteristic of *apilāpana,* which has been taken by commentaries to mean "not floating away," but which Gethin (2001, pp. 37–40) sees as better analyzed as having the sense of reminding one to bear certain qualities in mind. Having helped one recognize certain helpful and harmful aspects of one's behavior and thought, mindfulness also *remembers* what one has thus learnt, so as to apply it in the present. Mindfulness can either remain in the "here and now" or remember accurately, without self-serving distortions. Moreover, when one has finished a meditation "sit," it is good to mindfully recollect how it went, to help understand and consolidate what one has seen and developed.

In these respects, mindfulness has an aspect which Kuan (2008) called "introspective awareness." This identifies unskillful states that may have arisen, and calls to mind, and thus calls into play, counteractive qualities, as in the *Sutta* on the "Removal of Distracting Thoughts" (Bucknell and Kang 1997; *MN*.I. pp. 118–122; Soma 1981). It has the characteristic of "calling to mind" or "bearing in mind" (*Miln.* pp. 37–38). This is in fact the most usual way in which the word mindfulness has traditionally been used in English: "mindful of the fact that…, we have decided to do…," a politician might say: here it means bearing something in mind as relevant to a task at hand—being "on the ball." The *Milindapañha* sees *sati* as recollecting wholesome/skillful (and unwholesome/unskillful) states of mind, like a treasurer reminding a king of his treasures, and so it naturally embraces and resorts to the wholesome ones, that is, it remembers things in relationship to each other and so tends to know their value and widen one's perspective. It is, thus, a quality that sees and bears in mind connections between things.

Mindful recollection of a wholesome state one has previously experienced also makes an active connection to it and lets it flow into and arise in the present. Thus, mindfulness also has the characteristic of "taking hold of" the genuinely beneficial (*Miln.* pp. 38)—it follows the course of beneficial and unbeneficial states, like an adviser observing things on behalf of a king and so naturally takes up the beneficial ones and lets go of the unbeneficial ones.

7.5 Mindfulness as Calling to Mind Certain Concepts

A final aspect of mindfulness is what Kuan (2008) called "deliberately forming conceptions": the recollection *(anussati)* and contemplation of certain salutary things. Buddhaghosa's *Visuddhimagga* (Chaps. VII and VIII), drawing on the Pali *Suttas,* lists ten recollections: of the qualities of the Buddha, *Dhamma* or *Saṅgha,* of moral virtue, generosity, the gods and their bright realms, death and its inevitability, the unlovely organs and liquids making up the body, in and out breathing, or the peace of Nirvana. The *Mettā Sutta* (*Sn.* pp. 143–152) also describes the cultivation of loving kindness as a kind of mindfulness. All these mindful recollections help to undermine unskillful states and cultivate skillful ones. They recall and contemplate certain good qualities, or things as not being worthy of clinging to, so that they have a vivid presence, leaving a lasting and beneficial impression.

7.6 Mindfulness as a Kindly and Light Type of Awareness

Mindfulness is a patient, kindly observation, which gives space for things to be what they are, and then to gradually change and pass. This is very helpful when applied, for example, when one feels low, irritated, worried, or afraid. It helps one to acknowledge these states, but then to let go of them.

Mindfulness also lets one be less serious and heavy about things; it is a way of observing that can take a sideways look at our habitual actions and see their humorous side: this can sometimes take the form of "mindfulness of being a prat!"

7.7 Everyday Mindfulness

Mindfulness conduces to a simple, natural, non-habitual state. When one starts the day with more mindfulness, things tend to flow better: one is more alert to things, even subliminally, so that things tend to fall into place more easily. During the day, mindfulness can be used either to periodically notice what the breath is doing or how the mind is reacting. One can pause to check out how one feels: feeling one's contact with the ground through the feet, noting any tensions in the body, and then note one's emotional state.

In everyday settings, mindfulness also plays a role, alongside concentration, in good driving skills. It also helps one listen more carefully to what other people are saying, so one does not miss things or only hear what one assumes they are saying.

7.8 The Four *Satipaṭṭhānas*

The key canonical Pali texts on the cultivation of mindfulness are the *Satipaṭṭhāna Sutta* (*MN*. pp. 155–163; Anālayo 2003, pp. 3–13; Shaw 2006, pp. 76–85; Soma 1998) and its expanded version, *Mahā-satipaṭṭhāna Sutta* (*DN*.II. pp. 290–315). These contain what can be seen as the earliest summary of appropriate foci of Buddhist meditation and associated meditation methods. They concern the "application to mindfulness" *(satipaṭṭhāna)* to body *(kāya)*, feeling *(vedanā)*, mind-states *(citta)* and reality-patterns *(dhammas)*. Under mindful contemplation of the body are mindfulness of:

- What sustains it: breathing in and out
- What it does: postures (walking, standing, sitting, and lying down) and various bodily movements
- What it is composed of: its various solids (organs, bones, etc.) and liquid components, and the four elements (earth/solidity, water/cohesion, fire/heat, and wind/motion) composing it and the physical world
- Its stages of its decomposition after death

Beyond the body, mindfulness observes:

- Feeling: the pleasant, unpleasant, and neutral feeling-tones that arise, whether from body or mind, or from ordinary worldly causes or spiritual ones, such as the joy that may arise in meditation.
- Mind-states: the presence or absence of unwholesome states of mind and of one's degree of mental development and concentration.
- Reality-patterns as delineated in the Buddha's *Dhamma:* the five hindrances to meditative calming; the five bundles of processes making up the body and mind *(khandhas);* the senses and their objects and how, between them, fettering attachments can arise or be avoided; the seven factors of awakening, and how to perfect them; the four True Realities for the Spiritually Ennobled *(ariya-saccas*: usually translated as 'Noble Truths'*).*

These encompass a broad range of phenomena that need to be carefully observed, understood, and be appropriately responded to if liberation is to be attained.

7.9 *Samatha* and *Vipassanā*

Perhaps the most succinct way of summarizing the qualities needed for awakening/enlightenment is as: *samatha* (Pali, Skt *śamatha*)—calm, peace, tranquility—and *vipassanā* (Pali, Skt *vipaśyanā*)—insight (*SN*.IV. p. 360). It is said that both *samatha* and *vipassanā* are aspects of liberating knowledge: if *samatha* is cultivated, the heart/mind *(citta)* is developed, which leads to the abandonment of attachment/lusting after *(rāga);* if *vipassanā* is cultivated, wisdom (Pali *paññā,* Skt *prajñā*) is developed, which leads to abandonment of spiritual ignorance (*avijjā*, Skt *avidyā*; *AN*.I. p. 61, cf. *AN*.II. pp. 93–95). Here, one sees that the spiritual path involves work on both affective and cognitive aspects of the mind: attachment-rooted emotional reactions for and against things, and how one sees and understands things. These are interrelated, for emotional turbulence makes it difficult to see clearly, and confusion and misperception feeds emotional turbulence. Working together, *samatha* and *vipassanā* bring about a state in which direct knowledge can arise in a calm, clear, peaceful mind (see Harvey 2013, pp. 318–344; Shaw 2009, pp. 18–40, 111–139).

The two classical forms of meditative *bhāvanā,* or cultivation of the path, in Buddhism, respectively, aim particularly to develop the above two qualities and are named after them. The inner stillness *samatha* comes from developing a mental composure arising from sustained concentration. This lessens and suspends the driving force of craving and clinging attachment. *Vipassanā,* based especially on strong mindfulness, is clear seeing of the nature of reality as a flow of interacting mental and physical processes that are impermanent, *dukkha*—physically or mentally painful, stressful (especially when grasped at), unsatisfactory—and impersonal. This can in time destroy craving and delusion through flashes of right view and direct seeing.

Wise attention *(yoniso manasikāra)* plays a pivotal role in both *samatha* and *vipassanā. Samatha* trains attention so as not to be captured by passing thoughts and gives it a greater ability to focus in a sustained way. *Vipassanā* trains attention to note and be attuned to the aspect of things as changeable, *dukkha* and so unworthy of clinging to, and not something worthy of building an identity upon. Both kinds of wise attention nurture mindful attunement to and bearing in mind aspects of reality that support wholesome/skillful states of mind. We need to attend to, recognize, and bear in mind how mind and behavior are conditioned, so that we can direct the flow of mental energy down a wholesome/skillful channel rather than an unwholesome/ unskillful one.

Samatha and *vipassanā* are both needed for the arising of the noble eight-factored path that immediately leads up to stream-entry, the first crucial spiritual break through, which begins the destruction of spiritual fetters. Hence, it is said (*AN*.II. pp. 156–158) that one can go on to become an *Arahat* (liberated person) once the Path arises from one of (i) *vipassanā* preceded by *samatha;* (ii) *samatha* preceded by *vipassanā;* (iii) *samatha* and *vipassanā* yoked together; (iv) the mind being "gripped by *Dhamma* excitement" but then settling down and attaining concentration. As *samatha* and *vipassanā* naturally became terms for the methods which respectively cultivated these qualities, the above four approaches came to be seen as different sequences in which such methods might be practiced (Cousins 1984). As understood in Theravāda Buddhism: (i) is the vehicle *(-yāna)* of *samatha,* which develops deep calm, then adds insight; (ii) is the vehicle of *vipassanā,* which on the basis of preliminary calm, develops insight then deeper calm (full *samatha*); and (iii) is the yoked method, which has alternating phases of progressively deeper levels of calm and insight. Method (iv) seems to have referred to insight leading to the arising of various pleasant experiences to which there is excited attachment—later called the "defilements of insight" (*Vism.* pp. 633–638)—then a return to composure and concentration (*Patis*.II. pp. 100–101). In time, it came to be seen as the way of the "dry/bare *(sukkha)* insight worker *(vipassaka)*" (*Vism*. p. 666, 702): insight without the explicit need for the cultivation of *samatha.*

Both *samatha* and *vipassanā* meditation utilize mindfulness, though *samatha* has an equal emphasis on one-pointed concentration *(samādhi)*. In *samatha* meditation, one develops states of increasing composure and stillness by mindfully focusing on one object, such as breathing, to, in time, attain various levels of mental absorption, *jhāna* (Pali, Skt *dhyāna*). In these, mental chatter falls away, as do the "five hindrances": desire for sense-pleasures, aversion, dullness and lethargy, restlessness and worry, and vacillation. There is developed a state of gathered attentiveness and mental brightness, with qualities such as joy and easeful happiness arising which are later allowed to fall away as the mind becomes even stiller.

Vipassanā meditation may be done either after a strong degree of calm and concentration has been developed or just a preliminary level of it, with deeper levels coming via *vipassanā* itself. In *vipassanā,* the aim is not to be concentrated on one object, but to open out mindfulness and become attuned to a small range of pervasive features of *all* mental or physical phenomena:

- That they are impermanent (Pali *anicca,* Skt *anitya*) as they constantly arise and cease from moment to moment, and on a larger time scale change and pass away
- That they are obviously or subtly painful, stressful, unsatisfactory (Pali *dukkha,* Skt *duḥkha*)
- That they are non-Self (Pali *anattā,* Skt *anātman*) "empty of self and what belongs to Self": impersonal, not something one can rightly identify with as any kind of permanent self or "I," and not something that is any kind of fixed possession.

The aim of *samatha* is to school the mind in letting go of unsubtle levels of mental operation by tuning the mind to more a subtle level, and then letting go of that level to allow subtler levels of stillness and gathered awareness to develop. Beyond the four *jhānas*, in *samatha's* four "formless" (Pali *arūpa,* Skt *ārūpya*) levels—the spheres of infinite space (the dimensions of space without any physical content), infinite consciousness (the basis of any object sensing and sense of a subject), nothing-ness, and neither perception nor non-perception—normal mental processing is progressively suspended, which thus enhances mindfulness of these processes by making them more noticeable. The aim of *vipassanā* is to develop greater depths of wisdom and understanding, including by using all these kinds of calm, clear mental space, to observe things in a very direct way and thus cut through layers of delusion, thus digging out the cognitive distortions that are the roots of suffering.

Defilements such as greed, hatred, and delusion are expressed at three levels: in overt actions of body and speech, as conscious thoughts and emotions, and deep-rooted latent tendencies in the mind. Overt defilements are restrained by moral virtue (Pali *sīla,* Skt *śīla*); conscious defilements are stilled by the *samādhi,* meditative concentration, induced by *samatha* meditation; latent defilements lurking in the unconscious are dissolved by wisdom, *paññā,* induced especially by *vipassanā* meditation.

7.10 *Samatha* Meditation

The most common way of developing meditation has been to practice the *samatha-yāna,* as described in such *Suttas* as the *Sāmaññaphala* (*DN*.I. pp. 47–85). In the *samatha* aspect of this, an object is chosen, mindfulness is applied to it, and concentration is developed focused on specific aspects of the object. As concentration strengthens, mindfulness is further developed as an adjunct which is increasingly aware of the subtle states of mind which arise from deep concentration. This might be compared to careful examination down a microscope. Thus arises a state of tranquil, focused alertness, with concentration and mindfulness developed to high degrees, in lucid trances known as *jhānas*, after the "access concentration" *(upacāra-samādhi)* that is on the brink of attaining the first of these. In the *Visuddhimagga* and commentaries, access concentration is the state attained when the five hindrances have been suspended, and the mind is focused on a vivid *nimitta*—a visual or tactile mental impression of the object of concentration—but the qualities needed for *jhāna* are not yet at full strength. In the *Suttas,* though, there is no apparent distinction between the state in which the hindrances are first suspended and the first *jhāna.* They describe entry to the first *jhāna* thus:

> And when he knows that these five hindrances have left him, gladness (*pamujja*) arises in him, from gladness comes joy (*pīti*), from the joy in his mind his body becomes tranquil, with a tranquil body he feels pleasure (*sukha*) and with (easeful) pleasure his mind is concentrated. Completely secluded from sense-desires and unwholesome qualities, he lives having attained the joy and pleasure of the first *jhāna*, which is accompanied by mental application (*vitakka*) and examining (*vicāra*), and born of seclusion (*viveka*). And with this joy and pleasure born of seclusion, he so suffuses, drenches, fills and irradiates his body that there is no spot in his entire body that is untouched by this joy and pleasure born of seclusion. (*DN*.I. p. 73)

In the vehicle of *samatha,* deeper levels of *jhāna* are developed before *vipassanā* is developed in earnest. In the method of "*samatha* and *vipassanā* yoked together," one level of *jhāna* is developed, then its impermanent and unsatisfactory nature is examined with *vipassanā,* then a deeper level of *jhāna* is developed, then seen with *vipassanā*, etc. Moreover, at the time of stream entry, when the mind gains its first glimpse of Nirvana, there is a brief or sustained experience of a "transcendent" *(lokuttara)* level of *jhāna* (e.g., *Dhs*. p. 277) rather than one with a conditioned object. For those starting with a more *vipassanā* approach, this may be the first, and perhaps only, experience of *jhāna.*

Buddhaghosa's *Visuddhimagga* describes in detail 40 possible objects of meditation (*Vism.* pp. 110–111, detailed in *Vism*. IV–X; Conze 1972; Shaw 2006, pp. 86–194), which primarily, but not exclusively, pertain to *samatha.* They can lead to different levels of *samatha,* and are especially helpful for different personality types, who may be more affected by greed, hatred or delusion or, more skillfully, by faith, intelligence, or discursiveness (*Vism.* pp. 101–110) :

- Mindfulness of breathing, which best suits the delusion and discursive types→any of the four *jhānas*
- The four divine abidings: loving kindness, compassion, empathetic joy, and equanimity; hate type→third *jhāna*, or fourth by equanimity
- The ten *kasiṇas* or "universals": prepared examples of things which represent the elements (earth, water, fire, wind), light, or limited space—all of which suit all types; or colours, for the hate type: blue, yellow, red, white; these→any of the four *jhāna*s. A *kasiṇa-maṇḍala,* or "universal-circle," such as a blue disc, a circle of earth, or a bowl of water is focused on until it can be seen clearly in the mind's eye as a mental image, representing such a universal quality as blueness, the solidity of earth, or the cohesion of water (*Vism.* pp. 123–125).
- The four formless states: four subtle levels of existence, known from the fourth *jhāna,* and suitable for all types
- The ten kinds of unloveliness or foulness (*asubha,* Skt *aśubha*): ten stages of the decomposition of a corpse; for the greed type, to counteract lust→first *jhāna*
- Mindfulness of the 32 parts of the body; intelligent type→first *jhāna.*

- Mindfulness of the inevitability of death, recollection of the peaceful qualities of Nirvana, perception of the repulsiveness of food, or reflection on the four elements composing the body; intelligent type→access concentration.
- Recollections of the qualities of the Buddha, *Dhamma* or *Saṅgha,* the benefits of moral virtue or generosity, or of the various types of god/*devas;* for the faith type→access concentration.

7.11 Mindfulness in *Samatha* Meditation

Since the twentieth century popularizing of Burmese methods of practicing according to the *Satipaṭṭhāna Sutta* (see below), mindfulness has often come to be equated with the practice of *vipassanā,* and *samatha* seen as only involving concentration (Anālayo 2003, pp. 67–91, discusses this view); *samatha* is even sometimes, wrongly, translated as "concentration." Given that a central *samatha* method is mindfulness of, or with, breathing, this is a curious narrowing. Mindfulness has a range of aspects and uses, and we should bear these in mind, that is, be mindful of them!

Samatha mindfulness of breathing takes a look at something seemingly very ordinary, always under one's nose. It is the steady watching and clear awareness of a smooth, natural breath, with its varying length, and heedfully noting the flow of sensations and related feelings. This allows one to feel what it is actually like, rather than just thinking about it: as if feeling it for the first time.

Mindfulness's quality of careful observation helps one not be confused about the breath, and its quality of alertness prevents "switching off" from the breath into a dull staring attitude, as when the mind stops taking things in when reading.

It remembers that the aim is to stay with the breath in the present moment, so it guards against losing concentration and switching away from the breath, wandering away into the past, future, daydreams, worries, and sleepiness.

It carefully notices when attention nevertheless wanders onto such things, so that it can be gently brought back to the breath, so as to again mindfully feel it and know where one is in the process.

If annoyance arises in the mind, whether directed at one's own wandering mind, external noises, or their source, mindfulness recognizes this, but helps one step back from involvement in the irritation, so one can let go of it and return to the breath. The same applies, for example, with any anxiety on "am I doing this right?"

Once a good pattern of breathing has been established (some forms of *samatha* breathing mindfulness work with a slow breathing adjusted to various different lengths/depths), mindfulness observes it without interference, so one can let the breath be, and not be anxious, as one nears the end of the in-breath, about when the out-breath will start, or vice versa; it will happen naturally.

The *Ānāpānasati Sutta,* the Discourse on Mindfulness with in and out Breathing (*MN.*III. pp. 82–88; Bucknell and Kang 1997, pp. 26–28; Shaw 2006, pp. 146–158) describes 16 phases, grouped into four sets, with these sets respectively developing the four *satipaṭṭhānas:* the applications of mindfulness to body, feeling, mind-states, and basic patterns in experience:

1. Breathing in long, he knows, "I am breathing in long"; or breathing out long, he knows, "I am breathing out long."
2. Or breathing in short, he knows, "I am breathing in short"; or breathing out short, he knows, "I am breathing out short."
3. He trains himself, "I will breathe in sensitive to (*paṭsaṃvedī*) the whole body (of breath)." He trains himself, "I will breathe out sensitive to the whole body (of breath)."
4. He trains himself, "I will breathe in calming (*passambhayaṃ*) the body-conditioner (*kāya-saṃkhāraṃ:* at *MN*.I.301, in-and-out-breaths (*assāsa-passāsā*))." He trains himself, "I will breathe out calming the body conditioner."

5. He trains himself, "I will breathe in sensitive to joy (*pīti-*)." He trains himself, "I will breathe out sensitive to joy."
6. He trains himself, "I will breathe in sensitive to (bodily and perhaps mental) pleasure/ease (*sukha-*)." He trains himself, "I will breathe out sensitive to pleasure/ease."
7. He trains himself, "I will breathe in sensitive to the mind-conditioner (*citta-saṃkhāra*: at *MN*.I.301, perception (*saññā*) and feeling (*vedanā*))." He trains himself, "I will breathe out sensitive to the mind-conditioner."
8. He trains himself, "I will breathe in calming the mind-conditioner." He trains himself, "I will breathe out calming the mind-conditioner."

9. He trains himself, "I will breathe in sensitive to the mind (*citta-*)." He trains himself, "I will breathe out sensitive to the mind."
10. He trains himself, "I will breathe in satisfying/gladdening (*abhippamodayaṃ*) the mind." He trains himself, "I will breathe out satisfying/gladdening the mind."
11. He trains himself, "I will breathe in concentrating (*samādahaṃ*) the mind." He trains himself, "I will breathe out concentrating the mind."
12. He trains himself, "I will breathe in releasing (*vimocayaṃ*) the mind." He trains himself, "I will breathe out releasing the mind."

13. He trains himself, "I will breathe in contemplating the impermanent (*anicc'ānupassī*)." He trains himself, "I will breathe out contemplating the impermanent."
14. He trains himself, "I will breathe in contemplating dispassion/fading away (*virāga*)." He trains himself, "I will breathe out contemplating dispassion/fading away."
15. He trains himself, "I will breathe in contemplating cessation (*nirodha*) [of specific items of experience, or even of one's whole conditioned 'world' of experience]." He trains himself, "I will breathe out contemplating cessation."
16. He trains himself, "I will breathe in contemplating letting go (*paṭinissagga*)." He trains himself, "I will breathe out contemplating letting go."

The *satipaṭṭhānas* developed by the above are in turn said to develop the seven "factors of awakening" (Pali *bojjhaṅga,* Skt *bodhyaṅga*): mindfulness, discrimination of *dhammas,* vigor, joy, tranquility, concentration, and equanimity, which culminate in clear knowing and release *(vijjā-vimutti).*

Here, while the fourth set of the four phases clearly pertain to *vipassanā,* the second set includes mindfulness of two of the factors of the first two *jhānas*, as developed by *samatha*: *pīti,* joy, and *sukha,* easeful bodily pleasure that later becomes purely mental happiness (*SN*.V. pp. 213–216 says that the faculty of pleasure *(sukhindriya)* is absent in the third *jhāna,* yet *somanassa,* happiness, is still present there; that is, bodily *sukha* is replaced by mental *sukha* (*SN*.V. p. 209)). Moreover, mindfulness is described as a basis for suspending the five hindrances and entering the first *jhāna* (*DN*.I. pp. 71–73) and is seen as especially strong in the third and fourth *jhānas* (*DN*.I. pp. 75–76):

> Again, a monk with the fading away of joy remains imperturbable, mindful and clearly aware, and experiences in himself that happiness of which the Noble Ones say: "Happy is he who dwells with equanimity and mindfulness," and he enters and remains in the third *jhāna*. And with this happiness devoid of joy he so suffuses his body that no spot remains untouched....
> Again, a monk, having previously given up (physical) pleasure and pain, with the disappearance of mental pleasure and pain, remains in the fourth *jhāna* which is beyond pleasure and pain, and purified by equanimity and mindfulness. And he sits suffusing his body with a mind thoroughly purified and cleansed, so that no part of his body is untouched by it.

So, mindfulness is used in *both vipassanā* and *samatha,* but in different ways.

The seventh path-factor, right mindfulness—identified as the four applications of mindfulness (*SN*.V. pp. 9–10)—is the natural support for the eighth factor, right concentration, identified as the four *jhānas* (*SN*.V. p. 10). With mindfulness an aid to all the path-factors (*MN*.III. p. 71), it also naturally aids the insight/*vipassanā* of right view, whose wisdom also aids all the factors (*SN*.V. p. 2). Hence, *jhāna* is also associated with wisdom:

> There is no *jhāna* for him who lacks wisdom, and no wisdom for him who lacks *jhāna*. He in whom are found both *jhāna* and wisdom, indeed, is close to Nirvana. (*Dhp*. p. 372)

We also see how in the list of the five faculties—trustful confidence, vigor, mindfulness, concentration (the four *jhānas*: *SN*.V.198) and wisdom—mindfulness feeds into qualities particularly associated, respectively, with *samatha* and *vipassanā.*

7.12 Mindfulness and Concentration/Mental Unification *(samādhi)*

Samatha meditation aims to cultivate the power of concentration till it can become truly one-pointed, fully focused on a chosen calming object. In such a state, the mind becomes free from all distraction and wavering, in a unified state of inner stillness: mental unification.

In meditation, "concentration" *(samādhi)* refers not so much to the gentle effort of concentrat*ing,* though this is also needed, as to the concentrat*ed* state(s) of mental unification that this leads to. *Samatha* teacher Sarah Shaw (unpublished) said:

> The word concentration does not necessarily mean the kind of rigid application of mind that occurs when the maths teacher at school enjoins us to "concentrate"! Here it is more akin to its earlier English sense of bringing together, as in a concentrate. *Samādhi* is like a pooling of the resources of the mind when faced with a pleasing and intricate problem, that absorbs all one's interest—a state which interest in a mathematical problem can bring of course, or working out and digging a rock garden. Attention is governed not so much by one's own effort, but by the object itself, which changes and influences the nature of the mind that considers it. The object starts to be perceived without "wanting" or rejection, but for its own sake. This is the kind of concentration which, according to the *abhidhamma* can and indeed is in a small part present in daily consciousness. When this is developed in *jhāna*, the mind is made unified and one-pointed, capable of seeing without distractions or hindrances.

Concentration yokes the mind onto an object or project, be this good, bad, or indifferent. It is a state of being focused, whatever the level of one's alertness/awareness. It is possible to be quite focused, but not very mindful: for example, Sir Isaac Newton boiling his watch instead of an egg, when concentrating on an intellectual problem. It is possible to be very mindful without necessarily focusing on any one object, though if there is good mindfulness, this makes concentration easier. When concentration is combined with mindfulness and focused on a simple object such as the breath, it becomes "right concentration" and integrates the mind's energies so as to bring about mental stillness, tranquility, and peace: a quiet yet positive state of mind. As Shaw (2009, p. 10) said:

> Right concentration…is the stilling of the mind in concentration. By concentration, the Buddhist path means the state of mind when attention is fully engaged, aroused by an object of interest, such as a flower, a view of a wide area of sea or countryside, or a pattern of frost on a window pane. Where there is interest that is accompanied by mindfulness, so that there is neither excessive fascination nor indifference, this can be deepened in a meditation practice, set apart from other activities in the day. The texts do warn that concentration can arise in a lot of negative situations, so that it is wrong concentration: it is possible to be very focused when having an argument. When it is right concentration, it is said to be characterized by mindfulness and an absence of any wish to harm or spoil. This happens when the mind comes to rest on an object with interest and mindfulness, and without hindrance. It becomes then an alert attention that can be deepened to take the mind into a refreshing and restorative meditation, known as *jhāna*.

Right concentration is a wholesome one-pointedness of mind: a wholesome state of mind steadily focused on a calming object. It is an intensified steadiness of mind, a state where the mind is like a clear flame burning in a windless place or the surface of a clear, undisturbed lake. It is a state of steady focus, mental composure, and stillness, which unifies and harmonizes the mind's energies in a way which is an internal parallel of the situation where a class of children are all intently listening to a good teacher, not fidgeting or looking out of the window. It is experienced as a state of tranquility and clarity and comes about when there is a state of happiness that allows the mind to contentedly stay on the object, as one has developed a natural interest in it.

In *samatha* meditation on the breathing, *mindfulness* establishes a link between the mind and the breath, knowing its length and how it feels, while concentration is the state of being well focused on the sensations known by mindfulness, initially aided by some system of counting, such as counting up to a certain number on the in-breath, and from that number back to one on the out-breath. At any time in the meditation, *mindfulness* will give awareness of:

- The length of the breath, its speed, smoothness, and whether it is an in or out breath
- The subtle sensations which arise along the path of the breath and subtle feelings that come when one attends carefully to the flow of the "breath body"
- Where one is in the process, such as the stage of practice one is in, and what one is supposed to be doing
- Aspects of posture that may need retuning
- Whether the mind has wandered.

Concentration is the quality of remaining generally focused, centered, on the breath, including the sensations in a particular part of the path of the breath. At first, this is particularly aided by attention to the numbers one is counting as one breathes. The counting aids both mindfulness and concentration.

When the mind wanders, this is because, first of all, mindfulness slips and one forgets what one is supposed to be doing. Concentration is then lost as the mind becomes distracted and loses its focus. If one then becomes involved in a long wandering thought, there may be concentration on *this*, but no mindfulness. When one notices that the mind is not on the breath, this marks the return of mindfulness, which then allows one to reestablish awareness of the breath, then the concentration on it.

Samatha practice starts to work well when there is a balance of a high degree of both mindfulness and concentration, so as to bring about a state of alert stillness.

7.13 Mindfulness in *Vipassanā* Meditation

The way of *vipassanā* then *samatha* became popular in Burma in the twentieth century and from there spread elsewhere (Cousins 1996; King 1980, pp. 116–124). The same applies for the way of *dry vipassanā,* which sees the deliberate cultivation *jhāna* and even access concentration as unnecessary for awakening, momentary concentration being sufficient; though Buddhaghosa saw concentration as briefly at the level of first *jhāna* at the time of stream-entry (*Vism.* p. 666). *Vipassanā* meditation uses a high degree of mindfulness, plus right effort and a degree of concentration: how much depends on the teacher. Typically, the breath is used as a home base for the attention to keep returning to, so as to keep the mind calm and uncaptured by distractions. The insight that develops also naturally brings about deeper stillness and calm due to strong momentary concentration and the detachment which insight brings.

The practice of the four *satipaṭṭhānas* is the key basis of *vipassanā* meditation. Rather than focusing on one chosen object, as in *samatha, vipassanā* opens out the attention so that mindfulness calmly observes each passing sensory or mental object, to systematically notice certain pervasive characteristics of experience. The conditioned states that make up body and mind, of "oneself" or "others," are seen to constantly arise and pass away and be unsatisfactory and impersonal processes to which it is inappropriate to become attached. When not doing sitting meditation, the meditator may carefully observe the sensations involved in movements, such as bending and stretching the arms, eating, washing, and going to the toilet. "Mindfulness of walking" is a specific kind of practice, also used by *samatha* practitioners to strengthen their mindfulness. In this, a person walks back and forth along a path with the mind focused on the sensations in the feet and calf muscles, and the various phases of walking may be mentally noted with terms such as "lifting," "moving," and "putting." This develops a light, open feeling of spaciousness, and may even lead to the "foot" disappearing into a flow of sensations.

During seated meditation, the breath is usually investigated, for it is through this rising and falling process that the body is kept alive. *Vipassanā* meditation is more analytical and probing than *samatha* meditation, though, as it aims to investigate the nature of reality, rather than remaining focused on one relatively stable object and feelings that arise from doing this. Thus what might become a distraction within *samatha* meditation can become an object for *vipassanā*. Thus the mind does not remain focused on the breath, but also observes various physical sensations as they occur, such as itches and the release of previously unnoticed tensions. As the body is more easily perceived, mindfulness takes this as its object first, so as to build up its power before observing the more fleeting and subtle mental processes, starting with feelings. These are observed as they arise and pass away, noting simply whether they are pleasant, unpleasant, or neutral, born of the body or of the mind, ordinary or more spiritual. No significance is attached to them; however, they are viewed simply as passing phenomena. Mindfulness then moves on to the states of mind, noting moods and emotions as they arise and are allowed to pass. Finally, mindfulness investigates *dhammas,* significant reality-patterns, up to and including the True Realities of the Spiritually Ennobled, noting when they are present, when they are absent, how they come to arise, and how they come to cease. (An element of this may arise incidentally within a mainly *samatha*-type practice, but it is not the main focus.)

While investigating the processes described above, the aim is to experientially recognize their shared features: the "three marks." Their constant arising and ceasing demonstrates that they are impermanent. That they are ephemeral, unstable, and limited, not the kind of thing that one can rely on, shows that they are unsatisfactory, obviously or subtly painful. That they rise according to conditions cannot be controlled at will, and thus, do not truly "belong" to anyone, shows that they are non-Self, "empty of Self or what belongs to Self." Investigation shows that the appearance of "oneself" and external "things" as substantial self-identical entities is a misperception. These insights are not of a conceptual, intellectual nature, but arise as flashes of penetrative understanding or wisdom. Once these have occurred during meditation, they may also arise in the course of the day, as things are observed with mindfulness. This process, then, combines gradual cultivation and progressively deeper, and sudden, flashes of insight.

When the whole panorama of experience is seen to be made up of processes—mental or physical, internal or external, past, present or future, subtle or gross—that are non-lasting, unreliable, and insubstantial, then there can be a disenchantment (Pali *nibbidā,* Skt *nirvidā*) with, a letting go of these processes. As a person thus comes to recognize all that he or she has fondly identified with as "I" or "mine" as actually changing, conditioned, and subtly unsatisfactory, it is directly known that these cannot be truly "possessed" as "mine," or be a true identity as "I," an essence, "my self." As each thing is seen in this way, this allows a relinquishing of any attachment to or identification with it, which leads to a sense of lightness, a spacious accommodation of whatever happens to arise and joy. This will be the more complete, the more it is realized that *everything* is non-Self; that "Self" is an empty concept. Not only an empty concept, but a harmful one: for taking something changeable as a permanent "I" can only lead to suffering when that thing changes. And to protect "I," we often cause suffering to others. Thus, *vipassanā* comes to lead the meditator beyond the limiting habit conditions that are rooted in I-centered-ness, hence strengthening compassion. Ultimately, it allows a glimpse of that which is totally *un*conditioned—Nirvana—beyond change, limitation, and suffering: deathless, unborn, beyond all thought of "I."

Vipassanā meditation thus aims to dissolve the kind of views that nourish the unskillful states of mind. If body and mind are simply changing, impermanent, *dukkha*, conditioned processes, which cannot be adequately controlled by "me," and are insubstantial products of other such processes, mental or physical, then: Why crave or be greedy for them?; Why hate others, for we are all equally tied up with *dukkha*?; Why continue with the delusion of protecting an essential "me" that cannot be found?; Why build up I-centered conceits (*I* am superior, *I* am inferior, or *I* am just as good/bad as anyone else) around physical and mental processes which are subject to moment-to-moment change?; Why be tied by any fixed view that identifies with things as "me" or "mine," or viewing them as "my real self," as substantial, solid? Let go and be free.

Recent Burmese methods of *vipassanā* have included the following. U Ba Khin (1899–1971; King 1980, pp. 125–132; Kornfield 1995, pp. 235–256) taught a method that emphasizes awareness, from a concentrated mind, of the impermanence of mental and physical phenomena, particularly by attention to feelings arising from the sense of touch. Attention is given to atom-like "clusters" *(kālapa)* of examples of the four material elements, plus of color, odor, taste, and nutritive essence, seen to be basic constituent elements of anything physical. Mindful awareness of the jingling buzz of the *kalāpas* is seen to bring insight into all of the "three marks." One gains enough concentration from mindfulness of breathing to perhaps gain a *nimitta,* then works on mindfulness of impermanent and *dukkha* feelings in different parts of the body, so that these feelings build up. The aim is for the mind to calmly observe these and let them, and incipient reactions, fade away, so as to leave a peaceful space in which ingrained mental habit patterns have been dissolved.

S. N. Goenka (1924–2013), an Indian raised in Burma, taught U Ba Khin *vipassanā* at many centers around the world (www.dhamma.org).

Like the approach of U Ba Khin, that of Mahāsī Sayadaw (1904–1982) is one in which *vipassanā* in time leads to deep *samatha* with Nirvana as its object, though the former seems to put more overt emphasis on an initial phase of *samatha* as a platform for *vipassanā,* and the Mahāsī method is sometimes presented as one of "dry *vipassanā*" (Anālayo 2003, pp. 64–65). The Mahāsī method emphasizes constantly observing and analyzing the flow of experience, bodily and mental, aided by labeling what is perceived, starting with the rising and falling of the abdomen as one breathes (Bucknell and Kang 1977, pp. 133–22; King 1980, pp. 132–137; Kornfield 1995, pp. 51–82; Nyanaponika 1996, pp. 85–113). The method is perhaps akin to slowing down a film to gain awareness of each frame, by a process of incessantly cutting up experience into segments and labeling them in an impersonal way.

7.14 Secular Mindfulness and Buddhist Mindfulness

The term "mindfulness" is now a popular one, both in Mindfuless-Based Stress Reduction (developed from 1979 by Jon Kabat-Zinn at the University of Massachusetts) and Mindfulness-Based Cognitive Therapy (developed by Zindel Segal, Mark Williams, and John Teasdale), and as seen with a host of popularizing books of varying quality. The UK National Health Service recommends certain mindfulness treatments as a way to help people who suffer from depression from relapsing back into it through falling back into negative thought patterns. The Buddhist influences on Kabat-Zinn were Nyanaponika's *Heart of Buddhist Meditation,* which was influenced by Mahāsi's *vipassanā* approach, his practice of the latter, and of Korean Zen, and a reading on Japanese Zen, Vedānta and Krishnamurti (Kabat-Zinn 2011, p. 289).

How, though, does secular mindfulness relate to full-spectrum Buddhist mindfulness, what is their degree of overlap, and what aspects of Buddhist mindfulness may perhaps be being neglected or overlooked in secular mindfulness? Secular mindfulness has been explained– as an operational guide to practice, rather than a definition– by Kabat-Zinn (1994, p. 4) as, "Mindfulness means paying attention in a particular way: on purpose, in the present moment, and non-judgmentally." Another explanation, by Bishop et al. (2004, p. 232), is:

> Broadly conceptualized, mindfulness has been described as a kind of non-elaborative, non-judgmental, present-centered awareness in which each thought, feeling, or sensation that arises in the attentional field is acknowledged and accepted as it is.

I note that this kind of definition is more in line with the use of mindfulness in *vipassanā* than in *samatha* meditation, as it concerns mindfulness applied to whatever arises. That said, *samatha* should surely have an important role in the therapeutic use of mindfulness, through its bringing calm to a troubled mind.

The above descriptions also talk as if mindfulness only concerns attention to the immediate present. The practice of Buddhist mindfulness certainly has aspects which emphasize this, strengthen the ability to do it, and learns much from it. Yet mindfulness can also be applied to past experiences or used to "bear in mind"—be mindful of—certain qualities or things one has previously learnt or understood, as they pertain to the present. Indeed the Pali word *sati,* which is translated as "mindfulness," also has the sense of "recollection."

The quality of being non-elaborative is certainly a strong feature of Buddhist mindfulness. The aim is to develop and retain a direct and immediate awareness, a lucid awareness of something in its vivid and distinct presence, including a clear memory: to keep things simple, and not go off at a tangent into fantasies, stories about oneself, or get lost in plans and stray memories.

The term "non-judgmental" is potentially misleading, though. From my understanding, while Theravāda Buddhist mindfulness is not judgment*al,* it is not free of *judgment*. It aims to see things as they really are, and to do this one needs to suspend reactions of like or dislike, attachment or aversion, self-blame or self-praise. One needs to quieten me-centered reactions and commentaries. Simply doing this, being non-judgmental, is helpful and valuable and is an important skill to learn, especially in the early stages of practice. But the greatest value is that this stance of observant equanimity allows one a clearer view of how certain inner states are wholesome/skillful and certain other ones are unwholesome/unskillful. This wise judgment or discernment then helps one to naturally incline towards the wholesome and away from the unwholesome and to learn from mistakes and successes in doing this. It also helps in recognizing the *dukkha* quality of things. This means that "accepted as it is" in the above quote needs reflecting on. To fully acknowledge and accept the reality of something need not also entail accepting that this thing is okay. For example, in the teaching on the four True Realities for the Noble Ones, all of which need to be acknowledged and understood, the second, the origin of *dukkha,* needs to be *abandoned* (*SN*.V. p. 422). That said, Kabat-Zinn (2011, pp. 291–292) has been influenced, in his emphasis on aiming to let go of being judgmental, and what he calls "non-dual awareness," by Chan and Zen.

In early Buddhist literature, though, there is no criticism of "discrimination" as problematic. It occurs in no list of fetters or hindrances! Moreover, one of the seven factors of awakening, listed immediately after mindfulness, is *dhamma-vicayo,* "discrimination of *dhamma*s," which is seen as directly related to wisdom (*SN*.V. p. 111), and *vīmaṃsā*, "investigation," is an aspect of one of the four *iddhi-pādas,* or "bases of success" on the path.

It is quite clear that the distinction between *kusala* (Pali, Skt *kuśala*), skillful/wholesome, and *akusala/akuśala,* unskillful/unwholesome, actions and states of mind is fundamental to early and Theravāda Buddhism. At first, the cultivation of skillful states may lead to attachment to these and aversion to their opposites—so that one may perhaps become proud of one's skillful states, look down on those with less of them, or irritated at other people's "needless" unskillful states—but then it will be increasingly realized that these reactions are themselves unskillful and thus must be abandoned. Later, more subtle forms of unskillfulness will remain and will require even more skillful forms of discrimination to identify and undermine. In all of this, mindfully recognizing, undermining, and not feeding the unskillful is far more effective and skillful than trying to fight against the unskillful as an opposing enemy. All of this is clear spiritual psychology. It is learning to be more skillful in developing wholesome skillfulness.

7.15 Mindfulness in the Theravādin and Sarvāstivādin *Abhidhammas*, and Whether It Is a Universal Feature of the Mind

Abhidhamma is a kind of systematic catalogue of mental states, their qualities, and how they condition each other. In Theravādin *Abhidhamma,* mindfulness is seen to always occur along with certain other qualities (Bodhi 1993, pp. 85–88). Hence, the nonoccurrence of these qualities is a sign that, in that moment, true mindfulness is also absent, though it may soon return.

Mental states present, to some degree, in all wholesome states, are seen to be: faith/trust/confidence, mindfulness, self-respect, regard for consequence, non-greed (generosity, non-clinging), non-hate (loving kindness), equipoise, plus these state of mind and (experienced) body:

- Stilling/tranquility: a calm, contented state, opposed to restlessness and unease
- Lightness: buoyancy, lack of heaviness, being unencumbered, when there is ease of action; opposes dullness and lethargy
- Softness: when body and mind are pliable and receptive, opposed to fixed views and self-importance.
- Readiness: when body and mind are workable and wieldy, like refined gold; opposed to desire for sense-pleasures (when the mind is too "runny," i.e., not "together") and ill-will (when mind is too "brittle")
- Competence: being fit for any task; opposed to vacillation
- Straightness: simplicity, directness, uprightness; opposed to unnecessary complexity, craftiness, or deceit.

At least according to the Theravādin *Abhidhamma*, the presence of mindfulness is a key determinant of a mental state being wholesome—when it is present, the mind is in a wholesome state, and mindfulness of a wholesome state strengthens such a state. Moreover, when one is truly mindful of an *un*wholesome state in one's mind, one has already left it, if only for a moment. Unwholesome states "melt" under the gaze of mindfulness and require a lack of it. This is an almost magical aspect of mindfulness! Its gaze naturally supports positive states of mind and undermines negative ones. That said, being mindful in one moment does not guarantee being mindful in the next moment. Other qualities that mindfulness works with can help it be more sustained, though.

Concentration is seen as present to some degree in *any* state of mind, be this the momentary focus on a passing object, or even the sustained concentration of a sniper, whose lack of concern for his target is a sign of lack of mindfulness.

In the Sarvāstivādin *Abhidharma*, which had a continuing influence on Mahāyāna traditions, *smṛti,* the Sanskrit equivalent of Pali *sati,* is seen rather differently than in the Theravāda. This is because *smṛti* is seen as a universal mental quality, present in all states of mind, including unwholesome ones (*AKB*.III. 24; Chapple 1996, pp. 86–87, 227; Dhammajoti 2009, p. 36). The Sarvāstivāda seem to have used the term "*smṛti*/mindfulness" for a mental quality that, at least in its weakest form, is more rudimentary and general type of mental quality—a lower-grade mental function, as basic memory—than the Theravāda. It is explained thus:

> *Smṛti* is non-failing with regard to the object; a *dharma* by virtue of which the mind does not forget the object, by virtue of which it cherishes it in order to so express it (*abhilaṣatīva*). (*AKB*.II. p. 24)

For the Sarvāstivāda, a distorted memory, occurring as part of an unskillful mental state, would still be *smṛti,* while for the Theravāda such a memory would be a form of *saññā, or* perceptual interpretation: one of the universal mental qualities accepted by both it and the Sarvāstivāda. A memory would only count as *sati,* for the Theravāda, if it was clear and undistorted and part of a skillful mental state (Gethin 2001, pp. 40–44).

However, the Sarvāstivāda see one of the qualities present in all *wholesome* states as *apramāda* (*AKB*.II. 25; Pali *appamāda*), heedfulness, which is close to what the Theravādin tradition means by *sati.* Accordingly, the Sarvāstivāda see *pramāda* (Pali *pamāda*), heedlessness, as an ingredient of unwholesome states (*AKB*.II. 26). Of course, while the Theravāda does not see mindfulness as always present in the mind, it sees it as a state that everyone experiences from time to time.

In a similar way, the Sarvāstivāda saw *prajñā* (Pali *paññā*) as an ingredient in all mental states, including unwholesome ones (*AKB*.II. 24). This was because they saw it, at least in a weak form, as a basic kind of understanding or knowledge, which can be either conventional or transcendent, impure or pure, with only stronger forms of it being a kind that can count as "wisdom" (*AKB*.I. 2a, *AKB*.VII. 1).

That said, given the generally positive image of *smṛti/sati* and *prajñā/paññā* in Buddhism, the view that they are features of *all* mental states may have fed into the view, common in the Mahāyāna, that the basic nature of mind is not just something with a simple level of memory and understanding, but as having *alert mindfulness* and *wisdom* in it—a view found in some versions of the *Tathāgata-garbha* or Buddha-nature doctrine.

Clearly, these higher-level qualities can only arise in a mind that has basic memory and understanding, and delusion can only arise in a mind with some level of understanding. Only something that can understand can *mis*understand, and an insentient thing such as a stone cannot experience delusion. Basic memory and understanding is a necessary condition for mindfulness and wisdom; but does that mean that the former are implicit in the latter…? Buddhists seem to have had different views on this. As Anālayo (2013, p. 160) said:

> Alongside considerable overlap in meaning, the early Buddhist conception of mindfulness shows features that are distinct from how this quality is perceived in later Buddhist traditions as well as from the way mindfulness is defined in modern day clinical usage. Needless to say, each of these particular definitions has its rationale and significance within its particular context, hence distinguishing these different "mindfulnesses" does not imply a value judgement of any kind.

A parallel issue is on the nature of the *pabhassara/prabhāsvara citta,* the "brightly shining mind." A famous and influential passage on this states: "This mind, monks, is brightly shining, but it is defiled by defilements which arrive" (*AN*.I. p. 10). *Theravādins* see it as a bright level of mind equivalent to *bhavaṅga,* the resting state of mind that is constantly flicked in and out of, with the radiance uncovered in *jhāna* (Harvey 1995, pp. 155–179). This uncovered radiance is seen as a good basis for going on to attain enlightenment. The Tathāgata-garbha tradition of the Mahāyāna saw it as either (a) a potential for enlightenment that needs to be uncovered then matured, rather like the Theravādin view, or (b) actual enlightenment that just needs to be uncovered (Williams 2009, pp. 103–128). A potential danger in the latter view is that subtle defilements, or at the least the potential for them to arise, can be left unchallenged. The radiant mind of the fourth *jhāna* is an ideal springboard from which Nirvana can be experienced, but it is not the same as Nirvana. One phase of the cycle of cosmic eons described in the *Suttas* is that in which all beings are reborn in a heaven, that of great fruit (Pali *Vehapphala*), at the level of the fourth *jhāna* (*Vism*.XIII. p. 62; Gethin 1997, pp. 198–205; 1998, pp. 123–125), but most later leave this to further wander in *saṃsāra.* If a state of great calm and strong mindfulness should not be mistaken for the liberation that it *can* open the door to, how much more should one beware of mistaking non-judgmental attention for the full-spectrum mindfulness that it can open the door to.

7.16 Conclusion

The quality of *sati,* or mindfulness, is rich and multifaceted, and one needs to mindfully explore its qualities, and mindfully recollect and bear these in mind. The benefits of certain aspects of it are being made widely available through secular applications of mindfulness. The main *vipassanā* forms of Buddhist meditation that secular mindfulness has drawn from use mindfulness to contemplate the qualities of impermanence, painfulness, and impersonality in any experience that arises: the three marks. In *samatha* meditation, mindfulness is paired with the quality of concentrated mental unification to focus on particular phenomena such as the breathing process. This is in order to take the mind into stilled and subtle states in which there is a progressive letting-go of ordinary states of mind and their limitations and a quiet space in which insight has a great opportunity to see clearly that the three marks apply to both the states of ordinary consciousness and also to altered states of consciousness that can arise in spiritual practice.

Abbreviations

AKB. *Abhidharma-kośa-bhāṣya,* (tr. L.M.Pruden, from L. de La Valleé Poussin's French translation), *Abhidharmakośabhāṣyam,* 4 volumes, Berkeley, Asian Humanities Press, 1991)
AN. *Aṅguttara Nikāya*
Dhp. *Dhammapada*
Dhs. *Dhammasaṅgaṇī*
DN. *Dīgha Nikāya*
Miln. *Milindapañha*
MN. *Majjhima Nikāya*
Patis. *Paṭisambhidāmagga*
Skt Sanskrit
SN. *Saṃyutta Nikāya*
Sn. *Sutta-nipāta*
Vism. *Visuddhimagga*

All the above except *AKB.* are cited from their Pali Text Society versions, using page or volume and page numbers, but section numbers for *Dhs.* and verse numbers for *Sn. AKB.* references are to book and section.

References

Anālayo. (2003). *Satipaṭṭhāna: The direct path to realization.* Birmingham: Windhorse.
Anālayo. (2013). Mindfulness in early Buddhism. *Journal of Buddhist Studies, XI,* 147–173.
Bishop, S. R., Lau, M., Shapiro, S., Carlson, L., Anderson, N., Carmody, J., Segal, Z., Abbey, S., Speca, M., Velting, D., & Devins, G. (2004). Mindfulness: A proposed definition. *Clinical Psychology: Science and Practice, 11,* 230–241.
Bodhi, B. (1993). *A comprehensive manual and Abhidhamma: The Abhidhammattha Sangaha: Pali text, translation and explanatory guide.* Kandy: Buddhist Publication Society.
Bucknell, R., & Kang, C. (1997). *The meditative way: Readings in the theory and practice of Buddhist meditation.* Richmond: Curzon.
Chapple, C. K. (1996). Abhidharma as paradigm for practice. In F. J. Hoffman & M. Deegalle (Eds.), *Pali Buddhism* (pp. 79–101). Richmond: Curzon.
Conze, E. (1972). *Buddhist meditation.* London: Allen and Unwin.
Cousins L. S. (1984). Samatha-yāna and Vipassanā-yāna. In D. Dhammapala, et al. (Eds.), *Buddhist studies in honour of Hammalava Saddhatissa* (pp. 56–68). Nugegoda.
Cousins, L. S. (1996). The origins of insight meditation. In T. Skorupski (Ed.), *The Buddhist forum* (vol. 4, pp. 35–58). London: School of Oriental and African Studies.
Dhammajoti, B. K. L. (2009). *Sarvāstivāda Abhidharma.* Hong Kong: Centre of Buddhist Studies, The University of Hong Kong.
Gethin, R. (1997). Cosmology and meditation: From the Aggañña Sutta to the Mahāyāna. *History of Religions, 36,* 183–219.
Gethin, R. (1998). *The foundations of Buddhism.* Oxford: Oxford University Press.
Gethin, R. (2001). *The Buddhist path to awakening.* Oxford: Oneworld.

Harvey, P. (1995). *The selfless mind: Personality, consciousness and nirvana in early Buddhism*. Richmond: Curzon.
Harvey, P. (2013). *An introduction to Buddhism: Teachings, history and practices* (2nd ed.). Cambridge: Cambridge University Press.
Kabat-Zinn, J. (1994). *Wherever you go, there you are: Mindfulness meditation for everyday life*. London: Piatkus.
Kabat-Zinn, J. (2011). Some reflections on the origins of MBSR, skillful means, and the trouble with maps. *Contemporary Buddhism, 12*(1), 281–306. (This issue of this journal later appeared as a book: Williams, M., & Kabat-Zinn, J. (2013). *Mindfulness: Diverse perspectives on its meaning, origins and applications*. London: Routledge.)
King, W. L. (1980). *Theravāda meditation: The Buddhist transformation of yoga*. University Park: Pennsylvania State University Press.
Kornfield, J. (1995). *Living Dharma: Teachings of twelve Buddhist masters*. Boston: Shambhala.
Kuan, T-f. (2008). *Mindfulness in early Buddhism: New approaches through psychology and textual analysis of Pali, Chinese and Sanskrit sources*. London: Routledge.
Nyanaponika, T. (1996). *The heart of Buddhist meditation: A handbook of mental training based on the Buddha's way of mindfulness*. Newburyport: Red Wheel/Weiser.
Nyanaponika, T. (1997). *The power of mindfulness: An inquiry into the scope of bare attention and the principal sources of its strength*. (Wheel booklet 121–122). Kandy: Buddhist Publication Society. (Access to Insight website: http://www.bps.lk/olib/wh/wh121.pdf)
Shaw, S. (2006). *Buddhist meditation: An anthology from the Pāli Canon*. London: Routledge.
Shaw, S. (2009). *Introduction to Buddhist meditation*. London: Routledge.
Soma, T. (1981). *The removal of distracting thoughts: Vitakka Santhana Sutta*. (Wheel booklet 21). Kandy: Buddhist Publication Society. (Access to Insight website: http://www.bps.lk/olib/wh/wh021.pdf). Accessed 1 Feb 2015.
Soma, T. (1998). *The way of mindfulness: The Satipaṭṭhāna Sutta and its commentary* (6th ed.). Kandy: Buddhist Publication Society. (Access to Insight website: http://www.accesstoinsight.org/lib/authors/soma/wayof.html). Accessed 1 Feb 2015.
Williams, P. (2009). *Mahāyāna Buddhism: The doctrinal foundations* (2nd ed.). London: Routledge.

Peter Harvey is emeritus Professor of Buddhist studies at the University of Sunderland, UK. His research focuses on early Buddhist thought and practices and Buddhist ethics. He edits *Buddhist Studies Review,* journal of the UK Association for Buddhist Studies, having founded the Association in 1995 with Ian Harris, and from 2002 to 2011 ran an online MA Buddhist Studies program. He is author of *An Introduction to Buddhism: Teachings, History and Practices* (University of Cambridge Press, 1990, 2nd edn., 2013), *The Selfless Mind: Personality, Consciousness and Nirvana in Early Buddhism* (Curzon Press, 1995), and An *Introduction to Buddhist Ethics: Foundations, Values and Practices* (University of Cambridge Press, 2000). He teaches mindfulness of breathing meditation according to the method of the Samatha Trust (http://www.samatha.org/).

Chapter 8
Mindfulness and the Six Perfections

Karma Lekshe Tsomo

8.1 Introduction

The Buddhist path to awakened awareness is a process of practicing the *pāramitās* (Pāli: *pāramī*). The term *pāramitās* is generally translated as "perfections," and also as *transcendental virtues* (Dayal 1932), *supreme virtues* (Edgerton 1970), and *particular ideals of human character that guide human behavior* (Wright 2011). The term is also understood to mean primary, surpassing, or most excellent. An etymology based on the Pali tradition defines *parami* as the culmination of one's moral cultivation.

The perfections also provide one of the few reliable ways of measuring the accomplishments of one's life. "Accomplishments" in the realm of work and relationships have a way of turning into dust, but perfections of the character, once developed, are dependable and lasting, carrying one over and beyond the vicissitudes of daily living. Thus, they deserve to take high priority in the way we plan our lives. These two facts are reflected in the two etymologies offered for the word perfection *(parami-):* They carry one across to the further shore *(param-)* and they are of foremost *(parama)* importance in formulating the purpose of one's life. (Thanissaro 2010).

The *pāramitās* are called perfections because it is through their practice that one perfects the cultivation of these supreme virtues. The ultimate achievement of the *pāramitās* is accomplished through mindfulness, compassion, and wisdom, without pride or self-concern. Extrapolating from the Tibetan etymological rendering (*pha rol tu phyin pa*, or "going beyond"), Willis (1979) defined the term as "transcendent action."

Right mindfulness *(sammā sati),* the seventh step of the Noble Eightfold Path, is the path of practice that leads to the cessation of suffering and dissatisfaction

K. L. Tsomo (✉)
Department of Theology and Religious Studies, University of San Diego,
Maher Hall 276, 5998 Alcalá Park, San Diego, CA 92110, USA
e-mail: tsomo@sandiego.edu

E. Shonin et al. (eds.), *Buddhist Foundations of Mindfulness*,
Mindfulness in Behavioral Health, DOI 10.1007/978-3-319-18591-0_8

(dukkha): right view, right thought/intention, right speech, right action, right livelihood, right effort, right mindfulness, and right concentration. Mindfulness *(sati)* is thus integral to the achievement of liberation from cyclic existence, or *nirvana*. Mindfulness is also integral to the practice of the six perfections and to the attainment of perfect awakening, or *samyak sambodhi*. The word "mindfulness" *(sati)* denotes a single-pointed awareness that helps ground one's attention totally in the present moment and thereby liberates one from habitual actions and responses. Nyanaponika (1973) understood *sati* to mean "bare attention," a clear and single-minded awareness that is "a purely receptive state of mind." He noted that *sati* frequently appears in conjunction with *sampajañña,* meaning clear comprehension and active observation.

Traditionally, the Four Foundations of Mindfulness are taught as a method of mental cultivation that includes mindfulness of four categories of objects: body, feelings, mind, and other phenomena (Silananda 2002). These four categories appear in a number of texts, for example, in the *Anapanasati Sutta*. Nyanaponika (1973) interpreted these four "instructions for practice" as contemplations, or objects of mindfulness: contemplation of the body, contemplation of feelings, contemplation of the mind, and contemplation of mind-objects. In the modern world, mindfulness is associated with increased awareness of physical, verbal, and mental actions.

8.2 The Path to Perfection

In 1978, when I was studying Buddhist philosophy and Tibetan language at the Library of Tibetan Works and Archives in Dharamsala, India, the well-known Tibetan physician Yeshi Dhonden explained the practice of medicine in terms of the six perfections (Dhonden 1986, 2000). He said that a physician practices all six perfections every day when treating patients and proceeded to describe each one. Generosity is a frame of mind of wishing to give health to each patient, including medicine, advice, and solace. Ethical discipline is avoiding harm, deceit, and other moral transgressions in one's practice of medicine. Patience is practiced by remaining calm and avoiding anger, no matter how stressful or aggravating the situations one must face. Joyful effort is applying oneself diligently to relieving the ailments and sufferings of the patients. Concentration is giving one's complete, undivided attention to each patient and each prescription. Wisdom is understanding the patients' physical, psychological, and spiritual needs. By implementing the six perfections in one's medical practice, a physician is practicing on the *bodhisattva* path and progressing on the path to perfect awakening.

The many different schools of Buddhist philosophy and practice that developed over 2500 years in India and in countries throughout Asia are generally subsumed into two major branches: Theravāda and Mahāyāna. As Samuels (1997) pointed out, the usefulness of these categories may be questioned, as they oversimplify certain distinctions, including variant soteriologies and the nature of the *bodhisattva* ideal.

Nevertheless, for our discussion of the six perfections, it is convenient and necessary to give an overview of these two branches.

The Theravāda ("path of the elders") school flourishes today in Sri Lanka and Southeast Asia. It is based on the Pali Buddhist canon, or *tripitaka* ("three baskets") canon consisting of three divisions: *vinaya* (monastic discipline), *sūtra* (discourses of the Buddha), and *abhidharma* (higher knowledge, or commentarial literature). Theravāda is often referred to as the earliest school of Buddhism, though in fact it is one of some 18 early schools of the śrāvakayāna (vehicle of the hearers or learners) and is the only one of the 18 to survive until today. The goal of these schools is to attain liberation from all destructive emotions or mental defilements, especially greed, hatred, and ignorance—a state of mind known as nirvāna. To be liberated also means that one becomes free from *duhkha* (suffering and dissatisfaction) and from *samsara* (cyclic existence entailing repeated birth, death, and rebirth). A person who becomes liberated in this way, by purifying the mind of defilements, is an *arhat* ("foe destroyer"). An *arhat* generally continues a life of virtue and meditation, sharing the teachings until reaching the end of his or her life. What the *arhat* experiences after death is one of the questions the Buddha pointedly did not answer.

The Mahāyāna schools are based on a canon that includes both the earlier Buddhist literature and the *prajñāpāramitā* ("perfection of wisdom") literature that began to appear in India during the early centuries CE. Based on this literature, a variety of Buddhist schools developed in India and subsequently throughout central and East Asia, where they flourish until today. Practitioners of these schools aspire to achieve the perfect awakening of a Buddha. They set out to accomplish this by practicing the path of the *bodhisattva.* Three prerequisites are required for entering the *bodhisattva* path: renunciation of cyclic existence; *bodhicitta,* the altruistic aspiration to become a perfectly awakened Buddha in order to liberate all sentient beings from suffering; and direct insight into emptiness *(sunyata)*.

The attainment of perfect awakening does not come easily, however; to achieve this noble goal, extensive practice over immense expanses of time is required. Liberation from cyclic existence *(samsāra)* may be attained (hypothetically at least, assuming an immense accumulation of merit from past lives) in just one or two lifetimes; the attainment of the perfectly awakened state of a Buddha, on the other hand, is said to require three incalculable aeons of the accumulation of merit and wisdom. To follow this path, one first becomes a *bodhisattva,* "a being of awakening." Out of great compassion, the *bodhisattva* resolves to achieve the perfectly awakened state of a Buddha, rather than the more easily attainable state of *nirvana,* in order to liberate all sentient beings from suffering. It is not the case, as repeatedly claimed, that the *bodhisattva* postpones liberation indefinitely, for the obvious reason that, if all *bodhisattva*s postponed their own liberation until all sentient beings achieved liberation, none of them would become liberated. Some *bodhisattvas,* "like a shepherd," guide other sentient beings ahead to liberation; some, "like a king," attain liberation ahead of the citizenry; and others, "like a person who rows a boat," attain liberation together with their passengers. In any case, the determination to liberate infinite sentient beings is a serious commitment that will require a great deal of time.

8.3 Perfection by Numbers

Sets of six perfections are found in the texts of both branches: generosity, ethical conduct, patience, joyful effort, concentration, and wisdom. Sets of ten perfections are also found in the texts of both branches, but the four additional perfections vary. Both the sets of six and the sets of ten are regarded as practices that are essential for achieving the perfect awakening of a Buddha. A variety of Buddhist paths were set forth, for beings of different capacities and inclinations, even from earliest times, and different interpretations resulted in a variety of texts and formulations of the perfections and other teachings.

In the early centuries after the Buddha's passing away, as Buddhism became a popular religion, the idea was formalized that there were three paths to awakening to choose from: the path to awakening as a disciple of a Buddha *(sāvaka);* the path to awakening as a solitary Buddha *(pacceka-buddha),* that is, one who attained awakening on his own, but was not able to teach the path of practice to others; and the path to awakening as a rightly self-awakened Buddha (sammā *sambuddha).* Each path was defined as consisting of perfections *(paramī)* of character, but there was a question as to what those perfections were and how the paths differed from one another. The Theravādins, for instance, specified ten perfections, and organized their Jataka collection so that it culminated in ten tales, each illustrating one of the perfections. The Sarvāstivādins, on the other hand, specified six perfections, and organized their Jataka collection accordingly (Thanissaro 2010).

The ten perfections listed in the Theravāda texts in Pāli are: generosity *(dāna),* ethics *(sīla),* renunciation *(nekkhamma),* wisdom *(paññā),* energy or effort *(viriya),* patience *(khanti),* truthfulness *(sacca),* determination (*adhitthāna*) loving kindness *(mettā),* and equanimity *(upekkhā)*. The practice of these virtues is expressed as aspirations:

1. May I be generous and helpful! (Generosity)
2. May I be well-disciplined and refined in manners! May I be pure and clean in all my dealings! May my thoughts, words and deeds be pure! (Ethics)
3. May I not be selfish and self-possessive but selfless and disinterested! May I be able to sacrifice my pleasure for the sake of others! (Renunciation)
4. May I be wise and be able to see things as they truly are! May I see the light of Truth and lead others from darkness to light! May I be enlightened and be able to enlighten others! May I be able to give the benefit of my knowledge to others! (Wisdom)
5. May I be energetic, vigorous and persevering! May I strive diligently until I achieve my goal! May I be fearless in facing dangers and courageously surmount all obstacles! May I be able to serve others to the best of my ability! (Energy)
6. May I be ever patient! May I be able to bear and forbear the wrongs of others! May I ever be tolerant and see the good and beautiful in all! (Patience)
7. May I ever be truthful and honest! May I not hide the truth to be polite! May I never swerve from the path of Truth! (Truthfulness)

8. May I be firm and resolute and have an iron will! May I be soft as a flower and firm as a rock! May I ever be high-principled! (Determination)
9. May I ever be kind, friendly and compassionate! May I be able to regard all as my brothers and sisters and be one with all! (Loving kindness)
10. May I ever be calm, serene, unruffled and peaceful! May I gain a balanced mind! May I have perfect equanimity! (Equanimity; Narada 1982, p. 29).

The ten perfections listed in the Mahāyāna tradition in Sanskrit are: generosity *(dāna),* moral virtue *(śīla),* patience *(kṣānti),* effort *(vīrya),* meditation *(dhyāna),* wisdom *(prajñā),* skillful means *(upāya),* aspiration *(praṇidhāna),* power *(bala),* and knowledge *(jñāna)*. Mahāyāna texts explain the ten perfections as the practices of a *bodhisattva,* one who has generated the altruistic aspiration to become a Buddha in order to liberate all living creatures from suffering. These ten perfections are the qualities that a *bodhisattva* cultivates while traversing the ten stages *(bhūmis)* on the path to perfect awakening. In order to become a fully awakened being, a *bodhisattva* must accumulate enormous quantities of both merit and wisdom. This is not the instantaneous enlightenment made famous by Buddhist legends and hagiographies, but a painstaking process that reportedly requires three countless aeons *(kalpas)* to accomplish.

Mahāyāna texts and traditions also speak of the six perfections (Conze 1967; Dayal 1932; Powers 1995b; Rinchen 1998; Sopa and Patt 2005). The Sanskrit scholar Dayal (1932, p. 168) is of the opinion that the shorter list of six "evolved after a process of selection and experimentation." He contended that a list of five perfections existed at one time, but gradually the list of six became the most common formulation and has subsequently assumed a central role in Mahāyāna philosophy and practice. In his commentary on the Tsongkhapa's *Lamrim Chenmo* (graduated path to enlightenment), Geshe Lhundub Sopa and Patt (2005, pp. 178–79) described the six perfections as "the core of the Mahāyāna path." Further, he explained:

> The first four of these perfections (*pāramitā*) are the cause for attaining a Buddha's *rūpakāya*, or *body of form*. The first is the perfection of giving, which becomes the cause of attaining the unlimited resources of the Buddha-field. The second is the perfection of ethical conduct, which becomes the cause of the Buddha's perfect body. The third, the perfection of patience, become the cause of the Buddha's perfect retinue. The fourth perfection is persevering effort, which becomes the cause of a Buddha's perfect activity; this means that Buddha's act spontaneously in the most meaningful way, and whatever activity a Buddha undertakes is brought to the best possible completion. (The last two perfections, concentration and wisdom, result in the *dharmakāya* or *truth body* of a Buddha, whose nature is perfect knowledge, or omniscience, and freedom from all obscurations.)

In the *Samdhinirmocana-nāma-mahāyāna-sūtra,* the Buddha explained the six perfections in a variant way: "Avalokiteśvara, know that the first three are trainings in surpassing ethics. Concentration is a training in surpassing mind. Wisdom is a training in surpassing wisdom. I explain that effort is omnipresent." (Powers 1995b, p. 237). When Avalokiteśvara asked which of these "six bases of training" can be categorized, whether as the accumulation of merit or as the accumulation of wisdom, the Buddha replied, "Avalokiteśvara, training in surpassing ethics belongs to the accumulation of merit. Training in surpassing wisdom belongs to the accumulation of wisdom. I explain that effort and concentration are omnipresent." (Powers 1995b, pp. 237–239).

The practice of the six perfections not only constitutes the core of the *bodhisattva*'s path to perfect awakening but is also said to yield tangible results, for example, freedom from birth in unfortunate states of existence. From another perspective, however, the results of these core practices may not be easily measurable. The current trend toward classification, quantification, and analytical evaluation of the results of contemplative practices is worthy of note and interrogation (Mind and Life Education Research Network 2012). Studies of the effects of meditative practices that contribute to greater powers of concentration, reduced stress, and so forth are useful for documenting the measurable results of cultivating mindfulness, but in terms of mental cultivation and personal transformation, the results of contemplative practices are not so easy to categorize and quantify (Roth 2008).

Two important factors need to be kept in mind in the exploration of mindfulness and the six perfections. The first is mindfulness of one's motivation and the second is mindfulness of the goal of one's practice. From the perspective of motivation, one may practice mindfulness for the benefit of oneself or for the good of humanity, for the benefit of this life or for the benefit of future lives. From the perspective of one's goal, one may practice mindfulness in order to become a more effective businessperson, mother, soldier, or spiritual adept. From a Buddhist perspective, to practice for the benefit of this life is not considered a spiritual goal, to practice for the benefit of achieving a fortunate rebirth is an inferior goal, whereas to practice toward the goal of achieving liberation or perfect awakening is a superior goal.

8.4 The Perfection of Generosity

The first of the six perfections is *dāna,* which denotes "generosity" or "giving." The term has also been translated as "liberality," "charity," and "munificence" (Dayal 1932, p. 172). This practice is paramount in all schools of Buddhism and takes on central importance in the Mahāyāna tradition, where it is a defining characteristic of the *bodhisattva*. The practice of *dāna* is a means to develop freedom from attachment (to possessions, body, and life). The three types of generosity are giving (1) material goods, (2) Dharma teachings, and (3) protection from fear. The giving of material goods serves many purposes. The example that Tibetan masters commonly use is offering someone a cup of tea. In Buddhist cultures, offering a cup of tea is symbolic of friendliness, which is a virtuous attitude. Although a cup of tea is not very expensive, it provides warmth and comfort and expresses loving kindness to loved ones and strangers alike. If someone is hungry, we can offer a bite to eat to ease their discomfort. If a person is cold, we can offer warm clothes or shelter. If a student is poor, we can offer books or writing materials. These small gifts help to create an atmosphere of caring and demonstrate the values of loving kindness and compassion. When a person is hungry or cold, it is difficult to focus on spiritual teachings or abstract ideas. People with fundamental problems or requirements for daily survival need these resolved before they can realistically be interested by philosophical wisdom. Offering some small material thing to fulfill that need can set the person's mind at rest and create space for the person to open up to spiritual knowledge.

No matter how many material possessions a person may have, however, there is no substitute for the Dharma. When the time of death approaches, all the material wealth in the world will not be able to prevent the inevitable end. The same reasoning applies to loved ones. When the time of death arrives, neither friends, relatives, nor other loved ones, including our beloved teachers, can do anything to stave off the inevitability of death. In the transition from this life to the next, only our merit and mental cultivation will be of any use whatsoever. Attachment to our material possessions and loved ones may even act as an obstacle in effecting a smooth transition to whatever comes after death. Mindfulness of death and impermanence is realistic and a wise way to live. It helps to prevent us from stockpiling possessions, from frittering away time on unessential activities, and from living a superficial life; instead, mindfulness of death channels our attention and energy toward the cultivation of virtues such as generosity, thereby accumulating wholesome attitudes and actions that help propel us on the path to liberation. Based on an awareness of death and impermanence, many Buddhist practitioners live a simple life and make a conscientious effort to donate time and resources to the less fortunate. Since material possessions will be useless at the time of death and our attachment to them an obstacle in the process of transitioning to whatever awaits us after death, Buddhists may decide to give away whatever valuables they have to monasteries, temples, renunciants, or the poor as they approach the moment of death. With a realization of the transitory nature of worldly possessions, a good practitioner will "walk lightly on the earth" and, free from entanglements, be more mindful of the beauty and potential for awakening that exist in every moment of life.

Generosity is an antidote to stinginess, greed, and attachment. It transforms self-concern into concern for others and prevents rebirth in the realm of hungry ghosts *(preta)*. As a result of being generous and giving, in future lives one will become prosperous and live in comfortable circumstances. Appearing first, both among the six perfections and the ten perfections, generosity is given pride of place among the virtues that a *bodhisattva* must practice on the way to awakening. The Vessantara Jataka tells the story of Buddha Sakyamuni in a past life as a *bodhisattva* was a prince named Vessantara who gave away his wife and children. This story has become an emblematic act of generosity (Jory 2002). Not only are generous people assured of a prosperous rebirth but they will also have wealth to donate to those who are in need (Conze 1973).

Generosity is such an important practice that merely the thought of giving is said to be good and to accrue merit. The practice of generosity is epitomized in the image of the monk or nun who goes for alms. By receiving alms, members of the monastic community *(sangha)* serve as a "field of merit," since each act of giving to a renunciant is akin to sowing virtuous seeds. The seeds that are sown through the practice of generosity, especially to monks and nuns, are said to give rise to future happiness and well-being, including material prosperity. In modern times, the fact that monks have culturally been regarded as somehow inherently more worthy of merit than nuns, despite Buddhist theoretically egalitarian ideals, has come under increased scrutiny (Falk 2008; Tsomo 2004).

The attitude of the giver is critical in the practice of generosity. The most excellent practice is to give unconditionally, without attachment and with no thought of reward, free from partiality. The Indian-Burmese meditation master S. N. Goenka used to say that if we expect something in exchange for our generosity, that is a business deal and not the pure practice of giving. If we hope or expect to receive some recognition or reward for our generosity, our motivation is not purely to benefit others, but is tainted by self-interest. The best practice of generosity is done with an attitude of loving-kindness and compassion: "May all beings be happy and free from suffering." Even if someone has nothing to give, it is possible to rejoice in another person's practice of generosity and the merit accumulated is said to be equivalent.

Although the perfections that are taught in the Theravāda and Mahāyāna traditions vary, the practice of giving *(dāna)* appears as the first perfection on every list. To perfect the practice of generosity is regarded as a primary virtue to be cultivated in working toward liberation or enlightenment. It is not difficult to understand why this is so. Every time we give something away, we divest ourselves of attachment. No matter how small the item may be, the practice of giving releases some reliance on that item or some deluded expectation that an external object can bring happiness. If we relinquish that item without attachment and without any expectation of recognition or reward, we affirm, however slightly or unconsciously, that happiness does not depend on external objects. Gradually, the practice of giving reinforces an awareness that well-being depends primarily on being content with what is available in the present moment. Mindfulness of the ultimately satisfactory nature of each present moment serves to balance and correct the constant neediness that causes an endless sense of dissatisfaction *(dukkha)* and therefore liberates the practitioner, moment to moment, from the dis-ease that attends dissatisfaction.

Training in the practice of generosity is a process. It is recommended that one begin small and develop one's capacity for giving gradually. In the beginning, one can practice giving small things and gradually expand the scope of one's generosity over time. For example, in the Tibetan cultural sphere, it is customary to offer water bowls on the altar. The offering of water is significant, because water is thought of as pure; therefore, one's offering of water is symbolically pure. The offering of water is symbolically pure in another way too. Because water is virtually free of cost, the giver has no attachment to the offering and can offer it freely, without regret. If one offers something of value and later generates regret, the effectiveness or merit of the action is eroded. The practice of generosity begins with the thought of wishing to give. In the Mahāyāna tradition, it is taught that one can accumulate merit by repeatedly making offerings mentally. In the Vajrayāna tradition, one practices generosity by preparing a *mandala* that represents all the most excellent things in the universe and presenting it to the guru, Buddhas, *bodhisattva*s, *arhat*s, and all accomplished beings.

The perfection of giving, coupled with mindfulness, would be the attentive awareness in the mind of the giver, the nature of the gift, and the well-being of the recipient.

In the later texts, the perfection of generosity, like the other nine perfections—virtue, renunciation, wisdom, energy, patience, truthfulness, determination, loving-kindness, and equanimity—is clearly classified into three levels and explained in more detail, namely, *Dana-parami, dānapāramī, dānaupapāramī,* and *dānaparamatthapāramī.* Generally, each level is classified by the things given: (i) the first level, *dāna-pāramī*—the gift of belongings, children, wife; (ii) the medium level, *dāna-upapāramī*—the gift of limbs; and (iii) the ultimate level, *dānaparamatthapāramī*—the gift of life (Sheravanichkul 2008).

Suh (2014, p. 138) discussed the ethics of performing acts of giving as portrayed in a particular *jataka* tale:

> A series of such dramatic bodily performances are found in the past-life stories (*jataka* tales) of the historical Shakyamuni Buddha that are used as narrative didactic techniques and, as Ranjini Obeyesekere puts it, lessons on "how to be good Buddhists." In one such previous lifetime, the Buddha was born as the bodhisattva Rūpāvatī (Beautiful Woman), a self-sacrificing woman who slices off her own breasts as a gift of food for a starving mother so that she won't devour her newborn son. Transforming herself into nourishment for the suffering mother, Rūpāvatī's act of compassion and gifting of herself signifies a profound understanding of the suffering of all sentient beings as well as the depth of her commitment to save others. Upon saving the poor mother from the act of murder and infanticide, Rūpāvatī's body is restored anew and she is predicted to full enlightenment in the future.

Over the course of Buddhist history, such tales as these have not simply remained portrayals of ethical ideals in literary tomes, but have conveyed ethical values that are to be put into practice in everyday life. Rūpāvatī's "gifting of herself" as an "act of compassion" itself raises ethical questions. The sacrifice of one's body may be interpreted literally or figuratively. As Suh (2014, p. 138) remarked,

> Such stories of the radical acts of somatic compassion performed by *bodhisattvas* indicate that bodies can indeed be used for positive ends in Buddhist traditions. Yet, must bodies always be sacrificed in the quest for salvation? Is there a way to imagine a somatic compassion that has far more to do with the gift of the living body through intimacy than with the giving away of one's body through self-sacrifice? Can such intimate expressions of compassion themselves be the grounds for enlightenment and spiritual maturation?

In the Tibetan tradition, there are two practices that epitomize the practice of generosity. The first is *chö* (*gcod,* also spelled *chod,* literally "cutting"), a meditation practice in which one visualizes offering one's body parts to satisfy the needs of sentient beings. In the visualization practice of *chö,* one perfects the virtue of generosity by donating one's own severed limbs and internal organs to hungry ghosts and spirits, accompanied by the rhythm of drums and lyrical chanting. *Chö* practice presages the physical dissolution that awaits all sentient beings at death and helps nurture both detachment and compassion for the needy (Tsomo 2006, p. 82).

The second is the custom of "sky burial," a method of disposing of a dead body by offering it to birds and wild animals (Powers 1995a). "This kind of sky burial is the most common mode of disposing of the dead in Tibet, since the frozen ground and the lack of trees make both burial and cremation impractical. The time for disposing of the body is chosen through divination, conducted either by a *lama* (lit., teacher, a religious specialist), or an astrologer who determines when the consciousness has left the body. The rite serves as a stark reminder of the impermanence and interconnectedness of all life and is regarded as a final act of generosity by close relatives on behalf of the deceased" (Tsomo 2006, p. 16).

Sentient beings, both human beings and other animals, are intimately attached to their bodies. Overcoming the attachment to the body is a major step in overcoming the notion of an independently existent self. In making the decision to donate parts of one's body, whether in a process of visualization, such as in *chö* practice, or in the process of deciding to donate one's entire body to wild birds and animals after death, one gradually severs attachment to the corporeal form and, by extension, attachment to the self. The practice of generosity thereby reinforces one's awareness of the non-corporeal dimensions of human experience and nurtures insight into the true nation of the self.

8.5 The Perfection of Ethical Conduct

The second of the six perfections is *śīla,* translated variously as "ethics," "ethical conduct," "morality," "moral conduct," and "virtue." The practice of *śīla* includes refraining from unwholesome actions, engaging in wholesome actions, and working for the welfare of sentient beings. Although certain ethical principles are basic to all Buddhist schools, over many centuries, a variety of interpretations have developed in the Theravāda, Mahāyāna, and subsequent Buddhist schools. Goodman (2009) provided a useful analysis of Buddhist ethics in relation and juxtaposition to virtue ethics, consequentialist ethics, and other theories. Buddhist theoretical analysis of bioethics, neuroethics, and other issues of contemporary relevance is still in the initial stages (Tsomo 2012).

The practice of ethics is said to be the foundation for all other practices, the legs without which one cannot proceed on the path. Through the practice of ethics, one avoids being reborn as an animal. The practice of ethics is said to result in a perfect body and good complexion. The practice of ethical conduct requires mindfulness, in the sense that attentive awareness is necessary to maintaining disciplined conduct. An unruly, unfocused mind will find it difficult to make well-considered decisions in ethically challenged situations. At the same time, the practice of ethical conduct fosters mindfulness, in that maintaining specific ethical guidelines helps to focus one's concentration in the present moment. The practice of mindful awareness is therefore critical to maintaining one's practice of moral conduct.

The Buddha delivered teachings to audiences from a variety of different social and religious backgrounds for four and a half decades. Consequently, it is not surprising that the ethical injunctions that infuse the Buddha's teachings are framed differently for different audiences. Chronologically, the first formulation seems to have been the Noble Eightfold Path, which was taught in the context of the Four

Noble Truths that were expounded in the Deer Park (Sarnath) soon after the Buddha's awakening. According to tradition, after sharing his realization that life is beset by *dukkha* (suffering and dissatisfaction), he explained the cause of *dukkha* and the possibility of ending *dukkha,* which is achieved by following eight measures that will lead to that goal: right view, right intention, right speech, right action, right effort, right livelihood, right mindfulness, and right concentration. These well-known injunctions provide guidelines for actions of body, speech, and mind. These guidelines are categorized in terms of the three trainings in ethical conduct, concentration, and wisdom. Right speech, action, and livelihood are explained as pertaining to ethical conduct. Right effort, mindfulness, and concentration are explained as pertaining to right concentration. Right view and intention are explained as pertaining to right wisdom.

Another way in which the perfection of ethical conduct is explained is by means of precepts. There are several formulations of precepts, depending on one's status in society; for example, the 5 precepts of a layperson, the 10 precepts of a novice monk or nun, the more than 200 precepts of a fully ordained monk, and the more than 300 precepts of a fully ordained nun. A householder who has taken refuge in the Three Jewels (Buddha, Dharma, and Sangha) may undertake to live by the five precepts of a Buddhist layman or laywoman (*upāsaka* or *upāsikā*): to refrain from taking the life of a human being (murder), taking what is not given (stealing), sexual misconduct, false speech, and intoxicants. A person who wishes to renounce the household life may undertake to live by the precepts of a novice monk or nun. The first five of these precepts are the same as those of the Buddhist layperson, except that the precept to refrain from sexual misconduct is to refrain from sexual conduct altogether, plus five more precepts: to refrain from ornaments, entertainments, high seats or beds, untimely food, and handling silver or gold. After living by the 10 precepts for some time, a novice monk or nun who has reached the age of 20 may undertake to live by the more than 200 precepts for a fully ordained monk *(bhikṣu)* or the more than 300 precepts for a fully ordained nun *(bhikṣuṇī)*. The precepts for ordained monastics are included in the *pratimoks.a,* the code of monastic discipline found in the *vinaya* section of the Buddhist canon. The most serious transgressions are the four *pārajika*s ("defeats"), which entail expulsion from the *sangha*, the monastic community: sexual activity, taking the life of a human being, taking what is not given, and false speech.

Whether a person undertakes the lay, novice, or full monastic precepts, it is clear that these rules of training are an aid in the development of mindfulness and an understanding that mindfulness is essential for maintaining the precepts purely. The full component of monastic precepts regulates three areas of life: moral decision-making (e.g., to refrain from taking life), interactions with the monastic community (e.g., to refrain from removing another monastic's sleeping mat and replacing it with one's own), and interactions with the lay community, or proper deportment (e.g., to refrain from talking with a mouth full of food). To regulate the actions of one's body, speech, and mind, the practice of mindfulness is essential. Conversely, by undertaking to live by a set of precepts, one is fostering the practice of mindfulness.

Ultimately, the practice of precepts is conducive to avoiding suffering for both oneself and others. This is most obvious in the first precept for laypeople, which is to abstain from taking the life of a human being. This precept can be interpreted more broadly to avoid any sort of harm or injury to any living creature. In his Fourteen Wonderful Precepts, the Vietnamese monk, poet, and peace activist Thich Nhat Hanh extends the first precept beyond simply not killing to the protection of all life and to the protection of the whole planet. He frames this as the first mindfulness training:

> Aware of the suffering caused by the destruction of life, I am committed to cultivating compassion and learning ways to protect the lives of people, animals, plants, and minerals. I am determined not to kill, not to let others kill, and not to support any act of killing in the world, in my thinking, and in my ways of life. (Hanh 1993, pp. 13–19).

He links compassion not only with feeling but also with action in the world, and emphasizes the importance of mindfulness in countering our tendency to forgetfulness and the destructive emotions that often divert us from living mindfully and joyfully.

Another formulation of ethical conduct taught by the Buddha is the ten unwholesome actions: three of body, four of speech, and three of mind. The three actions of body are taking life, taking what is not given, and sexual misconduct. The four actions of speech are lying, harsh speech, divisive speech, and idle gossip. The three actions of mind are covetousness, ill will, and wrong views. Refraining from these unwholesome actions results in greater happiness and contentment in this life and rebirth in a higher state of rebirth, hopefully a human rebirth, in future lifetimes.

Chappell (1996) pointed out that, although academic discussions of Buddhist ethics have focused largely on Theravāda texts, numerous lists of moral regulations are found in some 200 Chinese Mahāyāna texts, most of which have yet to be translated. Based on the work of Hōdō Ono, he observed that there are many overlapping categories of precepts in the Theravāda and Mahāyāna texts (Ono 1954). He wisely warned, however, that "a distinction must be made between a list of moral rules and the framework of interpretation that provides their meaning and that guides practitioners in handling conflicting values" and noted that the Chinese Mahāyāna texts may represent different worldviews (e.g., Pure Land, Yogacāra, and Huayen) and variant ethical frameworks (Chappell 1996).

One may also take compassion as an ethical framework. For example, in considering the ethical treatment of animals, no harm is clearly a guiding principle, based on compassion for the suffering of all sentient beings. In this connection, mindfulness is essential to the practice of compassion, in several respects. First, it is vital to be mindful of the fact that living creatures have feelings and hence are capable of feeling pain and suffering. Second, it is important to be mindful that sentient life is precious, has a limited lifespan, and is liable to destruction. Third, it is important to be mindful that all living beings have the potential to achieve the fruits of the path—liberation as the goal of the *sravakayana* path and full awakening as the goal of the *bodhisattva* path. In either case, an awareness that each sentient being is equally vulnerable to suffering and equally precious, from the perspective of that being's potential to reach the highest goals of the path, inclines one to act with compassion and to refrain from harming any living being, so far as possible.

8.6 The Perfection of Patience

The third of the six perfections is patience *(kṣānti)*, also translated as "forbearance," "endurance," and "tolerance." (Chandragomin 1985). To be patient means that one does not retaliate or respond with anger and enmity when someone reviles, abuses, or insults one. Instead of exacerbating tensions and conflicts, one acts to diffuse them. Instead of giving in to habitual tendencies to react with irritation or indignation, one is able to bear the indignation or slight. Through the practice of patience, one remains bright, is not lured by sense pleasures, and develops supernormal powers.

The perfection of patience is an antidote to anger and hatred, two emotions that are considered highly destructive from a Buddhist perspective. Not only do anger and hatred cause misery to oneself and others but they also are said to destroy one's roots of merit. Anger causes both physical and emotional responses that, if uncontrolled, can result in unwholesome actions, including violent acts. For this reason, Buddhists speak of understanding the root causes of our actions: the destructive emotions *(kleśas),* also known as emotional afflictions or poisonous delusions. Mindfulness is key to becoming aware of the destructive emotions—greed, hatred, ignorance, primarily, and pride, jealousy, fear, and so forth—and bringing them under control, before they result in unwholesome actions. If one has trained sufficiently in the practice of patience, in conjunction with mindfulness, then it will be possible to calm or transform these destructive emotions as soon as they begin to arise and before they lead to destructive or nonvirtuous acts. If we are able to recognize unwholesome mental states as they arise, we can consciously transform them and bring the mind under control before the destructive emotions take control over us and lead to malevolent actions or misdeeds and their unfortunate results. By training conscientiously, we can learn to recalibrate our responses to unpleasant experiences. We can learn to control our reactions to perceived threats and insults and thereby avoid averse and inappropriate responses.

Mindfulness entails gaining control over one's mind, both when things are going well and also when things do not go our way. People, like other animals, do not find it difficult to be patient and pleasant when everything goes their way. The difficult matter is learning to be patient when things are not going our way. The true test of one's practice of mindfulness is to be able to refrain from reacting in inappropriate ways in circumstances that are unpleasant, aggravating, or difficult.

8.7 The Perfection of Joyful Effort

The fourth of the six perfections is joyful effort *(vīrya),* also translated as "vigor," "energy," (Dayal 1932; Wright 2011) and "zeal." The word *vīrya* might also be translated as "ardor," the adverbial form of which the Buddha used to describe the practice of the Four Foundations of Mindfulness:

> What are the four? Herein [in this teaching], bhikkhus, a bhikkhu dwells contemplating the body in the body, ardently, clearly comprehending and mindful, removing covetousness and grief in the world ….
> He dwells contemplating the feeling in the feelings, ardently, clearly comprehending and mindful, removing covetousness and grief in the world ….
> He dwells contemplating the consciousness in the consciousness, ardently, clearly comprehending and mindful, removing covetousness and grief in the world ….
> He dwells contemplating the dharmas in the dharmas, ardently, clearly comprehending and mindful, removing covetousness and grief in the world. (Silananda 2002, pp. 10–15)

The type of effort required to develop clear comprehension and eliminate all covetousness and suffering is not only clear and mindful but also skillful, energetic, and persistent.

The perfection of joyful effort serves as an antidote to laziness. The perfection of effort is exceedingly important, considering that real progress on the path to liberation or awakening is possible almost exclusively in the form of a human being and the fact that a human lifetime is both brief and fragile. Under the circumstances, one must put aside the things of this world and invest one's energy wholeheartedly in the path.

8.8 The Perfection of Concentration

The fifth of the six perfections is concentration *(samādhi),* also translated as single-pointed concentration. The perfection of concentration involves developing single pointedness of mind. The term *samādhi* is also sometimes translated as "meditation" (Wright 2011), although the term *dhyāna* is more accurate as a generic term for meditation. As a specialized term, *dhyāna* also refers to the four states of mental absorption: (1) detachment from desires, (2) single-pointedness, (3) mindfulness and equanimity, and (4) pure mindfulness and complete equanimity.

Learning to concentrate means learning to bring the mind under control and mindfulness is key to this process. As Conze (1967, p. 52) noted, "Etymologically 'mindfulness' *(smṛ-ti)* is derived from the root for 'to remember'"; hence the practice of mindfulness is a process of remembering to bring our attention back to the present moment, which "prevents ideas from 'floating away'." The perfection of concentration has many practical and spiritual benefits, which for Buddhists translates to mental cultivation. By being fully concentrated in the moment, the practitioner is able to recognize unwholesome mental states as they arise and avoid acting on them. Single-pointed concentration is said to be the foundation of all higher practices, since without firm concentration it is impossible to steady the mind. If "the wild monkey of the mind" is allowed to jump here and there, it will be impossible to focus even on a simple object, such as the inflow and outflow of one's breathing, much less the complicated visualizations and other advanced meditation practices that are a staple of the Vajrayāna tradition.

The practice of *shamathā* (tranquility or calm abiding meditation) is a method for developing *samādhi.* This method involves placing one's attention on a particular object repeatedly and for continually longer periods of time. By placing the mind again and again on the object, utilizing mindfulness and alertness, and lengthening the duration of one's attention on the object, one gradually develops single-pointed concentration *(samādhi)*. When one has achieved *samādhi,* it is said that one is able to focus the mind with full attention on a given object for up to 20 minutes at a stretch. Once one has achieved *samādhi* and is able to focus on the object for 20 minutes without any distractions, it is said that one is able to place the mind on the object indefinitely, without any wavering or mental distractions and without sloth and torpor. In this way, the practice of *shamathā* serves as an antidote to mental agitation and dullness and thereby facilitates the achievement of *samādhi,* single-pointed concentration.

Many different methods are used for developing *samādhi*. For example, in the Soto Zen tradition, there is a practice of "just sitting" *(shikantaza)*—a method of cultivating awareness through which one gains direct insight into the true nature of things. In the Rinzai tradition, one may focus on a *koan* as a method to spark direct insight. In the Vajrayāna tradition, there is a practice of "deity yoga"—visualizing oneself as an enlightened being as a means to achieve awakening. In this practice, one uses a "meditational deity" *(yidam)*—a particular Buddha or *bodhisattva*—as the object or focus of one's meditation practice. Initially, one visualizes the *yidam* in front of oneself, then gradually, after receiving an empowerment *(wang)* from a qualified master, one is initiated into a practice that involves merging with the *yidam* and ultimately embodying all the enlightened qualities of that Buddha or *bodhisattva.*

8.9 The Perfection of Wisdom

The sixth of the six perfections is wisdom *(prajñā)*. In the Buddhist traditions, wisdom *(prajñā)* denotes understanding, especially understanding regarding the path that leads to liberation. Through the cultivation of wisdom, one comes to understand the true nature of phenomena. The benefit of training in wisdom is that, by understanding the true nature of things, one is able to cut through the distortions that ordinarily cloud one's perceptions, such as greed, attachment, jealousy, pride, and so forth. The problem with distorted perceptions is that they may cause one to react in inappropriate or unwholesome ways, resulting in unpleasant consequences, for oneself and others. The cultivation of wisdom gradually enables one to perceive things more accurately, undistorted by ignorance and other destructive emotions *(kleśas)*. Perceiving things more accurately enables one to avoid reacting in inappropriate or unwholesome ways and helps one avoid the unpleasant consequences of unwholesome actions. The conscious application of wise and mindful attention is beneficial both karmicly and in the present moment, allowing one to perceive and appreciate objects and experiences without the disruption of distorted perceptions and destructive emotion, and ultimately. Conscious and mindful attention thus enables one to enjoy a more pleasant and trouble-free life now, in the present and also, from a Buddhist perspective, avoids unpleasant states of existence in the future.

In the view of most Buddhist schools, consciousness is defined as "knowing and awareness"; being conscious of an object is simply being aware of it. There is no need for a separate perceiving consciousness. To be conscious of an object is to perceive it, either with one of the five sense faculties or with the mental faculty. When one of the five sense faculties—the eye, ear, nose, tongue, or body faculties *(indriya)*—comes in contact with its appropriate object—a sight, sound, smell, taste, or touch—this results in a moment of conscious awareness—visual, auditory, olfactory, gustatory, or tactile, respectively. In the case of mental perception, similarly, when the mental faculty comes in contact with its appropriate object—for example, an image, memory, or idea—this results in a moment of conscious mental awareness. Once sense perceptions are conveyed to the mental faculty for processing, to be labeled and evaluated, as is habitual for human beings, these perceptions then become objects of mental awareness. To perceive an object with mindfulness means to be aware of this process, at least intellectually, in broad strokes. Because the initial experience of pure perception lasts only for a moment and the process of transmitting the data gathered through the sense faculties to the mental faculty occurs very rapidly, to develop an awareness of perceptions from moment to moment requires extensive training in mindfulness.

Philosophically speaking, wisdom is an understanding of the nature of phenomena. To understand things "as they are" refers to insight into the three characteristics of existence: distress and dissatisfaction *(duḥkha),* change and impermanence *(anitya),* and the lack of substantial existence or no-self *(anātman)*. This understanding is cultivated through meditation, using the body, feelings, consciousness, and other phenomena as the objects of awareness. An understanding of the nature of phenomena acts as an antidote to stupidity, foolishness, and ignorance. To practice the perfection of wisdom thus helps cut through mental defilements such as greed, hatred, pride, jealousy, and so forth.

In the Mahāyāna Buddhist schools, wisdom further denotes direct insight into emptiness *(śunyatā)*. This is the ultimate wisdom that directly understands the nature of phenomena as being empty of independent or true existence. This understanding is cultivated through meditation: first, through an intellectual process of analyzing a phenomenon to discover its true nature; and second, by focusing directly and single pointedly on the emptiness of that phenomenon. These two stages—intellectual analysis and single-pointed awareness—are practiced alternately until direct insight into emptiness arises.

For exalted beings directly perceiving reality, no difference is experienced between the subjective awareness apprehending emptiness and the emptiness which is apprehended. The analogy which is used to describe the experience is of water poured into water. Ordinary people apprehend emptiness by way of a mental image, and the apprehending awareness and what is apprehended are experienced as different (Rinchen 1998). This explanation of the wisdom understanding emptiness, given by the Tibetan scholar monk Geshe Sonam Rinchen in response to inquiries regarding the nature of the awareness that perceives emptiness, refutes the notion that there is a separate consciousness that is capable of perceiving consciousness.

Wisdom can be coupled with all the other perfections. For example, in the Mahāyāna tradition, there is a practice of understanding the "three circles of giving." In this practice, through meditation, one focuses on the empty nature of "the three circles": the giver, the gift, and the action itself. In the same way that the giver lacks independent existence, both the gift and the action itself are naturally devoid of true or independent existence.

According to the *Prajñāpāramitā Ratnaguṇasaṁcayagāthā,* wisdom is said to be supreme—foremost among the perfections—and integral to the first five:

> Just so do the five perfections of the *jina*s
> Have their name from the perfection of wisdom:
> When they are being turned over into all-knowledge,
> The name of enlightenment provides one single principle for all the six of them. (Conze 1973, p. 18)

Wisdom guides one in the practice of the first five perfections:

> All the qualities of enlightenment [that are in] the five perfections,
> They all grow from the perfection of wisdom. (Conze 1973, p. 16)

From this, Conze concluded that the first five perfections naturally culminate in wisdom, the sixth perfection.

In the Buddhist traditions, one who is deficient in wisdom has no hope of achieving highest enlightenment. Without the wisdom to see the true nature of things, one will be left adrift, tossed here and there by mental defilements such as greed, ill will, and confusion. It is therefore incumbent on the practitioner to cultivate the perfection of wisdom with focused attention in order to see things "as they are," rather than seeing them falsely, obscured by misconceptions and false imaginations. By taming the mind and training it in pure awareness, the practitioner awakens from the slumber of ignorance and accomplishes the perfect wisdom of all the Buddhas.

8.10 Practicing the Perfections

The foregoing discussion has explained the practice of the six perfections and how they are thought to accelerate liberation and perfect awakening. The practice of generosity *(dāna)* loosens one's attachment to the illusion of self and opens one's heart to the needs of others. Ethical conduct *(śīla)* creates a strong foundation of discipline and pure conduct that facilitates mental cultivation and all higher practices. Patience *(kṣānti)* strengthens one's tolerance and the restraint required to refrain from anger and retaliation even in the face of aggression. Effort *(vīrya)* enables one to overcome laziness and generates the energy needed to wholeheartedly engage in practices of body, speech, and mind. Meditation *(dhyāna)* is the generic term that encompasses numerous analytical and contemplative practices for cultivating the mind. Wisdom *(prajñā)* is the insightful awareness that understands phenomena clearly and directly, without obscurations or error. With insight and mindful awareness, these perfections have been practiced by seekers of enlightenment in

Buddhist cultures for centuries, as guidelines to achieving human perfection. Although the Theravāda and Mahāyāna formulations of the ten perfections may differ, the practice of each of the perfections strongly depends on the application of mindful awareness. Beginning with mindfulness of breathing *(ānāpānasati),* now being practiced by young children, hospice patients, and ordinary people around the world, the training in mindfulness can be used to perfect the achievement of virtue and liberate beings from suffering.

References

Chandragomin. (1985). *Difficult beginnings: Three works on the Bodhisattva Path*. Boston: Shambhala.

Chappell, D. (1996). Are there seventeen Mahāyāna ethics? *Journal of Buddhist Ethics, 3,* 44–65.

Conze, E. (1967). *Buddhist thought in India: Three phases of Buddhist philosophy*. Ann Arbor: The University of Michigan Press.

Conze, E. (1973). *The perfection of wisdom*. Monroe: Subterreanean Company.

Dayal, H. (1932). *The Bodhisattva doctrine in Buddhist Sanskrit literature*. Delhi: Motilal Banarsidass.

Dhonden, Y. (1986). *Health through balance: An introduction to Tibetan medicine*. Ithaca: Snow Lion.

Dhonden, Y. (2000). *Healing from the source: The science and lore*. Ithaca: Snow Lion.

Edgerton, F. (1970). *Buddhist hybrid Sanskrit dictionary*. Delhi: Motilal Banarsidass.

Falk, M. L. (2008). *Making fields of merit: Buddhist female ascetics and gendered orders in Thailand*. Seattle: University of Washington Press.

Goodman, C. (2009). *Consequences of compassion: An interpretation and defense of Buddhist ethics*. New York: Oxford University Press.

Hanh, T. N. (1993). *For a future to be possible: Commentaries on the five mindfulness trainings*. Berkeley: Parallax Press.

Jory, P. (2002). The Vessantara Jataka, Barami, and the Bodhisatta-kings: The origin and spread of a Thai concept of power. *Crossroads: An Interdisciplinary Journal of Southeast Asian Studies, 16,* 36–78.

Mind and Life Education Research Network (MLERN), Davidson, R. J., Dunne, J., Eccles, J. S., Engle, A., Greenberg, M., Jennings, P., Jha, A., Jinpa, T., Lantieri, L., Meyer, D., Roeser, R. W., & Vago, D. (2012). Contemplative practices and mental training: Prospects for American education. *Child Development Perspectives, 6,* 146–153.

Narada, M. (1982). *Buddhism in a nutshell*. Colombo: Buddhist Publication Society.

Nyanaponika, T. (1973). *The heart of Buddhist meditation: Satipatthna: A handbook of mental training based on the Buddha's way of mindfulness*. Kandy: Buddhist Publication Society.

Ono, H. (1954). *Daijō kaikyō no kenkyū*. Tokyo: Risōsha.

Powers, J. (1995a). *Introduction to Tibetan Buddhism*. Ithaca: Snow Lion.

Powers, J. (1995b). *Wisdom of Buddha: The Samdhinirmocana Sūtra*. Berkeley: The Dharma Publishing Company.

Rinchen, G. S. (1998). *The six perfections*. Ithaca: Snow Lion.

Roth, H. (2008). Against cognitive imperialism: A call for a non-ethnocentric approach to cognitive science and religious studies. *Religion East & West, 8,* 1–26.

Samuels, J. (1997). The bodhisattva ideal in Theravāda Buddhist theory and practice: A reevaluation of the bodhisattva-sravaka opposition. *Philosophy East & West, 47,* 399–415.

Sheravanichkul, A. (2008). Self-sacrifice of the Bodhisatta in the *Paññasa Jataka. Religion Compass, 2,* 769–787.

Silananda, U. (2002). *The Four Foundations of Mindfulness*. Boston: Wisdom Publications.
Sopa, G. L., & Patt D. (2005). *Steps on the path to enlightenment: A commentary on Tsongkhapa's Lamrim Chenmo (Vol. 2)*. Boston: Wisdom Publications.
Suh, S. (2014). *Silver screen Buddha: Buddhism in Asian and Western film*. London: Bloomsbury.
Thanissaro, B. (2010). *The ten perfections: A study guide*. http://www.accesstoinsight.org/lib/study/perfections.html. Accessed 18 Dec 2014.
Tsomo, K. L. (2004). *Buddhist women and social justice: Ideals, challenges, and achievements*. Albany: State University of New York Press.
Tsomo, K. L. (2006). *Into the jaws of Yama, lord of death: Buddhism, bioethics, and death*. Albany: State University of New York Press.
Tsomo, K. L. (2012). Compassion, ethics, and neuroscience: Neuroethics through Buddhist eyes. *Journal of Science and Engineering Ethics, 35,* 46–53.
Willis, J. D. (1979). *On knowing reality: The Tattvārtha Chapter of Asanga's Bodhisattvabhūmi*. New York: Columbia University Press.
Wright, D. S. (2011). *The six perfections: Buddhism and the cultivation of character*. New York: Oxford University Press.

Karma Lekshe Tsomo is a professor of Buddhist studies in the Department of Theology and Religious Studies at the University of San Diego, where she teaches Buddhist thought and culture, world religions, comparative religious ethics, and death and afterlife. She studied Buddhist philosophy in Dharamsala for 15 years and received a doctorate in comparative philosophy from the University of Hawai'i at Mānoa in 2000. She is a founder of Sakyadhita International Association of Buddhist Women and the founder and director of Jamyang Foundation, an innovative education project for women in developing countries. Her current research interests include Buddhist women and social change in Russia and Southeast Asia, Buddhism and bioethics, and Buddhist transnationalism.

Chapter 9
Mindfulness of Emptiness and the Emptiness of Mindfulness

Edo Shonin, William Van Gordon, Nirbhay N. Singh and Mark D. Griffiths

9.1 Introduction

Emptiness (Pāli: *suññatā,* Sanskrit: *śūnyatā*) refers to the fundamental Buddhist teaching that all phenomena are devoid or "empty" of an intrinsic self. The empty property of phenomena in Buddhism relates as much to animate constructs such as a tree, a car, or the human body, as it does to inanimate constructs such as the mind, space, or the present moment. If a primary objective of mindfulness practitioners is to become increasingly aware of the present moment, then logic dictates that at some point they must begin to apprehend the true and absolute mode in which the present moment exists. Buddhism teaches that for as long as mindfulness practitioners objectify the present moment and believe that it inherently exists, they will be prevented from perceiving the absolute nature of reality and from actualizing their goal of enlightenment (Shonin and Van Gordon 2013a). The purpose of this chapter is to draw upon various Buddhist philosophical systems of investigating reality in order to explicate the essential meaning of emptiness and to discuss the various ways that emptiness and mindfulness cooperate in order to foster spiritual awakening.

E. Shonin (✉) · W. Van Gordon
Awake to Wisdom, Centre for Meditation and Mindfulness Research, Nottingham, UK;
Bodhayati School of Buddhism, Nottingham, UK
e-mail: e.shonin@awaketowisdom.co.uk

E. Shonin · W. Van Gordon · M. D. Griffiths
Division of Psychology, Nottingham Trent University, Chaucer Building, Burton Street, Nottingham, UK

N. N. Singh
Medical College of Georgia, Georgia Regents University, Augusta, GA, USA

E. Shonin et al. (eds.), *Buddhist Foundations of Mindfulness,*
Mindfulness in Behavioral Health, DOI 10.1007/978-3-319-18591-0_9

9.2 Understanding Emptiness

One of the problems with attempting to explicate the principles of emptiness is that as soon as it is conceptualized as an object or construct, there occurs a betrayal of the essential meaning of emptiness and of how the Buddha intended his followers to realize and embody this teaching. This certainly does not mean that reading or listening to discussions concerning emptiness are fruitless endeavours (if this were the case we would not have committed the time to writing this chapter), but readers are requested to bear in mind that the only way to truly comprehend emptiness is by using a theoretical exposition (such as the one provided within this chapter) as the raw material that must be tested and transformed into insight during their day-to-day and moment-to-moment practice of meditation.

In our opinion, emptiness is one of the most poorly understood Buddhist teachings, and attempts by scholars or Buddhist teachers to impart an understanding of emptiness can sometimes end up creating further obfuscation as well as overcomplicating what is in effect a common-sense notion. For example, in our capacity as Buddhist teachers, we often receive comments from individuals conveying the same sentiments as those expressed in the following feedback from perplexed and/or distressed academic colleagues subsequent to attending a meditation retreat: "Emptiness is a very scary place to be. If I do not exist then who am I and what have I been doing all of my life? I need to be certain and confident that I exist in order to move ahead". Such feedback is consistent with recommendations that emptiness (and related Buddhist concepts such as *selflessness*) should be taught with caution and skill as well as an understanding of the individual's clinical, cultural, educational, and spiritual background (Michalon 2001).

In essence, emptiness means that nothing exists as a discrete entity and in isolation of everything else. For example, a tree in the garden manifests in reliance upon numerous causes and conditions, without which, it would not exist. Amongst innumerable others, the causes and conditions to which we are referring include the water in the earth and atmosphere, nutrients in the soil, respiratory gases carried by the wind, heat of the sun, and so forth. Thus, at the simplest level, it can be said that *interconnectedness* is a fundamental principle of emptiness. Phenomena do not exist in isolation of each other, and by logical default they are empty of an independent and inherently existing self. However, for the same reasons that phenomena are empty of an intrinsic self, they also are "full" of everything else that exists. Therefore, in the context that we are discussing emptiness here, one could actually employ the term *fullness* as a substitution to the term *emptiness*. In emptiness there is fullness and vice versa (Shonin et al. 2013).

Investigating emptiness through the lens of interconnectedness is a perfectly adequate means of becoming familiar with emptiness, but other lines of reasoning can (and ideally should) be followed. Indeed, one of the limitations of relying on interconnectedness to internalize the principle of emptiness is that interconnectedness still implies that phenomena inherently exist (otherwise it would not be possible for them to be connected to each other). Therefore, although interconnectedness can help to facilitate a basic understanding of emptiness, it is nevertheless based on a dualistic manner of perceiving and constructing the world. In Buddhism, even the slightest tendency towards perceiving reality dualistically (i.e. in subject–object terms) is understood to cement an individual's belief in the inherent existence of phenomena and to constitute a deviation from the direct path to enlightenment (Dalai Lama 2004; Urgyen 2000).

Now that reference has been made to the importance of maintaining a *non-dual* outlook in order to both accurately apprehend and appreciate emptiness, it is timely to include a further cautionary note regarding the potential drawbacks of formulating conceptions about emptiness. As different philosophical positions regarding emptiness and the nature of mind and reality are presented, there is a risk of reifying the inherent existence and/or supremacy of a given philosophical position. We have previously argued that this process of reification becomes problematic because it tends to restrict an individual's understanding of emptiness to theory rather than experience (Shonin and Van Gordon 2013a; Shonin et al. 2014a). Indeed, any theoretical or philosophical construction of emptiness is presented according to the norms and laws of conceptual thinking, and it can never accurately portray the profound nature of emptiness that exists outside the confines of conceptuality. For example, rejecting the position of duality in order to accept the position of non-duality is effectively another example of rejecting one erroneous concept in order to replace it with another. Duality is empty of inherent existence, but the same is true for non-duality in addition to the middle position between these two opposites.

This was basically the underlying message of the Indian *Māhāyana* Buddhist philosopher and saint Nagarjuna (2nd c. AD) who is credited as giving birth to the *Mādhyamaka* school of Buddhist thought. At the surface level, Nagarjuna advocated a middle way between the extremes of *inherent existence* and *nihilism*. However, the crux of Nagarjuna's message was to reject all conceptual positions, including that of a middle way. The reason for this is because if the extremes of existence and nihilism are both rejected, then a "middle way" that exists between these two contrary positions becomes an untenable notion (Shonin et al. 2014a).

In addition to Nagarjuna's *Mādhyamaka* school of Buddhist thought, an alternative means of investigating and understanding emptiness is provided by the *Yogācāra* school of *Māhāyana* Buddhism. Perhaps the easiest and most effective means of understanding the *Yogācāra* school's construction of emptiness and reality is via the analogy of a dream. Various psychosomatic sleep-state symptoms including anxious arousal, shouting and/or screaming, increased respiratory amplitude, and perspiration are associated with bad dreams and nightmare disorder (Zadra and Donderi 2000). Therefore, although common sense (and common human experience) provides adequate grounds for inferring that a dream is completely empty of intrinsic existence and constitutes an ephemeral creation of the mind, it is reasonable to conclude that dreamt phenomena that manifest during sleep are apprehended as "real" and "existing" by the dreamer (Shonin et al. 2014a). The *Yogācāra* school asserts that waking state reality occurs in much the same manner as a dream and that it unfolds entirely within the expanse of the mind.

Some Buddhist scholars (past and present) have asserted that the *Mādhyamaka* and *Yogācāra Māhāyana* Buddhist schools explicate conflicting constructions of reality and emptiness (for an overview of the key opposing arguments, see Williams 2008). These assertions are primarily based on the belief that the *Yogācāra* school expounds the view that all phenomena are empty of intrinsic existence and are effectively "mind made", but that the mind itself does actually inherently exist. In our opinion, the assertion or belief that the *Yogācāra* view posits an inherently existing mind are based on a poor understanding of the *Yogācāra* philosophical system (or on the works of certain (so-called) *Yogācāra* theorists that had a poor understanding of their own ontological position), and thus constitute only a partial representation of the *Yogācāra* grounding principles. Accordingly, and consistent with the view of the eighth-century Indian Buddhist philosopher Śāntarakṣita, we recently demonstrated (in a light-hearted Zen-style dialogue between a teacher and student entitled *Dream or Reality*—see below) that when the concept-belying approach of *Mādhyamaka* is followed to its conclusion, there remains no alternative but to accept the validity of the *Yogācāra* position. As demonstrated in the *Dream or Reality* dialogue shown below (Shonin and Van Gordon 2014a), *Mādhyamaka* reasoning ultimately validates the *Yogācāra* position that it is impossible to draw distinctions between the absolute nature of a "mind-created dream" and that of everyday reality:

Student: Professor?
Professor: Yes?
Student: Pinch me.
Professor: What are you talking about?
Student: It's just that we've been testing the *Shared Dream Inducer* (SDI) so frequently I can't remember if I set the *Dream Terminator*.
Professor: I hope you're joking.
Student: No, seriously. I know you've told me so many times, but I just can't remember.
Professor: You mean…
Student: Yes—there's no way of knowing whether we're currently in a dream or in waking reality! If we're dreaming, the SDI could keep us here indefinitely!
Professor: Can't we remedy this situation?
Student: We could activate the SDI and try to enter a dream. If the interface allows us entry then at least we'll know whether we're awake or dreaming.
Professor: That's way too risky. If we *are* already dreaming we could get stuck in a nested dream.
Student: Okay, I have another idea. In a dream, everything is the product of the mind, right? Things appear real to the dreamer, yet everything is an illusion.
Professor: Agreed. What's your point?
Student: So all we have to do is choose some objects around us and work out if they really exist. If they're real then we're awake, otherwise we're dreaming.
Professor: Interesting idea. Here you are, you can start with my fountain pen.
Student: Well, the pen certainly writes when I press it against the paper. Yes, I think it's real. I think we're awake.

Professor: So your criteria for reality is based on the function that an object performs?

Student: Of course.

Professor: I see. Now take away all of the components of the pen, so that you're left with only the nib. Go ahead.... Does the nib still write?

Student: Yes, it still works.

Professor: But the nib isn't the pen?

Student: Ah, good point. It appears my original premise was wrong. Although it performs the function of the pen, the nib is just a single pen component, and not all the parts that comprise the pen. And one thing cannot be another thing.

Professor: So is the pen real?

Student: Well, having just taken the pen apart and seen that all of its components are present, I would still conclude that the pen is real. I still think we're awake.

Professor: So you're saying that the pen exists as the sum of its component parts?

Student: Yes, that's right.

Professor: I see. But you've already said that something can't be two things at once. Yet now you seem to be saying that when the nib, cartridge, lid, and other pen components are put together, they stop being those components and become a new single entity?

Student: No, that's illogical. The component parts still exist in the pen, but the word "pen" is used to designate the collection of individual components that together form that object.

Professor: Right, so you're saying that "pen" is just a label?

Student: Well I guess so.

Professor: But if "pen" is just a label then the pen doesn't inherently exist. So are you now saying that we're currently dreaming?

Student: I'm a bit confused. Irrespective of whether we're awake or dreaming, although things certainly appear to exist, there now seems no logical basis upon which to make that claim.

Professor: Therefore your idea of investigating whether or not things are real doesn't get us any closer to working out whether we're currently dreaming or awake. Have you got any better ideas?

Student: If we're currently shared-dreaming, it means the SDI is keeping our brain patterns in synchrony. We could try to disrupt them and wake ourselves up by inducing an electric shock.

Professor: If you want to stick your finger in the electric socket go right ahead, but I'm certainly not joining you.... Any *more* ideas?

Student: *Hmm*... Well I don't remember ever bursting into laughter during a dream. So why don't I tell you a joke, and if it makes you laugh, that means we're not dreaming?

Professor: I'm not convinced about that: I don't think it concurs with findings from oneirology, for a start. But go ahead and tell your joke.

Student: What did the professor who always gave examples say when asked how many eggs he'd like for breakfast?

Professor: I don't know.

Student: Four eggs ample.

Professor: I thought you were going to try to make me laugh.

Student: Very funny.

Professor: Well, if you haven't got any more ideas, I have a suggestion. Let's just do nothing.

Student: I don't understand.

Professor: I built a fail-safe into the SDI so that even if the DT isn't activated, the dream automatically terminates after eight hours.

Student: What?! Couldn't you have told me that five minutes ago?

Professor: Well, haven't you learnt something?

Student: You're right, I've actually learnt a lot. A dream occurs within the expanse of the mind, and in a dream, there's the impression of coming and going, yet nothing really moves. Whilst dreaming, there is also near and far, but there is actually no distance. In a dream, although things appear, they are illusory and cannot be said to truly exist. However, composite objects perceived by the waking mind are also devoid of intrinsic existence. Are you saying that waking reality also unfolds within the expanse of the mind?

Professor: You'll have to work that out for yourself.

Student: We still haven't determined whether we're currently dreaming or awake.

Professor: Does it really matter? Can't you just relax and enjoy each moment of whichever reality you're currently in?

Student: Yes, I think I can.

The principal reasons for including the above dialogue in this chapter are to: (i) demonstrate that *Mādhyamaka* and *Yogācāra* philosophical outlooks ultimately converge at the same point, and (ii) further one of this chapter's primary objectives which is to help readers (and ourselves as authors) augment their understanding of emptiness. However, the *Dream or Reality* dialogue was also included to show that the process of discussing and investigating emptiness need not always be undertaken in an overly solemn manner, or in explicitly academic contexts. Indeed, as with the majority of Buddhist teachings, adopting an overly analytical or overly academic approach to investigating emptiness invariably inhibits the use and development of spiritual intellect (i.e. as opposed to cognitive intellect), and thus prevents an accurate comprehension of emptiness from manifesting (Shonin and Van Gordon 2014b). Furthermore, in our opinion, emptiness can be a wondrous, joyful, and exciting notion and as much as the English translation of the Sanskrit term *śūnyatā* (i.e. emptiness) could provoke negative associations (e.g. voidness, nothingness, nihilism), it also (for the aforementioned reasons) implies fullness, complete liberation from suffering, and the unity of everything that exists.

In essence, this is the underlying message of the *Heart Sutra* (Sanskrit: *Prajna Paramita Hrdaya Sutra*), a key *Māhāyana* Buddhist teaching on emptiness. As demonstrated below in what is our own translation of the *Heart Sutra,* it is by immersing themselves in emptiness (referred to in the sutra as the *perfection of wisdom* [Sanskrit: *prajna paramita*]), that the bodhisattvas and all Buddhas of the past, present, and future are able to enter the realm of deathless abiding and permanently liberate themselves from suffering:

> The Bodhisattva Avalokitesvara,
> whilst immersed in the perfection of wisdom,
> perceived that the five aggregates are empty,
> and overcame all suffering and anguish.
> Listen Shariputra,
> form is identical to emptiness,
> and emptiness is identical to form.
> Form is of the nature of emptiness,
> and emptiness is of the nature of form.
> The same applies to feelings,
> perceptions, mental formations, and consciousness.
> Listen Shariputra,
> all phenomena are sealed with emptiness.
> They do not arise or dissolve,
> are neither impure nor pure,
> they neither increase nor decrease.
> Thus, in emptiness, there is no form, feelings,
> perceptions, mental formations, or consciousness.
> There are no eyes, ears, nose, tongue, body, or mind.
> No sight, sound, smell, taste, touch, or object of mind.
> No eye consciousness and so forth until no mind consciousness.
> There is no ignorance and no cessation of it,
> and so forth until no old age and death.
> However, there is also no cessation of old age and death.
> There is no suffering, no cause of suffering,
> no cessation of suffering, and no path.
> There is no insight and there is nothing to attain.
> The Bodhisattvas who immerse themselves,
> in the perfection of wisdom,
> overcome all mental obstacles,
> and therefore they overcome all fear.
> They are forever parted from deluded views,
> and thus awake to Nirvana.
> All Buddhas of the three times,
> attain unsurpassed perfect enlightenment,
> by immersing themselves in the perfection of wisdom.
> Therefore know that the perfection of wisdom is:
> the great transcendent mantra,
> the great bright mantra,
> the highest mantra,
> the unsurpassed mantra,
> and the truth that eradicates all suffering.
> Thus, the perfection of wisdom mantra should be proclaimed as follows:
> Gate, gate, paragate, parasamgate, bodhi svaha
> Gate, gate, paragate, parasamgate, bodhi svaha
> Gate, gate, paragate, parasamgate, bodhi svaha. (Translated from the Digital Sanskrit Buddhist Cannon 2014)

The claim in the *Heart Sutra* that "form is identical to emptiness and emptiness is identical to form" is a spiritually profound statement (Shonin et al. 2014a). In very clear terms, it explicates that emptiness is not a mystical state of mind or an alternative non-worldly dimension, but constitutes the very nature and fabric of the reality in which we currently find ourselves (i.e. the present moment). According to Buddhist thought, when an individual awakens to this fundamental truth—that has always been right in front of their eyes—they move beyond the concept of *this* and *that,* of *existence* and *nonexistence,* and they encounter their indestructible Buddha nature (Norbu and Clemente 1999).

9.3 Mindfulness of Emptiness

Mindfulness is the process of regulating concentration and ensuring that it remains intact and does not deviate from the object of meditative placement (Van Gordon et al. 2015a). In the context that mindfulness was taught by the historical Buddha, the object of meditative placement refers to whatever primary activity the spiritual practitioner happens to be engaged in at a given point in time (Nhat Hanh 1999). This could be walking, talking, eating, sleeping, defecating, concentrating on a specific meditative object (such as the breath), or (at the other end of the scale) concentrating on the present moment more generally. Therefore, in literal terms, *mindfulness of emptiness* simply means that when an experience of emptiness arises in the meditator's mind stream, they should utilize mindful awareness in order to ensure that concentration remains focused on emptiness and that recognition of the emptiness experience is prolonged for as long as possible. The type of mindfulness required to effectively prolong the experience of emptiness is one where the individual embraces and bathes in each experienced moment of emptiness but does not conceptually elaborate upon that experience (Shonin and Van Gordon 2013a). In other words, during the practice of *mindfulness of emptiness* and as with all other forms of mindfulness practice, there should be no thought of emptiness, no feeling of emptiness, no mental formation of emptiness, and no self or I that experiences emptiness. There should only be emptiness.

Mindfulness of emptiness corresponds to the fourth type of mindfulness referred to in the seventh Dalai Lama's *Song of the Four Mindfulnesses* (not to be confused with the *Four Foundations of Mindfulness*). The preceding three types of mindfulness explicated by the seventh Dalai Lama were mindfulness of: (i) what is embodied by the Buddha and teacher, (ii) compassion, and (iii) the divine/subtle body. After having suitably prepared their mind (by cultivating the first three types of mindfulness), the seventh Dalai Lama directs his followers to practise *mindfulness of emptiness* by "not letting your mind stray" from the recognition of emptiness (Gelek 2009, p. 3). Repeated episodes of glimpsing emptiness, as well as the steady prolonging of such episodes, is understood in Buddhism to gradually lead to a stable realization of emptiness that eventually permeates all of the meditation practitioner's thoughts, words, and actions (Dalai Lama and Berzin 1997) .

A detailed discussion of the various meditative and/or spiritual strategies elucidated in the Buddhist teachings for cultivating an experience or glimpse of emptiness is beyond the scope of the present chapter. However, the following are some of the principal methods—all of which depend on mindfulness not only to preserve the emptiness experience when it arises but also to help bring about its manifestation:

1. *Emptiness via samatha–vipassanā meditation:* Arguably, the most traditional and well-documented means of cultivating an experience of emptiness is by utilizing *samatha* (Pāli, Sanskrit: *śamatha*) meditation in order to bring the mind into a state of tranquil abiding, followed by a period of *vipassanā* (Pāli, Sanskrit: *vipaśyanā*) meditation in order to perceive the underlying nature of phenomena (i.e. emptiness). Nevertheless, in our opinion, the practice of *vipassanā* meditation is poorly understood in the contemporary Buddhist and scientific (academic and populist) literature. Indeed, some researchers, scholars, and Buddhist teachers assert that *vipassanā* meditation is either (i) identical to mindfulness meditation (e.g. Bowen et al. 2006; Chiesa 2010) or (ii) an opening out of mindfulness in order to passively or calmly observe the three qualities that are understood in Buddhism to mark and underlie the existence of all phenomena (i.e. suffering, impermanence, and nonself; Harvey 2015). In our view, these accounts of *vipassanā* portray it as being a mostly passive process, and fail to emphasize the active and penetrative–investigative aspect of authentic *vipassanā* practice.

   A degree of meditative insight will certainly arise by being mindful of the present moment in order to passively observe the coming and going (and other characteristics) of phenomena (Kabat-Zinn 1990, 1994). However, this is very different and less potent than the ego-subduing insight that can be extracted via the practice of *vipassanā* and which can only arise when the practitioner moves beyond the idea of an identifiable present moment (Shonin and Van Gordon 2013a; Shonin et al. 2014a). According to Trungpa (2006, p. 47), *vipassanā* entails the meditation practitioner leaving behind their attachment to known concepts in order to perceive the "fourth moment" of reality (i.e. the fourth dimension of reality that exists beyond the notions of past, present, and future) .

   Accordingly, as implied by the record of the Buddha's teachings in the *Mahāvacchagotta Sutta* (*Majjhima Nikāya* [MN], 73), if one truly wishes to perceive the empty nature of phenomena, one literally has to penetrate them with the piercing wisdom induced via meditative serenity (i.e. *samatha*): "When these two things—serenity and insight—are developed further, they will lead to the penetration of many elements" (Ñanamoli and Bodhi 2009, p. 600). The insight of *vipassanā requires* hard work and will not arise by simply opening up mindfulness in order to observe phenomena and their underlying characteristics. If confusion is present in the mind of the person that mindfully observes the characteristics of phenomena, they will inevitably perceive those characteristics in a distorted manner. Put simply, *vipassanā* (or indeed any other form of Buddhist meditation) does not entail the Buddhist meditator "sitting on their backside" (both mentally and physically), becoming enthralled with (what they deem to be) the coming and going of their thoughts and feelings, and arousing conviction that they are engaged in some form of profound meditative practice. As demonstrated by the above *Dream or Reality* dialogue, in essence, phenomena exist only as mentally constructed labels. Therefore, since phenomena are the creation of the mind and are also of its nature, it follows that the mind is also the tool that must be utilized in order to actively deconstruct phenomena during *vipassanā meditation.*

Consequently, *vipassanā* involves making use of the tranquillity and concentration cultivated during *samatha* meditation in order to enter into a state of meditative analysis, whereby meditators actively search for an inherently existing self that resides within either themselves or another phenomenon. This is consistent with the wording of the *Mahāsuññata Sutta* (*Greater Discourse on Emptiness,* MN 971; Ñanamoli and Bodhi 2009) where, having brought the mind into a state of equanimity and concentration, the Buddha explains that the meditation practitioner must engage in *vipassanā* by actively (i.e. rather than passively) "giving attention to voidness" (p. 972) (voidness is another word for emptiness; see below for the full excerpt from the *Mahāsuññata Sutta*) .

Thus, the aforementioned claims that *vipassanā* corresponds to the practice of mindfulness meditation or an opening up of mindfulness meditation are effectively depicting practices that—whilst employing different breadths of attentional focus—are still located within the *samatha* spectrum of Buddhist meditative practice. Furthermore, the depiction of *vipassanā* as a practice that gives rise to insight via the opening up of mindfulness in order to allow the present moment to unfold *as it is,* more accurately describes the completion-stage practices of certain tantric Buddhist systems (e.g. *Māhamudrā, Dzogchen*). The insight that arises from such tantric practices goes well beyond the meaning of *vipassanā*, requires the individual to have traversed the necessary generation-stage practices, and more closely resembles the direct perceiving of, and unification with, a state of (or very close to) Buddhahood (Dalai Lama and Berzin 1997; Dalai Lama 2004; Urgyen 2000) .

Mindfully observing the coming and going of phenomena is a practice that still operates within the realms and limitations of duality, and it therefore prevents the meditating individual from truly letting go of self and becoming both the subject and object of their meditation (Shonin and Van Gordon 2014c). Thus, in sequential order, *vipassanā* requires the practitioner to: (i) introduce an appropriate degree of meditative serenity into their mind (i.e. via a prior period of *samatha* meditation), (ii) meditatively penetrate a given meditative object (or objects), (iii) actively search for an inherently existing self that abides within the object, (iv) identify and eliminate each layer of conceptual thinking that supports or presupposes the existence of an inherently existing self, and (v) abide in the profound experience that apprehends that all phenomena—including the meditating individual—are without an intrinsic self and are of a single nature and origin (Shonin and Van Gordon 2014c) .

2. *Emptiness via direct introduction:* Depending upon their level of realization and the spiritual capacity of the student, a very small number of Buddhist teachers are able to directly introduce (an even smaller number of) students to a fully authentic experience of emptiness (Shonin and Van Gordon 2015). Much like a lotus bud that feeds on the debris and grows out of the murky depths of a pond, this experience of emptiness will gradually consume the student's mental

poisons (e.g. greed, hatred, and delusion) and grow inside their mind stream until it defines the very essence of their being.

3. *Emptiness via renunciation and spiritual distress:* According to Buddhist thought, the average individual harbours a deeply embedded and erroneous belief that they and the world around them inherently exist (Van Gordon et al. 2015b). Consequently, as an individual enters the path of authentic Dharma practice and begins to gain insight into the ultimate nature of reality, they undergo a process of constant disillusionment. Each time a more gross aspect of ego is surmounted, a subtler aspect reveals itself and continues to corrupt their perception of reality. Despite their growing levels of spiritual insight and awareness, the mind of the aspiring Buddha has a tendency to try to position and reassure itself by forming attachments to its continuously changing understanding of reality (Trungpa 2002).

   The world (or *mandala*) created by the meditation practitioner's spiritual guide (who may or may not be in bodily form) comprises a cycle of allowing the practitioner to build up hopes and concepts, only to have them abruptly dismantled at some future point (Trungpa 2002). This process, which can often be quite painful or dramatic, eventually gives rise in the practitioner to the experience of a profound sense of renunciation. At this point, the individual knows from first-hand experience that any form of attachment to phenomena is futile and only incurs further suffering. In essence, the meditation practitioner is left with the feeling of having absolutely nowhere to go, nothing to do, nothing to accomplish, and of not needing to be somebody in particular (Shonin and Van Gordon 2014c). To all intents and purposes, they have been forced to perfect the practice of renunciation, and have "had their fingers burnt" so many times by forming attachments to phenomena that they default to a position of abiding in and becoming one with emptiness. Some of the best-documented examples of spiritual practitioners that have traversed this process and pattern of awakening are the lineage fathers of the Tibetan Kagyu Buddhist tradition (e.g. Naropa, Milarepa).

4. *Emptiness via sudden awakening:* The occurrence or practice of sudden awakening is most commonly associated with certain schools of Zen and *Vajrayāna* Buddhism (Shonin et al. 2014a). However, in truth, there are reports of individuals experiencing a sudden awakening across almost the entire collection of Buddhist practice traditions (including multiple examples throughout the Theravāda Pāli Canon; see, Van Gordon et al. 2015b). There are numerous scenarios and techniques that can trigger a sudden awakening including (but not limited to) (i) direct introduction by a fully realized teacher (see the third point above; Sogyal 1998), (ii) a *koān* (a question, scenario, conundrum, or dialogue intended to shatter conceptual thinking patterns and produce a *satori* experience (Japanese and Zen Buddhist terminology for awakening); Shonin et al. 2014a), (iii) a memory or situation that activates an "awakening key" established by the practitioner or their teacher in their current or a previous lifetime (Urgyen 1995), and (iv) locating a spiritual treasure (Tibetan: *terma*) hidden in their mind or in a physical location (similar to the forgoing technique of the "awakening key"; Shonin and

Van Gordon 2015). All of these methods appear to point towards the existence and feasibility of an "instant" path to spiritual awakening. However, in cases where awakening manifests suddenly, the breakthrough of realization invariably reflects the coming to fruition of spiritual momentum and insights accumulated during years (or even lifetimes) of diligent day-to-day practice (Trungpa 2006) .

As discussed earlier in the chapter, the practice of *mindfulness of emptiness* involves remaining fully aware of the emptiness experience after it has been induced (i.e. by utilizing a spiritual technique such as those outlined above). However, *mindfulness of emptiness* also requires additional attentional and intuitive resources on the part of the meditation practitioner. Indeed, the practice of *mindfulness of emptiness* is not only restricted to simply remaining mindful of emptiness when a recognition of the emptiness of phenomena becomes manifest but it also implies that there should be *mindfulness of emptiness* even when an experience of emptiness is not (deemed by the meditation practitioner to be) manifest in the mind.

Despite the view of certain Buddhist scholars that utilizing "memories from the past" (e.g. Thānissaro 2012, p. 15) is a central component of mindfulness, we have previously asserted that the recollection of past events is not a principal function of mindfulness practice (e.g. Shonin et al. 2014a; Shonin and Van Gordon 2013a). The reason for this is captured by the following record of the Buddha's teachings in the *Bhaddekaratta Sutta* (MN 131; Ñanamoli and Bodhi 2009): "Let not a person revive the past .... For the past has been left behind" (p. 1039). In other words, the past is history and life (in addition to spiritual practice) can only occur and be experienced in the present moment. In light of our prior assertion, it is perhaps useful or essential at this point to clarify what is meant and implied by our above suggestion that the practice of *mindfulness of emptiness* requires the meditation practitioner to continuously recognize or "recollect" the fact that phenomena are intrinsically empty of inherent existence.

When proposing that practising *mindfulness of emptiness* involves an awareness of emptiness even when an emptiness experience is not manifest in the mind, what we are essentially suggesting is that the practitioner becomes aware—in real-time terms—of the fact that in truth, there is never a time when an emptiness experience is not manifest in the mind. As stated in the *Heart Sutra*, in addition to form, each of the other aggregates (Pāli: *khandha*s; Sanskrit: *skandhas*) of feelings, perceptions, mental formations, and consciousness are also of the nature of emptiness. In fact, without exception, everything that an individual thinks, feels, or perceives is 100 % empty of inherent existence. This relates as much to the object of their thoughts, feelings, and perceptions as it does to the thoughts, feelings, and perceptions themselves.

Therefore, implicit within the practice of *mindfulness of emptiness* is awareness or knowing that the moment-by-moment experience of the ordinary and so-called deluded mind is actually of the texture and nature of emptiness. Indeed, a realization and embodiment of this very simple (but profound) principle is all that separates a fully enlightened Buddha from an ignorant sentient being that is still subject to samsaric wandering (and therefore suffering and delusion). This is very different from the practice of continuously trying to "remember" that mind and its contents are empty of existence. Remembrance of emptiness in this context becomes too much of a cognitive endeavour and effectively reifies emptiness into a construct that is separate from the individual that is attempting to realize it.

In essence, the practice of *mindfulness of emptiness* in the sense that we are currently discussing it relates closely to the Buddhist principle and practice of *right view* (Pāli: *sammā-ditthi,* Sanskrit: *samyag-drsti*). Knowing, without necessarily having directly perceived, the *empty, nonself,* and *non-dual* nature of reality is a fundamental aspect of right view. Indeed, having complete faith in the intrinsic emptiness of phenomena is a prerequisite for subsequently being able to glimpse emptiness (Shonin and Van Gordon 2015). In turn, this glimpse or intuition augments the quality and potency of the practitioner's conviction that due to emptiness, all things exist in them, and they exist in all things.

We are certainly not stating that there is no benefit to be derived from conceptually investigating emptiness and/or from trying to remember that phenomena are of the nature of emptiness. Indeed, such mental exertion can bring about a certain theoretical familiarity with the various principles of emptiness. However, in truth, no amount of investigation, analysis, or conceptualization will ever bring an individual into direct and irreversible contact with emptiness. Emptiness must be known, felt, lived, and breathed. Emptiness is what is—right here and right now. Meditation practitioners must simply be emptiness, and, for as long as they look for it outside of themselves, they will never find it (Norbu and Clemente 1999).

This is one of the key premises that the Buddha was attempting to convey in the extract below from the *Mahāsuññata Sutta.* As shown, the Buddha advised his followers that when, from a point of meditative concentration, they make an effort to give rise to an experience of emptiness (translated below as "voidness"), the very fact that they are objectifying emptiness and straining themselves in order to realize it prevents them from attaining their goal. However, if meditation practitioners loosen their attachment to the idea of experiencing emptiness and once again rest in meditative serenity, when they decide once more to engage in *vipassanā* meditation by actively giving attention to emptiness, it is easier for them to penetrate the underlying nature of phenomena:

> Here Ānanda, quite secluded from sensual pleasures, secluded from unwholesome states, a bhikkhu enters upon and abides in the first jhāna…the second jhāna…the third jhāna…the fourth jhāna, which has neither pain nor pleasure and purity of mindfulness due to equanimity. That is how a bhikkhu steadies his mind internally, quiets it, brings it to singleness, and concentrates it.
>
> Then he gives attention to voidness internally. While he is giving attention to voidness internally, his mind does not enter into voidness internally or acquire confidence, steadiness, and decision. When that is so, he understands thus: "While I am giving attention to voidness internally, my mind does not enter into voidness or acquire confidence, steadiness, and decision". In this way he has full awareness of that. …. Then that bhikkhu should steady his mind internally, quiet it, bring it to singleness, and concentrate it on that same sign of concentration as before. Then he gives attention to voidness internally. While he is giving attention to voidness internally, his mind enters into voidness internally and acquires confidence, steadiness, and decision. When that is so, he understands thus: "While I am giving attention to voidness internally, my mind enters into voidness internally and acquires,

confidence, steadiness, and decision". In this way he has full awareness of that. (Ñanamoli and Bodhi 2009, pp. 972–973)

9.4 The Emptiness of Mindfulness

Throughout this chapter, we have repeatedly made reference to the tendency of individuals to reify emptiness into a fixed construct and to form concepts regarding its nature and properties. The problem with doing so is that emptiness is also empty of inherent existence, and, as such, any conceptual understanding of what constitutes emptiness will necessarily be erroneous. In addition to the fact that emptiness is empty, the individual wishing to become adept at the practice of *mindfulness of emptiness* must also (experientially) understand that mindfulness is also empty of inherent existence.

The mental faculty of mindfulness that performs the function of regulating meditative concentration arises in dependence on numerous causes and conditions. For example, for *right mindfulness* (Pāli: *sammā-sati,* Sanskrit*: samyak-smrti*) to be aroused there must also be present (i) the faculty of right concentration (Pāli: *sammā-samādhi,* Sanskrit: *samyak-samādhi*), (ii) an animate or inanimate object upon which to focus this concentration, and (iii) a subject (i.e. a person) that decides to practise mindfulness. Other contributing factors for the arousal of right mindfulness are the experience of suffering (if the individual was already liberated from suffering, they would not need to practise mindfulness and spiritual development in order to transmute it), the fact that the meditator has a body (without one they would not be able to cultivate mindful awareness), and the fact that they are breathing and alive (being dead is not conducive to practising mindfulness). In fact, due to the law of interconnectedness, every single phenomenon in the universe (or multiverse) in some way plays a causal role in the arousal of right mindfulness (Shonin and Van Gordon 2014d). Consequently, apart from a mentally designated label, a construct or practice called mindfulness cannot be said to exist.

Realizing that mindfulness is empty of inherent existence is important for the following reasons:

1. *It helps to avoid spiritual materialism:* Trungpa (2002) utilized the term *spiritual materialism* to refer to the (common) occurrence of an individual engaging in (what they deem to be) spiritual and/or meditative practice that, rather than promote wisdom acquisition and spiritual growth, serves only to augment ego attachment and narcissistic behaviour. Understanding that mindfulness, as with all forms of spiritual practice, does not inherently exist is consistent with the Buddhist view that emptiness is an antidote to all factors that can obstruct or derail an individual's meditative and spiritual development (Gampopa 1998).
2. *It helps to avoid the pitfall of being "too mindful":* Related to the above point, we have previously noted that there is a tendency for individuals to either over-exert themselves in their meditation practice or develop a personality affectation due to them becoming "too mindful" (Shonin et al. 2014c). Being too mindful

refers to circumstances where a mindfulness practitioner or teacher makes excessive efforts to master the art of appearing to be mindful (e.g. adopting an overly pious demeanour, constant and/or inappropriate smiling, etc.) without actually having any presence of mind (Shonin et al. 2014c). Understanding that the mindfulness faculty is devoid of inherent existence helps to prevent individuals from becoming caught up in the idea of being a "meditator".

3. *It helps to prevent "meditation addiction":* We have previously reported (via both clinical case studies and personal observation) that it is possible for individuals to become addicted to meditation and/or mindfulness practice (e.g. Shonin et al. 2014b, c). *Meditation addiction* (a subcategory of what we have previously termed *spiritual addiction*) can manifest as both the positive or negative forms of addiction. It refers to an individual becoming dependent on meditation and/or mindfulness to the extent that they satisfy all six criteria for classification as a behavioural addiction according to Griffiths' (2005) component's model of addiction:

    a. Meditation/mindfulness becomes the most salient and preoccupying activity in their lives.
    b. It gives rise to mood modification.
    c. The individual's tolerance levels increase such that they engage in meditation for increasingly longer daily periods over time.
    d. They exhibit withdrawal symptoms if unable to engage in meditation.
    e. Meditation causes personal and interpersonal conflict (only in the case of a negative addiction), and intrapsychic conflict.
    f. The individual relapses and meditates as much as before following periods of abstinence from meditation.

5. *It is necessary for advanced meditative practice:* There has never been, and will never be, a Buddha that practises mindfulness. The words *practising mindfulness* implies that a subject is making a deliberate effort in order to keep its concentration fixed on a given object or objects. However, the state of Buddhahood is completely uncontrived and it transcends the limiting concepts of practising or making effort (Norbu and Clemente 1999). Furthermore, as referred to earlier in this chapter, at the ultimate level, there is absolutely no separation between subject (i.e. self), activity (i.e. mindfulness), and object (i.e. the present moment). Due to understanding that it is all things, an enlightened being knows that it does not need to isolate one part of itself so that it can be mindful of another part of itself. Progressing to the advanced stages of Buddhist meditation requires the meditation/mindfulness practitioner to be completely natural and spontaneous and to let go of the idea that they are practising something.

In essence, it can be argued that the ultimate purpose of mindfulness is to bring the practitioner to a point of spiritual awareness such that they no longer need to practise mindfulness. In this sense, mindfulness is very much an essential tool or stepping stone for awakening an individual's Buddha nature. However, as with everything else in Buddhist practice, mindfulness must ultimately be let go of. Realizing that mindfulness is empty of intrinsic existence goes hand in hand with realizing that the principal subject of mindful awareness—the present moment—is also devoid of an identifiable self. Therefore, in much the same manner that any attachment to concepts such as mindfulness and emptiness must be relinquished, the aspiring Buddha must also come to an experiential understanding that there are no logical grounds upon which it can be said that the present moment inherently exists. We have previously explicated the empty and ultimate nature of the present moment as follows:

> Imagine that you decide to take a trip to the countryside and have a picnic in your favorite tree-lined spot next to a river. From the time of your arrival until the time you pick up your picnic basket and start to make your way home, we are sure that it will not come as a surprise to you to hear that you have not been sitting in a static environment. At any given instant when you found yourself gazing at the river, you were observing a dynamic and continuously flowing phenomenon. Thus, between any given instant of time and the next, the river undergoes change. However, not only does the river change between two separate instances of time, but it also changes within the same instant of time. The reason for this is because time is a relative concept; it is a man-made construct that we human beings employ to try to add structure and order to our world.
>
> The truth is, any given moment of time can be continuously divided into ever smaller instants, and this process of division can continue ad infinitum. …not even for the most miniscule moment of time could we say that the river ever stands still. It is not just rivers that are subject to this continuous process of change, but every single phenomenon that we encounter. In many respects, we could actually view the present moment and all that it contains as one enormous flowing river: A graceful and swirling flood of interwoven mind and matter that continuously flows yet never actually goes anywhere…

If there is never a point in time when the river stands still, how can a thing that does not ever become static undergo any change? Change implies that something changes from one state or position to another. But since phenomena never truly come to rest in a fixed state, it is illogical to assert that such a transient and "permanently unfixed" entity can undergo change. That which never "is" cannot be said to change between one moment of time and the next (Shonin and Van Gordon 2013a, pp. 105–106).

9.5 Conclusion

Emptiness, which refers to the fact that all phenomena are devoid of intrinsic existence, is a fundamental principle upon which the Buddha based his teachings. Insofar as it can be said that Buddhist meditation constitutes a journey, then emptiness is the destination (but as explicated above, it is also the middle and start of the journey). Indeed, without exception, each individual aspect of Buddhist practice is either directly or indirectly orientated towards bringing about an internalization of emptiness. For example, although important competencies in their own right, the core Buddhist practices of generosity, loving kindness, and compassion also help the practitioner to adopt a humble demeanour. Due to becoming familiar with the practice of prioritizing other's needs and happiness over their own, this humble demeanour helps the meditation practitioner to loosen attachment to the belief in an inherently existing self (Shonin et al. 2014a). Attachment to the belief in an independent self-entity has been termed *ontological addiction* which is defined as "the unwillingness to relinquish an erroneous and deep-rooted belief in an inherently existing 'self' or 'I' as well as the 'impaired functionality' that arises from such a belief" (Shonin et al. 2014b, pp. 64). Emptiness is understood in Buddhism to be the most effective means for overcoming ontological addiction and for permanently transmuting the impaired functionality (i.e. suffering) that it causes.

Mindfulness is a fundamental faculty on the path to awakening. It serves to ensure that wholesome states of mind—in particular meditative concentration—are cultivated such that it becomes difficult for unwholesome states of mind (e.g. greed, hatred, delusion) to establish themselves in the mind (Thānissaro 2012). Mindfulness plays a vital role in helping to bring the meditation practitioner into intimate contact with the contents of their mind and with the happenings of present moment. Consistent with the Buddhist teachings, research demonstrates that mindfully attending to the *here and now* introduces focus, equanimity, and calm into the mind (Chiesa et al. 2011; Eberth and Sedlmeier 2012; Fjorback et al. 2011). When cultivated to an adequate degree, this attentional focus and mental quietude is essential for the subsequent arousal of insight—the primary objective of *vipassanā* meditation. It is during *vipassanā* meditation that the meditation practitioner seeks to mentally penetrate the absolute nature of phenomena in order to directly encounter the profound truth of emptiness.

In addition to being a prerequisite for cultivating this experience of emptiness, right mindfulness is also essential for preserving the emptiness experience after it has arisen. However, as elucidated in this chapter, the practice of *mindfulness of emptiness* goes well beyond the cultivation and maintenance of an experience of emptiness. Indeed, the diligent spiritual practitioner should be constantly aware of the fact that not only are phenomena empty of inherent existence but their thoughts, feelings, concepts, and perceptions in relation to those phenomena are likewise empty in nature. Due to this realization, the practice of *mindfulness of emptiness* eventually brings the spiritual practitioner to the profound and logically sound realization that all things are of the nature of mind and that although they searched outside of themselves (for innumerable lifetimes) in order to locate it, they have never once left the domain of emptiness:

> Like the repose that follows, when waking from a nightmare.
> Like the reprieve of an isolated General, who recognizes the encroaching soldiers as his own troops.
> Like the relief that arises, when realizing that the snake, was, all along, just a piece of old rope.
> Like the rapture of the despairing treasure hunter, who returns to find the riches buried beneath his own home.
> Oh self who has enslaved me for so long, now I have shed the shackles of ignorance, and entered the non-returning blissful abode. (Shonin and Van Gordon 2013b)

References

Bowen, S., Witkiewitz, K., Dillworth, T. M., Chawla, N., Simpson, T. L., Ostafin, B. D., et al. (2006). Mindfulness meditation and substance use in an incarcerated population. *Psychology of Addictive Behaviours, 20,* 243–347.

Chiesa, A. (2010). Vipassana meditation: Systematic review of current evidence. *Journal of Alternative and Complementary Medicine, 16,* 37–46.

Chiesa, A., Calati, R., & Serretti, A. (2011). Does mindfulness training improve cognitive abilities? A systematic review of neuropsychological findings. *Clinical Psychology Review, 31,* 449–464.

Dalai Lama. (2004). *Dzogchen: Heart essence of the great perfection.* New York: Snow Lion.

Dalai Lama, & Berzin, A. (1997). *The gelug/kagyu tradition of Mahamudra.* New York: Snow Lion.

Digital Sanskrit Buddhist Canon. (2014). Located. at: http://www.dsbcproject.org/.

Eberth, J., & Sedlmeier, P. (2012). The effects of mindfulness meditation: A meta-analysis. *Mindfulness, 3,* 174–189.

Fjorback, L. O., Arendt, M., Ørnbøl, E., Fink, P., & Walach, H. (2011). Mindfulness-based stress reduction and mindfulness-based cognitive therapy—A systematic review of randmized controlled trials. *Acta Psychiatrica Scandinavica, 124,* 102–119.

Gampopa. (1998). *The jewel ornament of liberation: The wish-fulfilling gem of the noble teachings.* New York: Snow Lion.

Gelek, R. (2009). *The four mindfulnesses.* Ann Arbor: Jewel Heart Transcripts.

Griffiths, M. D. (2005). A components model of addiction within a biopsychosocial framework. *Journal of Substance Use, 10,* 191–197.

Harvey, P. (2015). Mindfulness in Theravāda Samatha and Vipassanā meditations, and in secular mindfulness. In E. Shonin, W. Van Gordon, & N. N. Singh (Eds.), *Buddhist foundations of mindfulness.* New York: Springer.

Kabat-Zinn, J. (1990). *Full catastrophe living: Using the wisdom of your body and mind to face stress, pain and illness.* New York: Delacourt.

Kabat-Zinn, J. (1994). *Wherever you go, there you are: Mindfulness meditation in everyday life.* New York: Hyperion.

Michalon, M. (2001). "Selflessness" in the service of the ego: Contributions, limitations and dangers of Buddhist psychology for western psychotherapy. *American Journal of Psychotherapy, 55,* 202–218.

Ñanamoli B., & Bodhi, B. (2009). *Majjhima Nikaya: The middle length discourses of the Buddha* (4th ed.). Massachusetts: Wisdom.

Nhat Hanh, T. (1999). *The heart of the Buddha's teaching: Transforming suffering into peace, joy and liberation.* New York: Broadway Books.

Norbu, C., & Clemente, A. (1999). *The supreme source: The fundamental tantra of the Dzogchen Semde.* New York: Snow Lion.

Shonin, E., & Van Gordon, W. (2013a). Searching for the present moment. *Mindfulness, 5,* 105–107.

Shonin, E., & Van Gordon, W. (2013b). A close truth. Located at: http://edoshonin.com/2013/04/11/a-close-truth/.

Shonin, E., & Van Gordon, W. (2014a). Dream or reality? *Philosophy Now, 104,* 54.

Shonin, E., & Van Gordon, W. (2014b). Can a person be ignorant and intelligent at the same time? Located at http://edoshonin.com/2014/06/11/can-a-person-be-ignorant-and-intelligent-at-the-same-time/.

Shonin, E., & Van Gordon, W. (2014c). Using mindfulness and insight to transform loneliness. *Mindfulness, 5,* 771–773.

Shonin, E., & Van Gordon, W. (2014d). False spiritual economy: Why an "I Want it All and I Want it Now" attitude doesn't promote spiritual growth. Located at http://edoshonin.com/2014/12/12/false-spiritual-economy-why-an-i-want-it-all-and-i-want-it-now-attitude-doesnt-promote-spiritual-growth/.

Shonin, E., & Van Gordon, W. (2015). The lineage of mindfulness. *Mindfulness*. doi:10.1007/s12671–014-0327-x.
Shonin, E., Van Gordon W., & Griffiths, M. D. (2013). Buddhist philosophy for the treatment of problem gambling. *Journal of Behavioural Addictions, 2,* 63–71.
Shonin, E., Van Gordon, W., & Griffiths, M. D. (2014a). The emerging role of Buddhism in clinical psychology: Toward effective integration. *Psychology of Religion and Spirituality, 6,* 123–137.
Shonin, E., Van Gordon, W., & Griffiths, M. D. (2014b). Cognitive behavioral therapy (CBT) and meditation awareness training (MAT) for the treatment of co-occurring schizophrenia with pathological gambling: A case study. *International Journal of Mental Health and Addiction, 12,* 181–196.
Shonin, E., Van Gordon, W., & Griffiths, M. D. (2014c). Are there risks associated with using mindfulness for the treatment of psychopathology? *Clinical Practice*. doi:10.2217/CPR.14.23.
Sogyal, R. (1998). *The Tibetan book of living and dying*. London: Rider.
Thānissaro, Bhikkhu. (2012). Right mindfulness: Memory and ardency on the Buddhist path. e-book available at: http://www.accesstoinsight.org/lib/authors/thanissaro/rightmindfulness.pdf.
Trungpa, C. (2002). *Cutting through spiritual materialism*. Boston: Shambala.
Trungpa, C. (2006). The fourth moment. *Shambala Sun, 14,* 44–45.
Urgyen, T. (1995). *Rainbow painting*. Hong Kong: Rangjung Yeshe.
Urgyen, T. (2000). *As it is*. Hong Kong: Rangjung Yeshe.
Van Gordon, W., Shonin, E., Griffiths, M. D., & Singh, N. N. (2015a). There is only one mindfulness: Why science and Buddhism need to work together. *Mindfulness*. doi:10.1007/s12671–014-0379-y.
Van Gordon, W., Shonin, E., Griffiths, M. D., & Singh, N. N. (2015b). Mindfulness and the four noble truths. In: E. Shonin, W. Van Gordon, & N. N. Singh (Eds.), *Buddhist foundations of mindfulness*. New York: Springer.
Williams, P. (2008). *Mahayana Buddhism: The doctrinal foundations*. London: Routledge.
Zadra, A., & Donderi, D. C. (2000). Nightmares and bad dreams: Their prevalence and relationship to well-being. *Journal of Abnormal Psychology, 109,* 273–281.

Edo Shonin has been a Buddhist monk for 30 years and is the spiritual director of the International Mahayana Bodhayati School of Buddhism. He is the research director of the Awake to Wisdom Centre for Meditation and Mindfulness Research and a research psychologist at the Nottingham Trent University (UK). He is in the International Advisory Board for the journal Mindfulness and is an editorial board member of the International Journal of Mental Health and Addiction. He is internationally known for his work and has more than 100 academic publications relating to the scientific study of mindfulness and Buddhist practice. He runs the Meditation Practice and Research Blog at www.edoshonin.com.

William Van Gordon has been a Buddhist monk for 10 years and is the operations director of the International Mahayana Bodhayati School of Buddhism. He is the cofounder of the Awake to Wisdom Centre for Meditation and Mindfulness Research and is a research psychologist based at the Nottingham Trent University (UK). He is currently a principal investigator on a number of randomized controlled trials investigating the applications of an intervention known as meditation awareness training (MAT) in clinical and occupational settings. He is a member of the editorial board for the International Journal of Buddhism and has more than 100 academic publications relating to the scientific study of Buddhism and associated meditative approaches.

Nirbhay N. Singh is a clinical professor of Psychiatry and health behaviour at the Medical College of Georgia, Georgia Regents University, Augusta, Georgia, USA. Prior to his current appointment, he was a professor of psychiatry, pediatrics, and psychology at the Virginia Commonwealth University School of Medicine and the director of the Commonwealth Institute for Family Studies, Richmond, Virginia. His research interests include mindfulness, behavioural and psychopharmacological treatments of individuals with disabilities, and assistive technology for supporting individuals with severe/profound and multiple disabilities. He is the editor-in-chief of two journals: Journal of Child and Family Studies and Mindfulness and an editor of three book series: Mindfulness in Behavioural Health, Evidence-based Practice in Behavioural Health, and Children and Families.

Mark D. Griffiths is a chartered psychologist and professor of gambling studies at the Nottingham Trent University, and the director of the International Gaming Research Unit. He has spent almost 30 years in this field and is internationally known for his work into gambling, gaming, and other behavioural addictions. More recently, he has published many papers on the practical applications of mindfulness with Edo Shonin and William Van Gordon. He has published more than 500 refereed research papers, four books, 120+ book chapters, and more than 1000 other articles. He has won 14 national and international awards for his work including the John Rosecrance Prize (1994), CELEJ Prize (1998), Joseph Lister Prize (2004), and the US National Council on Problem Gambling Lifetime Research Award (2013). He also does a lot of freelance journalism and has appeared on over 2500 radio and television programmes.

Part II
Integrating Mindfulness into Research and Applied Settings

Chapter 10
Dharma and Distress: Buddhist Teachings that Support the Psychological Principles in a Mindfulness Program

Lynette M. Monteiro

10.1 Introduction

This chapter explores the Buddhist teachings that inform and underpin the themes contained in mindfulness-based interventions (MBIs) using a mindfulness program as a template protocol. It begins with a Buddhist perspective of the general themes of a mindfulness program: self-concept, emotional regulation, and the causes of stress. Following sections unpack the contributions of the two primary *suttas* from the Pali Canon, the *Satipatthana* and *Anapanasati Suttas* (Analayo 2003; Bodhi 2005; Buddhadasa 1976; Goldstein 2013; Gunaratana 2012; Hanh 2006, 2009a; Silananda 2002) to the curriculum of secular mindfulness programs. While these two *suttas* are the primary supports of mindfulness programs, there are also subtle themes informed by Buddhist canonical teachings that are worthy of note. Theravada *Suttas* that elucidate the themes of emotions, interpersonal contact, ethics, and community are also explored (Germer 2009; Hanh 2007, 2011; Harvey 2000; Keown 2005; Neff 2011; Salzberg 2002). The contribution of the Mahayana teachings to mindfulness programs is also important to the subtle themes of a mindfulness program. Concepts of identity are explored through Zen stories and *koans* and the ox-herding pictures serve as a guide for the spiritual journey that is at the heart of any mindfulness program (Soeng 2006).

10.1.1 Themes and Variations of Mindfulness

The cultivation of mindfulness in Buddhist practice is a central component in the transformation of suffering or *dukkha*. The definition of mindfulness *(sati)* however is diverse reflecting the many different Buddhisms and their attendant

---

L. M. Monteiro (✉)
Ottawa Mindfulness Clinic, 595 Montreal Road, Suite 301, Ottawa, ON K1K 4 L2, Canada
e-mail: lynette.monteiro@gmail.com

E. Shonin et al. (eds.), *Buddhist Foundations of Mindfulness,*
Mindfulness in Behavioral Health, DOI 10.1007/978-3-319-18591-0_10

philosophy and psychology (Williams and Kabat-Zinn 2013). Common to all perspectives of Buddhist practice is mindfulness as right mindfulness, rich in meaning and one of the "folds" in the Eightfold Path. One definition of mindfulness is a mental quality that recalls the path by which *dukkha* occurs and can be caused to cease (Goldstein 2013; Thanissaro 2012). It is this role in the process of cessation of the cause of *dukkha* that gives mindfulness its potency and makes it a focus of Buddhist practice.

Because of its association with the cessation of suffering, mindfulness has become an important component in the treatment of illness in secular and clinical settings. Current secular applications of mindfulness share with its Buddhist origins the intention of transforming *dukkha* and teach its practice in nonclinical programs for wellness and as clinical psychotherapeutic interventions conducted in individual or group sessions (Baer 2005; Germer et al. 2013; Kabat-Zinn 2003). Although the intent of current mindfulness approaches is consistent with Buddhist practices (Monteiro et al. 2014), the manner in which Buddhist teachings infuse and support the secular conceptualization and delivery of mindfulness practice is not always made clear or explicit. This clarification plays an important part in understanding the complicated and easily misunderstood concept that Westernized mindfulness has become (Grossman and Van Dam 2011).

Understanding the links between Buddhist teachings and its secular applications is crucial in the delivery of mindfulness programs and in the training of professionals delivering such programs for three reasons. First, it ensures that wisdom and virtue are conveyed as integral to mindfulness in its secular application. Second, it creates a framework within which mindfulness can be communicated skillfully. Third, it provides a compass to navigate through the process and progress of the participants' practice. Moreover, without a clear understanding that the path of transformation is through the cultivation of wisdom, virtue, and meditation, mindfulness approaches run the risk of becoming a superficially applied method.

The need for understanding the complex Buddhist principles and models of distress or *dukkha* has been voiced in many clinical and Buddhist publications (Maex 2011; Sharf 2013; Williams and Kabat-Zinn 2013). Questions posed have ranged from assessing if secular and clinical views of mindfulness are consistent with Buddhist principles to the necessity for reappropriating mindfulness as a specifically Buddhist model of developing well-being (Purser and Loy 2013; Titmuss 2013). While the debate continues mostly unresolved, there are few discussions that examine the Buddhist teachings that underpin secular mindfulness treatment programs. This understanding is crucial if secular mindfulness programs are to convey the components of mindfulness in a way that enhances the potential for well-being.

Buddhist teachings of mindfulness practice are an elegant and complex process. The path that leads to the alleviation of suffering is direct (Analayo 2003) and drills down into the roots of the causes of suffering. The intention of this examination and diligent uprooting of the causes of suffering is to cultivate wisdom and compassion for self and others. That is, the path of transformation is not only to develop mindfulness so the suffering ends but also to nurture the mind of love or *bodhicitta*

(Gethin 1992/2001). In order to develop a practice that encompasses these two factors of transformation, mindfulness programs are enriched when approached from an understanding of the key teachings of Buddhism.

Before beginning to examine the relevance of these important teachings to mindfulness treatment programs, two points are necessary to hold in mind. First, the landscape of Buddhism, its philosophy, and psychology is vast and complicated. The intent in this chapter is not to engage in the intricacies of establishing authority or authenticity of secular and clinical forms of mindfulness, but rather to examine the Buddhist teachings that underlie the principles of contemporary mindfulness. Second, the landscape of Westernized mindfulness is still in the process of being sculpted; definitions, mechanisms, and suitability to clinical populations are slowly being clarified (Baer 2003, 2011, 2005). Nevertheless, there are psychological themes that can be held up and viewed through the lens of Buddhist principles and psychology so that this growing edge of Buddhism and Western psychology can be better understood.

It is useful therefore to establish first the composition of current clinical mindfulness programs and the core principles of Buddhist thought on the generation of psychological distress. MBIs have developed over the past 35 years as the *sine qua non* of psychological treatments. While mindfulness-based stress reduction (MBSR), developed by Kabat-Zinn (2011, 2013) is accepted as the icon of stress reduction MBIs, many programs have been developed that differ in content and intent (Cayoun 2011; Monteiro et al. 2010; Segal et al. 2012). However, there are sufficient commonalities to allow a general discussion of their makeup. Although MBSR began with the influence of both Zen and *vipassanna* teachings, mention of Buddhism was avoided and its design strived to reflect the Dharma without Buddhist- or New Age-sounding terms that would distract from its intention (Kabat-Zinn 2003, 2011). Nevertheless, the definition of mindfulness offered by Kabat-Zinn has created a level of confusion and contradiction when assessed by Buddhist criteria (Davis and Thompson 2013; Dunne 2011). One rationale for downplaying Buddhist terminology in MBSR was to make the programs more accessible to non-Buddhists and to limit any negative reactions to being perceived as based in a religious framework (Kabat-Zinn 2011; Langer 1990). Another rationale was that the essence of Buddhist philosophy was universal and did not require explicit mention; this was also applied to the mention of ethics (virtue practices or *sila*), which was assumed to be embedded in the content and emerged from practice naturally. This latter deletion of a primary principle of Buddhist thought has been the focus of much criticism and debate in the mindfulness communities (Titmuss 2013).

Several Buddhist practitioners have addressed the difficulties with the way mindfulness is understood in Buddhism and will not be addressed here (see Williams and Kabat-Zinn (2013) for detailed discussion on Buddhist definitions of mindfulness). However, in order to fully appreciate the interconnection of Buddhist psychology and the clinical use of mindfulness principles, both the formulation of a mindfulness program and the commonly accepted Buddhist principles that support it are set out below.

10.1.2 Clinical Applications of Mindfulness Interventions

MBIs were developed to address mental health issues from a different standpoint than earlier historic might read smoother therapeutic approaches. Where before the focus was on what ailed the individual, MBIs shifted the attention to what was healthy. Through various meditative practices and interchanges with the facilitator of the program (inquiries) the healthy aspects of an individual's life are made accessible through a direct experience of that life. The approach drew from Buddhist principles such as impermanence, absence of a fixed, defined self, and the reality that suffering is a common experience. It developed awareness of these principles through technical skills such as various forms of meditations and yoga.

The secular and clinical application of mindfulness in Western psychology is attributed to both Langer (1990) and Kabat-Zinn (2013). Langer's mindfulness skills and interventions are based on a cognitive model that focuses on problem solving, developing creative perspective taking, and other outcome-focused procedures. The model of mindfulness developed by Kabat-Zinn and others relates to the experience that is unfolding for an individual. Initially called the stress-reduction and relaxation program (SRRP), the intervention developed to be the now-widely known model of mindfulness called MBSR. The prolific use of MBSR has resulted in the acronym taking on iconic proportions such that a program employing mindfulness and meditation is typically associated with it.

The clinical territory of mindfulness interventions, however, is widespread encompassing far more than stress reactions to physical and mental challenges (Eberth and Sedlmeier 2012; Fjorback et al. 2011). Its application has expanded to the treatment of numerous mental health issues such as depression, anxiety, addictions, and eating disorders to name a few. Various clinical treatment models have been integrated into the development of MBIs. Cognitive behavioral therapy (CBT) has fostered mindfulness-based cognitive therapy (MBCT; Segal et al. 2012) and mindfulness-integrated cognitive behavioral therapy (MiCBT; Cayoun 2011). Addiction models have fostered mindfulness-based relapse prevention (MBRP; Cowen et al. 2010). These have been beneficial integrations of traditional clinical approaches with mindfulness that enhance both protocols and resulting in a paradigm shift for the former and a new venue for application for the latter.

Mindfulness interventions are delivered in both individual and group formats. As an intervention for individuals, mindfulness can inform the therapist's approach to addressing psychological issues (Shapiro and Carlson 2009a); that is, it has incorporated into a preexisting therapeutic model the concepts of mindfulness such as impermanence, nonself and other Buddhist principles. Therapy can also be mindfulness based in that it reflects the principles of mindfulness and includes many of the practices such as meditation.

The more familiar format of MBIs is as a group program where the basic format tends to be consistent across applications (Cullen 2011; Kabat-Zinn 2013). It is composed of 2–2½-h classes offered in an 8–10 week session with an all-day meditation retreat about halfway through the course. Although this is a typical format, there are several adaptations in the length of each class or the overall number of weeks; this is typically dictated by the needs and capacity of the population seeking treatment. For example, in working with groups diagnosed with schizophrenia, Jacobs et al. (2014) have discussed how modifications may be necessary to be consistent with the individuals' ability to sit in silence for meditation. Other adaptations were explored by (Hickman et al. 2012) and summarized by Dobkin et al. (2013).

The specific content of an MBI varies along a continuum of experiential to cognitive approaches. MBSR and its variants tend to rely on experiential styles of interacting with the inquiry process leaning more towards shaving away intellectualization of our experience and creating a space in which sensations and emotions can be directly felt. Other programs balance more didactic styles with the experiential processing to offer both understanding of the disorder as well as experiential connection with the emotions arising at the moment. Although all programs have a curriculum, programs such as MBCT and MiCBT lend themselves to a more manualized approach.

The effectiveness of mindfulness interventions has been well established although the exact mechanisms by which it is achieved have yet to be elucidated fully (Coffey et al. 2010; Grabovac et al. 2011; Shapiro and Carlson 2009b). For example, MBCT has been demonstrated equivalent or superior to medication or treatment as usual (TAU) for depression (Kuyken et al. 2008; Piet and Hougaard 2011; Teasdale et al. 2000). Reduction in symptoms of anxiety disorders have been reported (Vøllestad et al. 2011). Pain and addiction symptoms have also been found to be responsive to mindfulness protocols (Cusens et al. 2010; Kabat-Zinn et al. 1987). Follow-up studies show maintenance of practice is an important part of sustained well-being (Bowen and Kurz 2012; Carmody and Baer 2008).

While clinical uses of mindfulness tend to focus on diagnosed psychological issues, secular applications target more generic issues such as generalized stress or a desire to improve the quality of life. Each mindfulness program will differ in specific content as an interactive and organic unfolding as the relationship between facilitator and participants drives it. However, the general principles of most programs follow the map of the original MBSR program and typically two central Buddhist *suttas* are referenced in these programs: the *Anapanasati* and the *Mahasatipatthana* (Cullen 2011). A number of other teachings from the Theravada and Mahayana/Zen traditions implicitly support themes in an MBI however have not been previously explored. They are included here as potentially fruitful sources for future examination.

10.1.3 The Dharma of Psychological Distress

Buddhism provides a twofold understanding of the universe: cosmological and psychological (Gethin 1998). Of interest to the discussion of mindfulness is the psychological model of the realities faced by all beings. The central tenet of those realities is that all experiences result in *dukkha* (Harvey 2013c). Current interpretations of this complex term reflect a sense of dissatisfaction with or of being off-balance in our life; for ease, the Pali term *dukkha* will be used throughout. The Buddha was emphatic that he taught only two things: the understanding of *dukkha* and its cessation (Bodhi 2008; Gethin 1998; Hanh 1998). These two teachings are contained in the four noble truths or true realities, which point to the realities that arise in a human life and form the base of the Buddhist perspective on distress. Conventionally referred to as a diagnostic protocol for determining suffering, its cause, the prognosis, and treatment, the four realities of all beings are elegant in their simplicity yet complex in their ministration. They begin with the first reality, the acknowledgment that *dukkha* exists. This suffering arises by three means: as an inevitable part of life, as a resistance to the reality that things change and often not to our liking, or as an outcome of learned and trained reactions in our relationship with self, others, and the world. The first step is to acknowledge that there is *dukkha* in our life; in fact, without seeing *dukkha* as present there is no motivation to investigate the causes and conditions that create it.

The second true reality of all beings is the recognition that there is a causal set of links that have resulted in *dukkha*. This cycle, interdependent co-arising, stands as the template for personal transformation and provides explanatory power regarding the development of psychological distress. Buddhist explanations of the cause of *dukkha* differ from other philosophical and religious systems in that they do not posit an external agent who causes *dukkha* or to whom we can appeal for the end of *dukkha* (Gethin 1998). Instead, Buddhist cosmology is consistent in that *dukkha* occurs at both the universal and individual levels and the cycle of interdependent co-arising *(paṭiccasamuppāda)* that governs the arising, enduring, and dissipating of *dukkha* is the same in each level. That is, as a general principle, it proposes that all things arise through causal links as consequences of multiple causes and conditions (Harvey 2013b). Specifically, it refers to the cycle from ignorance to birth, ageing, and death.

This is a key concept in the understanding of how distress is created and warrants a detailed discussion. The cycle of interdependent co-arising describes both a macro-level lack of awareness of the cycle itself and a microlevel one of repetitive, unskillful actions and their consequences. These links can be an individual arising of experiences or occur across lifetimes. As a cycle, it actually has no beginning point *per se* however ignorance of the cycle itself or of our mental state is typically taken as the origin and activation of the cycle (SN 2, 1-2; Harvey 2013c). From this follow mental formations, consciousness, form, the six senses, sense contact, feeling tones, craving, attachment, becoming, birth, and old age and death. Although seemingly linear, each link arises and can be transformed through a multiplicity of causes and consequences in and of itself. When moving in the direction from ignorance to death, it becomes clear in this second reality of life that nothing occurs by itself. The three poisons (root *kleshas*) of attachment, aversion, and delusion act as propellant of this cycle from ignorance to death. In colloquial terms, our desire for what we do not have, rejection of what we have, and confusion about the interconnectedness of intentions, *kleshas,* actions, and consequences reflect ignorance of reality and result in a never-ending spiral into dissatisfaction and distress.

McMahan (2008) noted that this traditional view of interdependent co-arising reflects a more dismal perspective of life with little hope to be found in its multiplicity of causes and conditions, a rejection of symptomatic relief from the travails of life, and its almost impossible goal of *nibbana/nirvana*. He pointed out that contemporary interpretations of interdependent co-arising emphasize the interconnections or web-like nature of the process. That is, where the traditional view counsels disentanglement from the vicissitudes of life, current Buddhist perspectives encourage an engagement with life in all its amazing complexity. These perspectives also emphasize interbeing, a term offered by Hanh (2005, 2007) and one which shifts attention to the relational rather than self-focused attempts at transformation. In fact, by seeing that all beings are connected through thought, word, and action, the practice of transformation of the *kleshas* becomes even more urgent as an ethical necessity. Furthermore, engagement rather than distancing parallels the intention of mindfulness programs to connect with life in its entirety rather than withdraw from its challenges.

The third true reality is the acceptance that there is a way out, a way to address *dukkha,* and that the prognosis is good. This path out of the eternal cycle of interdependent co-arising is through the practice of extinguishing the three poisons. Typically referred to as attaining *nirvana/nibbana,* it is sometimes misunderstood to mean we simply stop feeling for and about everything. In some cases, it is held as a condition we strive for to transcend the trials of the world, be a dispassionate observer of all phenomena. However, because we are never outside the world and continue to be challenged by its vicissitudes as well as the multifactorial outcomes of interdependent co-arising, the transformational process is one that must be sustained continuously.

The fourth and most intricate true reality is the treatment for the arising of *dukkha* and ministration of the treatment protocol. The Eightfold Path comprises practices that cultivate discernment among actions, thoughts, and speech leading to wholesome ways of being as opposed to those resulting in unwholesome ones. The steps in the path are view, intention, speech, action, livelihood, effort, mindfulness, and concentration. They are designed to cultivate mental faculties that transform the three poisons and reverse the cycle of interdependent co-arising. Conventionally, each step in the Eightfold Path is referred to as "right" view, intention, and so on. However, to avoid implying a singular way of having a view, more flexible descriptors are used.

The practice of the Eightfold Path begins with the development of clear thinking or view and cultivation of clear intention; this is the wisdom factor of the path *(prajna/pranna)*. This cluster of the Eightfold Path also forms a feedback loop to the first noble truth by training the mental faculties to see the problem clearly and approach it with appropriate intentions. The second cluster of the Eightfold Path is made up of skillful speech, appropriate or ethical livelihood, and skillful action; this is the path of ethical conduct *(sila)*. It would be fair to say that actual mindfulness practice resides in this cluster as we negotiate through relationships with self, others, and the world. Along with the cultivation of clear view and intention creates the conditions for wise choices in transforming *dukkha*. The third and final cluster is meditation *(samadhi)* and is composed of well-directed diligence or effort, well-trained mindfulness, and cultivated concentration. This factor of the Eightfold Path is the technical aspect of practice; it feeds into and underlies the development of the other clusters. It provides a mental state that is calm and focused so that the interconnected relationship can be seen clearly and managed wisely.

Implied in the four true realities is the necessity for cultivating a clear, steady mind in order to meet our distress, taking personal responsibility for examining the cause of that distress which may include seeing our role in creating the distress, accepting the help that is available, and finally engaging in the process that alleviates the distress. As an explanatory model of how psychological intervention works, the four true realities articulate the process in psychotherapy and the issues a psychotherapist could encounter.

Despite its apparent simplicity, each of the steps requires in-depth therapeutic work and is a cauldron for resistances and projections. Buddhist psychology expands each of the steps through models of cause and effect all of which are complex and beyond the scope of this chapter. Mindfulness practices are both the process and content of developing an ethical way of being that in turn reduces the occurrence of *dukkha*. Ultimately, the intention in understanding the complex and interconnected systems of how psychological distress arises, endures, and can dissipate is to cultivate ethical choices that enhance well-being of self and others.

10.2 A Buddhist Perspective of Psychological Components in Mindfulness Programs

Mindfulness programs set the path of cultivating a more intimate relationship with our experience as a proximal goal with the ultimate outcome being a more intimate relationship with others and the world (Wyatt et al. 2014). Based on the tenet that *dukkha* arises because of reactive tendencies (attachment, aversion, and delusion; Bodhi 2008), mindfulness practices take up the intention of clarifying wisdom, ethics, and stabilizing skills so that whatever is present can be seen, touched, heard, tasted, smelled, and perceived in ways that are unclouded by preconditioned self-concepts, emotional dysregulation, and overburdened sense systems. That is, we take up the practice of mindfulness so that decisions and choices are wholesome, useful, and beneficial. Mindfulness programs typically focus on opening up tightly held self-perceptions, stabilizing emotional reactivity, and clarifying how triggers set off the physical and psychological systems.

10.2.1 Self-concept

Self is an intricate term that encompasses awareness of who we are through our actions and external events, our interconnectedness through relationships with others, and our sense of agency over our inner and outer environments (Baumeister 2011). Our knowledge of who we are, how we are in external and internal states, is a lens through which we view and evaluate our experience of positive or negative outcomes. Physical and mental illness impact our self-concepts as functional, independent, and perhaps even invulnerable individuals (Thoits 2013). Depending on the degree to which these self-perceptions are affected, it can play a role in our recovery (Markowitz 2001; Tekin 2011). In Western psychology, the concept of self contains a sense of agency and the presence of an agent, a doer of deeds, thinker of thoughts (see Tuske 2013 for discussion of nonself and the issues it raises for Western philosophy). A cultural perspective of independence and individuality directs the factors of this inner self and attaining an independent, separate selfhood has been considered the mark of personal development. In the context of cognitive theories, identity is defined by schema or aggregates of worth, characteristics, relationships with others, and aspirations in the world. A challenge to any one of these schema sends ripples of disruption through the identity, and the closer the schema is to an aspect of self that is valued, the more impact these ripples will have. Traditionally, psychological distress is viewed as our response to these challenges, typically framed as a response to a threat to self-constructs. Well-being is the restoration of the sense of self as whole or repaired.

Buddhist psychology takes what initially seems to be a diametrically opposed view by holding that no absolute, agentic self actually exists (Gethin 1992/2001, 1998). The Buddha's teachings on "no-self" have been the source of many, many debates over what he meant and how congruent it may be with Western ideas of self (Tuske 2013). Gowans (2003) and Harvey (2013c) describe the Buddha's teaching of nonself as contextual rather than absolute. In the quotidian, we may speak of an empirical self as a convenience to communication. This empirical self has no reality beyond serving as a device for relating ones mental and physical state. Beyond this, there is no substantive self that exists independent of the five aggregates or channels through which the world is experienced and is permanent. Just as every event or experience arises from an innumerable and unknowable number of causes and conditions, no single event or feature can completely locate or define a fixed self (Harvey 2013a). The intricacies of causes and conditions that mitigate against seeing self as fixed and unitary are perhaps the most important and useful aspect of mindfulness as a means of addressing psychological distress.

Most individuals experiencing psychological distress present for treatment with a sense of self that was viewed as solid and unchanging (Wyatt et al. 2014). Following a negative life event, such as illness, injury, or loss, this self is seen as damaged or changed in ways that are unacceptable. The desire is for treatment to return them to the state before the precipitating event and to fully understand the cause and effect so that it can be prevented from ever happening again. In Buddhist terms, this stance is one of delusion or a resistance to seeing what reality now exists. Grief for what was lost, wanting what cannot be retrieved, or demands for compensation for the loss can be seen as types of attachment to what we believe defines our self. Refusal to acknowledge limitations from injury, a diagnosis of physical or mental illness, or a rejection of treatment for manageable diseases such as diabetes or chronic illnesses reflect aversion or anger. Regardless of which root *klesha* is activated as a defense against seeing the consequences of our current state, the motivation to respond is based in the delusional belief that what was lost is what defined who the person was.

In Buddhist terms, what is perceived as self is a compilation of five aggregates *(skandhas/khandhas)* or channels through which the world is experienced: form, feelings/sensations (assessment of experiences as pleasant, unpleasant or neutral), perceptions (recognition of object), mental formations (opinions, preferences, ideas), and consciousness (self-awareness; Bodhi 2008; Gunaratana 2012). For example, an individual may report that they are aware (consciousness) of pain (sensation) in their broken leg (form). They see the situation as unfair (mental formation) because they cannot walk well enough (perception) to work and will become bankrupt (mental formation). Out of this flow of experience, a self that is defined by the circumstances as worthless emerges. Aversion to their circumstances leads to *dukkha* as they struggle with accepting their situation and may not make discerning choices that lead to well-being (wholesomeness). Alternatively, the situation may be one that seems positive on the surface. An athlete may see their physique (form) as something extremely pleasing (feeling) and admire the strength and muscular features of it (perception). They may assess their state as valued in the eyes of others or gaining admiration (mental formations) and be aware of the way they are admired (consciousness). In this scenario, a self that is valued for its specific form emerges. This attachment to form as a defining aspect of self leads to *dukkha* when time and events result in the inevitable changes of the body.

Attachment, aversion, or misperception of any combination of these five aggregates results in *dukkha,* whereas viewing them as fundamentally impermanent results in the insight that nothing uniquely defines a self that is enduring and sufficient. This understanding further leads to seeing experience as a ceaseless flow of body, emotions, sensations, and thoughts. Self then becomes an ever-changing property of what causes and conditions are present. It emerges as conditional to the flow of events and is not attached to any singular aspect. Thus, in the Buddhist perspective, self is multidimensional, mutifaceted, and multidetermined. It is flexible, adaptive, and creative; *dukkha* arises when it is perceived as contingent on a single thing, experience, or capacity to perform.

In a mindfulness treatment program, attachments to the way things were, rejection of how things are now, and confusion about the whys and what ifs are explored through dialogue with the participants. Inquiring with curiosity into perceptions and consciousness as well as explorations of mental formations and perceptions about events and responses to them create the space in which faulty perceptions can be observed and mental formations can be shifted (Kabat-Zinn 2013). Clinging to ideas shifts to releasing the mental rigidity; aversion and anger shift to approach and kindness; delusion and confusion shift to clarification and a willingness to be with not knowing what the outcome will be. As the concept of self evolves from a fixed definition of "this-is-who-I-am" to "just-this," illness and wellness are contained simultaneously without contradiction.

10.2.2 Emotion Regulation

Mindfulness practices offer the opportunity to be present to arising emotional states and to shift our relationship to them (Segal et al. 2012). Emotions are an essential part of making decisions, organizing actions to achieve goals, and can be adaptive and useful (Fairholme et al. 2010). However, suppression, avoidance, or lack of awareness of emerging (typically unpleasant) emotional states can result in decisions that are not adaptive or beneficial. Ekman and Davidson (1994) conceptualize emotions as arising from a confluence of cognitive, behavioral, and physiological responses to an external event or an internal. Most models of emotions and their expression involve awareness of sensations, ability to attend or be present to the experience, an appraisal system to determine the meaningfulness of the experience, all of which finally generate a response based on prior learning, exposure, and situational factors. Lazarus and Folkman (1984) placed emotions (affect) as part of a multimodal determination of experience involving behavior, affect (emotion), sensations, imagery, and cognition. Buddhist psychological understanding of emotions is similar in viewing emotions as what may be evoked by feeling tones but arise from mental formations (Analayo 2003; Gunaratana 2012).

All experiences evoke emotional responses. Someone who loses his job, a woman whose partner or child dies, a couple whose marriage breaks up, or a student who fails an important final exam experience emotions to varying degrees of intensity and which may be considered understandable given such loss. The specificity of the emotions is linked to the individuals' interpretation of the meaning of that event to them. The person who lost the job may respond with understandable anger if he felt unfairly treated; the woman responds with sorrow and grief as her loved ones die; the couple feels confusion if they feel wronged or misunderstood; and the student reacts with helplessness if he believes he put in the best effort he could. These are typical responses and considered normal in the face of the circumstances.

Dukkha arises when emotions are dysregulated; that is, they are over- or under-controlled in response to loss, pain, and other human conditions. A corollary of the root *kleshas,* attachment, aversion, and delusion/ignorance is that they both are and lead to emotionally driven, reactive actions and that reactivity reflects a level of emotional dysregulation. When an individual is caught in what is called an afflictive mental factor, their mind is clouded and it results in a misperception of what is actually transpiring internally and externally. From a general psychological perspective, when caught in the turmoil of attachment, the focus is primarily on reducing the threat of losing the object of our attachment and not on the reality of what that object of attachment is. For example, the person who lost his job may feel his self-worth as a provider threatened and not see that the job was not beneficial to his well-being. Initially, emotional distress is normal in a case of losing a job;

however, his attachment to self-perception as being a provider can lead to intensifying the emotional experience (fear, anger, frustration) and can lead to behaviors that may not be helpful such as quickly taking another job that is just as harmful to his health. Similarly, suppressing grief after the loss of a loved one in order to seem strong or intensifying anger through blame in case of a relationship breaking down are examples of emotional dysregulation or afflictive mental factors.

In Buddhist terms, these reactions reflect continuing to cling to aspects of self. The root *kleshas* fuel these negative emotions which in and of themselves are not inappropriate but that the rationale for viewing them as threats to our identity is based in a misperception. The normal grief for the loss of a partner or child is suppressed because its expression is believed to reflect badly on the individual. Confusion becomes an obstacle to finding a new job because the individual believes he is being negatively judged. Anger interferes with letting go of the relationship because of a belief that others are to blame. Problem solving for the student is limited because of a loss of confidence, which is part of his sense of self.

Although it appears to be predominantly a cognitive process, the initial reactivity is sparked from an inner experience of discomfort. Internal experiences such as sensations of tension, numbness, flutteriness can evoke reactive behaviors if prior learning has associated clusters of sensations with a specific negative emotion. Essentially an avoidance of the internal experience, it signals low distress tolerance or difficulty staying with an uncomfortable inner experience (see Boulanger et al. 2010 for detailed discussion of experiential avoidance). While it may be that negative emotions have their source in clusters of arising internal sensation, traditional therapies have focused on the external expressions of aggregated sensations such as depression, anxiety, and anger. As Aronson notes, however, in Buddhist approaches, emotions are not typically addressed, and the focus is more on using our experience to realize impermanence, transform the *kleshas,* and reverse the cycle of interdependent co-arising (Aronson 2004).

Nevertheless, the ability to stay with the internal sensations of emotions does become the purview of a Buddhist model of distress in that meditations train equanimity for inner experiences by simply noting feelings such as pleasant, unpleasant, and neutral in tone are present. As well, the concept of no-self mitigates against personalizing unpleasant experiences thereby creating a space between the experience and allowing for a skillful response to the experience. An additional benefit to the practice of noting sensations is the likelihood they can dissipate before dysregulation is activated. This cultivation of presence to unpleasant experience becomes very relevant in addressing the physiological aspects of stress in reducing reactivity to the experience itself.

10.2.3 Stress Models

Buddhist and Western conceptualizations of stress and distress vary and differences may be more related to their level of inquiry than an actual disjunction in concept. In Buddhist terms, all phenomena result in *dukkha* or distress; in fact, life as it is, or samsara, is *dukkha*. The central model of the causation of *dukkha* is worth repeating here because psychological distress infuses the cycle and begins with a misguided thinking process (Gunaratana 2012). The cycle of interconnected 12 links are the initial lack of awareness of the way *dukkha* arises, mental formations, consciousness, form, the arising sense phenomena, contact, clinging, attachment, self-making, and inevitably the rounds of (re)birth, old age, and death. In Buddhism, escaping or being liberated from this cycle constitutes the reduction or better, the cessation of stress/distress. While it is possible to be liberated from the process of clinging and attachment and become someone able to live well, the commitment is to be fully liberated from the entire cycle. Western perspectives of stress/distress might be seen as addressing a section of the cycle of the generation of *dukkha,* that is, treating the connections from ignorance and mental formations to attachment while leaving issues of (re)birth, old age, and death to spiritual and medical practitioners.

Endocrinologist Seyle (1974) was among the first to investigate and define stress (he later noted it was better referred to as "strain") as the physiological response regardless of the positive or negative nature of the stimulus and that pathological outcomes occur when the stress is unremitting. Later models include McEwen's (2002) model of allostatic load, which more closely aligns with the idea that strain on an existing biological system results in its eventual breakdown. Porges' (2011) polyvagal theory posits a complex model of neural regulation of the autonomic system. Relevant to the earlier discussion of sensations and their evolution into *dukkha* is the proposal in the polyvagal theory of neuroception as the mechanism through which defensive stances are triggered. According to Porges (2007), external events and intentionality in social contexts are appraised via neuroception and discerned for their threat value, which activates the appropriate response, defense, or engagement.

The human system has evolved to be adaptive to both low- and high-threat environments, and the neural system is staged to appraise the degree of safety in a hierarchical manner with the higher cognitive functions able to override lower "primitive" systems in responses to threat. Tempering the upregulation of the nervous system when under stress or threat and activating the downregulation to reestablish homeostasis relies on a well-functioning feedback system. Typically, under prolonged stress, the lower appraisal system is reinforced to be highly active and the feedback provides what can be seen as misperceived levels of threat.

Although still being tested as a viable theory that supports a neurobiological role in emotional responses and a source for social engagement behaviors, Porges' theory offers several conceptual hooks to understand the cycle of stress and distress. Most important to this exploration of Buddhist principles that underlie clinical mindfulness is that an accurate appraisal of threat may not necessarily lead to a discernment of wholesome action. For example, neuroceptive appraisal of low threat can still result in activation of sensations that aggregate to anxiety-based responses, or high threat appraisals may not inhibit engagement in the situation (Porges 2007). In other words, visceral awareness is insufficient to make wise or wholesome choices if clear comprehension of the situation is absent.

Equally relevant to developing a Buddhist perspective on clinical mindfulness, polyvagal theory proposes that calming of the activated system and soothing behaviors can be elicited via the autonomic nervous system. This proposal suggests breath-related meditations play a role in calming and soothing, a state that is important at a physiological level so that cognitive processes have access to clear incoming information. A psychophysiological perspective also opens the door to viewing clinical issues as multifaceted and the need for integrating biological, physiological, and psychological factors as important contributors. Furthermore, it removes the implication that symptomatic relief through mindfulness practice is a shallow and ignoble goal; from the perspective of the polyvagal theory, addressing symptoms (or more precisely the sensations that arise as symptoms) plays an important role in reducing reactivity.

10.3 Foundational Dharma Teachings in Mindfulness Programs

The attainment of liberation depends on the realization of the causes and conditions that give rise to *dukkha*. That is, the crucial step towards liberation is to cultivate discernment of what is a fabrication of desire (clinging and attachment, aversion and anger). To set out on this path, we first begin to train the mind to calm and then to see clearly so that wisdom in the form of discernment can develop.

The cultivation of tranquil calm states is called *samatha* practice and the cultivation of wisdom is called *vipassana* practice. Together these form the foundational practices. However, it is important to be aware that there is an ongoing discussion whether *samatha* (single-pointed meditation developed in the first stages of the *Anapanasati Sutta*) and *vipassana* (cultivation of insight as in the later stages of the *Anapanasati* and the *Satipatthana Suttas*) together are required to attain *nivarna* or if *vipassana* is sufficient. Mills (2004) argued that the interaction of *samatha*-plus-*vipassana* are required otherwise true discernment and moral concern for others is not likely to arise. Turning to the Pali Cannon, we read of the Buddha using the simile of a crossroads at which sits the lord of the city (consciousness) who is approached by "a swift pair of messengers" (*samatha* and *vipassana*) conveying a message "in accordance to reality" (teachings on *nibbana*; SN 35.245; Bodhi 2000). While recognizing that such debates are important, for the purposes of this discussion, we will rely on the Buddha's teachings that both arrive at the same time to perform their duties.

The two primary *suttas* referenced in mindfulness programs are the *Anapanasati* and *Satipatthana Suttas,* awareness of breathing and four ways to establish mindfulness, respectively. Analayo (2013) raised some questions about the *Anapanasati Sutta*'s guidance with respect to their logic and intention; however, these intriguing inquiries are beyond the scope of this discussion (see Chap. 4). The *Anapanasati* and *Satipatthana Suttas* are typically read as working hand in hand to cultivate meditation through the awareness of the breath and mindfulness of body, feeling, mind, and phenomena as its full practice (see Chap. 5). Rarely mentioned or written about together as a practice framework, Hanh's (2006, 2009a) commentaries on the two sutras are likely the most accessible in both exploring and integrating them as a protocol of practice.

Mindfulness programs tend to focus on the principles of the *Satipatthana* primarily, and *vipassana* is the primary meditative approach (Cullen 2011). However, the content of the *Satipatthana* is not immediately obvious in most clinical programs. That is not to say a mindfulness program's curriculum should walk in lockstep with the *suttas;* the experiential and clinical aspects of such programs necessarily take precedence. Yet, it is important to hold these teachings in the forefront in order to understand how mindfulness is to be facilitated and to address issues that may arise in its subtly complex practice.

10.3.1 Anapanasati Sutta

The Buddha taught the *Anapanasati Sutta,* also called the *sutta* on mindfulness of breathing, as the base practice which brings the *Satipatthana* to fruition (Buddhadasa 1976; Hanh 2009a). Elegantly set up, the 16 stages beginning from awareness of the breath itself and ending with liberation from attachments and craving are organized as 4 tetrads of meditations that tuck into the 4 ways to establish mindfulness *(Satipattthana)*. There are several excellent commentaries available on the nuances and details of this important *sutta* (Buddhadasa 1976; Hanh 2009a). The following section is a synopsis of the tetrads and integrates the teachings into components of a mindfulness program.

The framework of the *Anapanasati Sutta* is deceptively simple; however, to assume the practice is equally simple would be a mistake. Despite appearing linear and steplike, the process is actually iterative with later stages doubling back on the first ones. The first and second tetrads, each consisting of four stages of meditation, develop awareness of the in- and out-breath, the length of breath, awareness of the body, and the perceptions and mental formations that arise from the body. Buddhadasa (1976) explained that this tetrad is the most crucial to the practice and should be explored in detail. Stages I and II of the first tetrad are considered the preparative stages for practice and the implication is that we are practicing ethics by virtue of restraint; the attention being on the breath prevents unwholesome actions, thoughts, and speech when in a meditative state. They invite the practitioner to be aware of the breath as it enters and exits the nostrils and then to be aware of the shortness and length of the breath.

The effect of the length of the breath on the state of mind and body is also observed. Buddhadasa (1976) noted that a normal state of mind is associated with easeful, long breaths, and the practice is on noting how the breath will change and be an indicator of our circumstances. This observation becomes useful in teaching mindfulness as it links the physiological, physical, and emotional states of the practitioner. In this stage of practice, the mind is trained to be "tethered" to the breath and weaned away from its typical distractions. The practice is primarily one of concentration training; nevertheless, it cultivates associated qualities of zeal, gladness in its realization, single-pointed mind, equanimity, full awareness of the experience, and the physical body.

In stages III and IV, awareness of the body is developed through the observation of the impact of breathing on the body and the arising insights to impermanence, *dukkha,* and no-self. The breath is seen as conditioning the physical body as the body sustains its mental states. This sense of fully knowing the in- and out-breath in the body is the first way to establish mindfulness of the body in the body (see section on *Satipatthana* below). Beginning with stage III and continuing to stage VIII, the cultivation of ethics, concentration, and wisdom comes to the fore.

In mindfulness programs, meditation instructions tend to be brief with the intention of allowing the participant to explore the process freely. However, it would be useful to address some aspects of stage I and II overtly to avoid misunderstanding or misdirection. When attending to the breath, for example, practitioners notice that the act of bringing attention to the breath results in a tension or a change in the length and depth of the breathing. The *Anapanasati Sutta* invites experimentation with placing attention on the breath and the expansion/contraction of chest and abdomen during the in- and out-breath cycles and observing the outcome. The mind in its untethered state is easily distracted and this often leads to frustration for beginning meditators. The metaphors of training a puppy to sit and stay, or guiding a friend back to the path, are helpful. It is also helpful to indicate that returning to the breath is an active choice to turn away from mental activity that is unhelpful. At this level of practice, the breath is also being connected to the body, as a conditioner of the body.

The second tetrad, stages V to VIII, follows the same formula and uses feeling tones (pleasant, unpleasant, neutral) as the object of meditation. It is a practice that leads knowing the nature and characteristics of experience. As awareness of feeling is trained, perception of that feeling being "my feeling" becomes connected to it and that is followed by thoughts of whether it is negative or positive. It is in these connections that the cycle of interdependent co-arising is relevant because the value given to the feeling gives way to craving and attachment. The connection of breath to feeling allows the observation of the cognitive process of perceiving what is felt and how preferences (wanting what is pleasant, aversion to unpleasant) arise and cease.

From a clinical perceptive, stages V–VII offer entry for practice to issues of distress avoidance and emotion dysregulation. These stages offer a mental processing model for the way in which the preferential mind arises and offers insight to the approach/avoidance tendencies. Revisiting the cycle, sense impressions (the contact of an object with the six senses) lead to feeling which in turn results in perception of the object typically as personal ("my"). This then results in a (cognitive) valuation of the experience as good or bad. In pain-related experiences, the sense impressions can project rapidly to a personalization of pain and an appraisal of pain being bad or unwanted. Aversion evokes various avoidance behaviors that may be temporarily helpful. However, these actions condition the body to react with tension and thereby sustain the cycle of distress avoidance.

Stage VIII is a practice of using the breath to disengage from a runaway thinking process or any experience of overwhelming perception or feeling. In effect, the practitioner cycles back to stage I and reconfirms the technique of breathing until the coarse breath becomes fine and subtle. The difference from the practice in stage I is that the object of meditation is the perception and feeling, not the breath. The feeling and perception are said to become calmed as well, by which is meant that their distractive capacity is reduced and they have less power to hijack thinking. This tetrad is folded into the second way to establish mindfulness of feelings in the feelings.

The third and fourth tetrads focus on the states of mind. The third tetrad, stages IX–XII, is practice in opening to the mind as being impermanent, *dukkha,* and having no-self. To accomplish this, the previous strategies are used for noting and conditioning the mind. As confidence in the process grows and results are experiences in terms of both concentration and calming the mind, a satisfaction of the mind arises. Insight arises as well in relation to the nature of our experience, its history, chronicity, and trajectory. It is important not to lose sight that this practice is consistently unfolding in the context of the Eightfold Path and that the cultivation of ethics, concentration, and wisdom are the base of practice. Ultimately, the full awareness of the mind results in liberating it from its own sense impressions and from ignorance that opens the cycle of interdependent co-arising. This stage of practice is also considered the culmination of the moral training, a transformation of the attitudes and behaviors that form an obstacle to mindfulness. This tetrad is connected to the third way to establish mindfulness of the mind in the mind.

The fourth tetrad, stages XIII–XVI, focuses on the development of the practitioner's mental state so that the nature of all phenomena can be understood. This tetrad is associated with the fourth way to establish mindfulness of phenomena. Here, the awareness is on the flow of experience and its aim is the cultivation of wisdom or insight to experience as impermanent, constantly fading, ceases, and can be let go. Through contemplation of the five aggregates, six internal sense bases, and interdependent co-arising, insight to the constantly changing nature of our experience is attained, not as an intellectual exercise but as an inner experience.

Hanh (2009a) described this stage as seeing the wave and the water. Although waves form and have many different sizes and shapes, they rise and fall, appear and disappear. Yet they do not lose their essence as water. He also points out that this final stage is a bittersweet one. We may feel pessimistic by its message of impermanence that to most of us means loss. We can also see the potential of joy in realizing that everything is interconnected and that we are not limited by and can be liberated from our concepts of status, possessions, or relationships. This insight facilitates letting go of anxiety, fear, anger, and all the things that form the basis of craving and attachment.

In the context of a mindfulness program with all its demands for alleviation of *dukkha,* it is important to note that there can be pressure to leap forward into content of the third and fourth tetrads by pointing to the "good news" of liberation from *dukkha* or to use that possibility as an enticement to practice. However, this distracts from and becomes an obstacle to practice. The iterations through breath, body, feeling, and mind are crucial building blocks from which insight to phenomena arises. These last two tetrads, being concerned with cultivating wholesome states of mind, require a process of observing the impact of negative states of mind. There can be a reluctance to turn towards such inner experience; however, it is important to convey that knowing these negative states are present is an important practice (*dhukkha,* the first true reality of all beings). Accepting the reality of depression, anxiety, grief, and so on are the first step to knowing what needs to be healed.

This is a complex *sutta* and, like most Buddhist teachings, is intricately intertwined with other teachings. To convey all of its complexity in a mindfulness program would be burdensome; however, familiarity—experiential and intellectual—with its intentions as it cultivates each stage of meditative capacity is important. Questions and experiences arise about the usefulness of meditation throughout a mindfulness program and, because there is a strong emphasis on sitting meditation, a facilitator needs to be reasonably versed in the intent and purpose of the *Anapanasati Sutta.*

10.3.2 *Satipatthana Sutta*

The *Satipatthana Sutta* is likely the central teaching on the cultivation of mindfulness in the Theravada tradition. Step by step, it cultivates awareness of the body, feeling, mind, and all phenomena of mind; each of these can be thought of as platforms on which mindfulness rests or ways in which to establish mindfulness (Goldstein 2013). However, the cultural use of this *sutta* is not without controversy. Sharf (2013) pointed out that this dominance of the *Satipatthana* is a recent phenomenon and related to attempts by Burmese meditation teachers to make Buddhism more accessible to lay persons. This attempt shifted the emphasis from *samatha* and developing higher levels of consciousness *(jhānas)* to "bare awareness" of the flow of our experience and the idea of living in the moment. Sharf and McMahan (2008) noted that these concepts form the foundations of Buddhist modernism and now is transcultural. Nevertheless, as the primary framework of current uses of mindfulness practice, it is important to examine the structure of the *sutta* and, perhaps more important, its approach in cultivating mindfulness.

Gunaratana (2012), Hanh (2006), Goldstein (2013), Silananda (2002), and Analayo (2003, 2013) have written several excellent commentaries; the books by the first three authors are accessible for the general practitioner, while the latter two authors present a scholarly approach. Hanh (2006) and Analayo (2003) have examined the terms *ekayana* and *Satipatthana. Ekayana* or *ekayano maggo* is determined as "one path" or the "direct path leading to one goal." *Sati* is translated as mindfulness or awareness with *upatthana* meaning attending. Mindfulness then is rendered as "attending to the current situation" (Analayo 2003, p. 29). Sharf (2013), drawing from a number of sources including Gethin (1992/2001), indicated that *sati* imparts a sense of "remembering," not as memory, but as a recall of an interconnectedness of all things skillful and unskillful. In that context, *sati* conveys a discernment of wholesome from unwholesome actions that are accessed in the vast web of recalled experiences. Important to practice yet rarely mentioned in mindfulness programs, the refrain of the *Satipatthana* fosters a positive environment for practice. It is a repeated reminder of the essentials of the practice: contemplate inner, outer, and both inner and outer experiences; contemplate the nature of impermanence; recognize what is unfolding in this moment without mental discourse; and let go of clinging to any one event that arises in our mental or physical realm of experience (Goldstein 2013). Drawing primarily from Analayo's (2003) translation and commentaries, we now examine the four ways to establish mindfulness and their relevance to contemporary interventions.

The first way to establish mindfulness is to cultivate mindfulness of the body. In the *Anapanasati Sutta,* this is the first tetrad, which focuses on breath and how it conditions the body. The practice as described in the *Satipatthana* cultivates mindfulness through awareness of breathing, body postures (sitting, lying down, walking), its activities, and details of its composition. One intention of this practice is to bring awareness of the physical aspects of our body, suspending preference and judgment. The purpose is not to separate body from mind but rather to see the body as an intricate set of related parts that function best when closely attended. A second intention of this practice, which can include some contemplations we might find unpleasant, is to bring into awareness all aspects of the body—pleasant, unpleasant, and neutral to our conception. It aims at reducing the desire for the pleasant parts and aversion to unpleasant parts of our physical nature. This in turn reduces the discursive thoughts, deepens concentration, and allows insight to arise.

In clinical mindfulness, bringing attention to the body is a trigger for aversion. Typically, participants in a mindfulness program are attending because they have met with significant physical challenges through physical or chronic illness or injury. They may also be disconnected with their body because of emotional experiences connected to the body. These can range from experiences of anger and anxiety to experiences of sexual or physical abuse resulting in post-trauma symptoms. The protective and defensive stance to their situation is to use distraction, denial, or an alternate hyperintense experience. Bringing attention to the source of their suffering with all its psychological issues (feeling betrayed by the body) may not feel like a possible or useful approach. The concept of equalizing pleasant and unpleasant aspects of the body is a beneficial practice for a less combative presence to it. Practice with the breath also offers insight to the ever-changing flow of physically based experiences and the observation of how the breath conditions the body is likely to be very useful. As noted in the *Anapanasati Sutta,* the breath becomes more fine and subtle, the body calms, and discursion diminishes along with its attendant distraction. We feel less yoked to our body and at its mercy; our concepts of the body as ill or globally malfunctioning are moderated by a view that is more balanced with aspects that are functioning well.

The second way to establish mindfulness is to cultivate mindfulness of feeling. In Buddhist terms, feeling *(vedana)* implies knowing or experiencing and includes bodily and mental feelings. It can be confusing initially because in Western terms "feeling" refers to emotions; here, it means pleasant, unpleasant, or neutral tones of an experience. Emotions are considered a state of mind and relegated to the next section of the *Satipattahana.* The practice is one of noting that initial moment of assessment: Is this pleasant? Is this unpleasant? Is this neutral? The intent is to capture that momentary experience before the appraisal system activates and our preferential mind creates a reaction. Analayo (2013) suggested this level of attention might allow access to our intuitive sense, that moment of "I knew (I felt there was something wrong)" which we tend to dismiss after the cognitive process takes over. Another intention is to discern whether the feeling is activating old habits that tend towards unhealthy choices. Again, this reflects the link of the cycle of interdependent co-arising where craving and attachment are activated based on pleasant or unpleasant feelings.

Working with unpleasant and pleasant feeling in a clinical context connects back to the tendency for emotional dysregulation discussed above. Avoidance of what is unpleasant and craving what was pleasant result in irritation, frustration, and generally negative emotions. Neutral feeling is of particular interest in clinical populations for two reasons. First, in groups who are disconnected or dissociated from their inner unpleasant experiences, most feelings may be relegated inaccurately to feeling nothing or numb. Not being aware of what is arising often leads to an experience only being felt when it is intense and therefore not immediately manageable, for example, anxiety and physical pain. This in turn triggers a cycle of overcontrolling the unpleasant experience, which only surfaces again unpredictably. Second, neutrality may not be seen as part of the overall experience. Most individuals who experience pain or anxiety report that their experience "comes out of the blue" or "comes and goes without reason." That is, the experience arises as an unpleasant one and then disappears (perhaps after hours of suffering) only to start again. They may note that the period in-between pain surges are spent in worry and tension, anticipating the next round. When they can note the full round of an experience in which unpleasant feeling arises, endures, dissipates, and then is followed by a brief moment of transition, a neutral space, impermanence is apparent. In this neutral zone, the breath is able to have a foothold and the opportunity for better choices arises.

The third way to establish mindfulness is by contemplation of the mind. There are intense debates about the definition of mind, its location, and its function. Mind here is defined as consciousness whose function is awareness (Gunaratana 2012) and it is present in every aspect of experience just as heat is present in every part of a chili pepper. It arises from contact between an object and the senses giving rise to a sense-consciousness. In other words, it arises from innumerable causes and conditions, is impermanent, and is only known by its impact on the body and feelings. In this stage of the *Satipatthana,* awareness of the quality of what arises as mental events is cultivated through the qualities of ardency, clear comprehension, mindfulness itself, and concentration. Also called forth in the previous two ways of establishing mindfulness, these mental qualities are likely most necessary in contemplating the mind with its tendencies to be colored by the five aggregates (of which it is a part as well) and veer towards attachment, aversion, and delusion/ignorance.

The third stage of the *Satipatthana* is perhaps the most obvious in its applicability and usefulness in a mindfulness program. Buddhist and Western psychology have a common ground in acknowledging the powerful role of mental events in physical and mental health. There is an important distinction however in where they enter to the aspect of mind. Cognitive-based therapies examine and work with the content of mind, that is, thoughts and thinking patterns. In the *Satipatthana,* the specific contents are viewed as impermanent and the focus of intervention is the quality of the contents or event in the mind. If the content leads to poor choices, negative outcomes, or further deepening the cycle of dependent co-arising, then the response is not to challenge the irrational nature of the mental event or its sequelae. It is to cultivate antidotes for the attachment, aversion, and delusion/ignorance they activate. The intervention is transdiagnostic and not limited by details of any individual's personal history or event. This is useful as a guide consistent with the principles of mindfulness programs, which cultivate the experience of the event and not the story woven about it.

The fourth way to establish mindfulness is to contemplate the ways in which experience arises. The five hindrances, five aggregates, six sense spheres are the focus of practice, and the intention is to clarify and transform the impediments to awakening. Buddhist psychology places primary value in the way our perception forms the entirety of our experiences including the experience of self. This cycle is conditioned by our desires and preferences and is, for the most part, distorted and preserving of a self. The intention of practice is to unwind from the initiating stimuli that lead to the cycle of conditioning and see reality.

In a mindfulness program, the five hindrances (desire, anger, sloth and torpor, restlessness and worry, and doubt) provide grist for the mill. The hindrances arise after the first week of home practice and endure in various ways providing a wealth of opportunities to encourage observation of how they trigger frustration, anxiety, and avoidance. The five aggregates also provide opportunity to examine our perceptions of who we are, who we think we are, and how that results in the choices we make for ourselves. This is the central context of a mindfulness program and fostering the qualities of ardency, clear comprehension, mindfulness, and concentration can be supportive and encouraging for participants.

The practice of *Satipatthana* establishes an ardent, concentrated mindfulness that cultivates clearly understanding our experiences and their outcomes. The Eightfold Path of wisdom, ethics/virtue, and concentration is embedded in each stage, and it is the focal point of the practice. The core of this teaching is that we are refining a way of remembering all in our past that brought about *dukkha* and its cessation, temporary as this latter may have been. The *Satipatthana* framework is quite explicit in noting that the intention and focus is the cultivation of discernment and the transformation of the three poisons. In other words, we are cultivating our ability to speak, think, and act in ways that do not perpetuate the creation of *dukkha* for others and ourselves. This development of a moral stance to our relationships is the practice of *sila* or virtue ethics (Harvey 2000; Keown 2005). In the contemporary use of mindfulness, there are many discussions specifically related to the cultivation of ethics (McCown 2013; Monteiro et al. 2014, 2010) and its seeming absence.

Hanh's version of ethics practice, the Five Mindfulness Trainings (Hanh 2007) and the Fourteen Mindfulness Trainings (Hanh 2005) for his formal students, are ways in which ethics can be practiced. Monteiro et al. (2010) and Cayoun (2011) describe other ways of integrating ethics into a mindfulness program.

10.4 Subtle Dharma Teachings in Mindfulness Programs

10.4.1 Teachings from Theravada

Two significant *suttas* play a role in mindfulness programs but are typically not prominently mentioned. The first addresses the misunderstanding about emotional states and how they are activated. In the discussion above on emotional dysregulation, it was noted to be an important rationale for cultivating mindfulness practices. The dyad of the *Theranamo* and *Bhaddekaratta Suttas* offer a framework by which to understand the intention of practice and how feelings are actually transformed in the context of human relationships. The second teaching is from the *Metta Sutta,* a popular practice however not always addressed in mindfulness programs as a cultivation of a moral conduct. Its role as one of the four *brahma-viharas* is also important in developing a balanced practice of mindfulness.

A Solitary Life The *Theranamo Sutta* (SN 21.10; Bodhi 1995) tells of the Buddha's instructions to an elder monk in the *sangha* who had a preference for living in isolation. When the *sangha* expressed concerns about the monk Theranamo, the Buddha spoke with him to inquire about his chosen way of life. Hanh's (2011) commentary draws together the *Theranamo* (SN 21.10), *Bhaddekaratta* (MN 131-14), and *Migajala* (SN 35.63) *Suttas* to expand the Buddha's teachings that living a solitary life, cut off from others does not result in peace or freedom from distress. The Buddha pointed out that even in such solitary conditions, we are in the company of our craving, attachment, and other mental states (SN 35.63; Bodhi 1995). We are still bound by our mental formations, delusions, and the six senses. Rather than rejecting the world, which we inaccurately assume causes our distress, a better way to live alone is to free ourselves from craving and attachment. In that way, we truly are living away from the source of our *dukkha.*

In the context of emotional regulation, these *suttas* address our tendency to control our external environment in order to feel emotional stability. It is not uncommon for participants to lay the source of their distress in the external aspects of their lives. It is the spouse, children, boss, traffic, illness, or life itself (viewed as something separate from themselves) that is the cause of anxiety, depression, anger, and helplessness. It is also common to hear that they would like to eradicate emotions, not feel so much, or be indifferent to the arrows that trigger pain and suffering. They would like to "get rid" of "their" anger, depression, panic attacks because these are the actual causes of their distress. Past and future are also seen as sources of distress.

Memories of painful events and worry about what might be painful events to come are powerful triggers of suffering in the present.

As their experiential tolerance increases through the course, this better way to live alone becomes more apparent. The cause of *dukkha* is no longer external to such an absolute extent. It is now experienced as internally generated or interactive. As the true source of suffering is understood and the capacity to be attentive to it in the present increases, past and future take their place as mental events. The liberation for participants in a mindfulness program is not only from the distress of feeling vulnerable to a world full of triggers but also from actual social isolation or desperate need to connect without discernment of the quality of relationships.

Metta and Its Companions The *Metta Sutta* or loving-kindness meditation is likely one of the most beloved practice in Buddhism. It is said that the Buddha taught *metta* to monks who were living in the forest and were afraid of tree deities who were trying to scare them out of the forest (Sn 1.8). The practice of *metta* was intended implicitly to cultivate moral conduct in the face of challenges. In other discourses, the Buddha's teachings address the impact of anger (AN 7:60), resentment and negative speech (MN 21 & 128) and the cultivation of good-will as their cessation (see Buddhaghosa 2010 for consolidation of discourses). Gunaratana (2001) described *metta* as loving-friendliness, a quality of mind that can only be cultivated when we relinquish our rigid views and confused thinking. Chodron (2001) connected aggression and suffering to ignorance, the first link in the cycle of interdependent co-arising. She noted that in order to transform *dukkha,* we need to recognize our interconnectedness to realize that what we wish for ourselves, others would also wish for themselves.

The practice of *metta* is sometimes a difficult one for mindfulness program participants to embrace. The sequential offering of *metta* to loved ones, neutral persons, those who have hurt us, and then to all beings can elicit resistance and feelings of frustration or confusion. Sometimes, the practice of offering *metta* to someone who has caused hurt is not included if there is reason to believe it would be a trigger for emotional reactivity. However it may be offered in the session, *metta* practice is fertile ground for teaching moments and discussions of self-care and other care. Participants discover that it is easier to offer to other than to themselves or that having offered it to themselves they touch the level of depletion they feel.

Metta is also one of the four *brahma-viharas* or "limitless qualities" of mind (Chodron 2001); the other three are compassion, equanimity, and resonant joy. It is important to practice all four *brahma-viharas* (SN 46.54; Bodhi 2000) as an interconnected set of moral stances. Compassion *(karuna)* is defined as the ability to be with one's own or another's suffering. It plays a significant role in cultivating a sense of connectedness; it is differentiated from empathy, which carries an implication of resonating with the other's suffering. Compassion has been related to the capacity to activate a sense of feeling safe (safeness) and the ability to tolerate distress (Gilbert 2005, 2009). A growing practice is one of self-compassion, which is the cultivation of our stance to ourselves as we suffer. It is also a mindfulness training program in and of itself (Germer 2009; Gilbert 2009; Neff 2011).

Equanimity *(upekkha)* is the capacity to see beyond the layers of perception and mental formation into the essential interconnectedness of all things. Young (2011) described equanimity as a stage of mind that does not impede the experience of pleasant or unpleasant feelings. Thus, the feelings retain their untainted ability to motivate, inform, and direct skillful actions. In mindfulness programs, this capacity is necessary to reduce reactivity not only to emotional distress but also to physical pain.

Unselfish joy *(mudita)* is the ability to feel joy in another's joy. In the cultivation of unselfish joy, Buddhaghosa (2010) recommended not beginning with a loved one because *mudita* is not intended to arise out of the experience of mutual care. He recommended beginning with a good friend, progressing to a neutral person and then a hostile one. This progressive mode of practice eventually cultivates impartiality towards categories of beings that have formed as a result of our mental formations and perceptions. Monteiro and Musten (2013) proposed that in order to appreciate others' joy regardless of the quality of relationship we have with them, we must first have cultivated the capacity to clearly know our own joy. In that sense, the term "resonant" joy coveys the idea that we understand the other person would feel joy and our understanding is independent of our feelings towards them.

10.4.2 Teachings from Mahayana

Kabat-Zinn (2011) described MBSR as rooted in the Theravada and Zen traditions (Soto and Rinzai). According to Kabat-Zinn, the teacher–student relational process of *koan* work was the inspiration for the teacher–participant dialogue of inquiry that occurs in mindfulness programs. Part Socratic, part verbal *akido,* the inquiry aims to clear away the detritus of the delusional thinking process to expose the clear knowing of our experience as it is happening. It strives to undermine an external authority, an expert who has the answers. Although there are no details of which teachings from Zen play a specific role in mindfulness programs, it is not difficult to see that some concepts addressed above in the Theravada teachings also have a Mahayana/Zen parallel. Rahula (1978), despite a somewhat argumentative stance towards Mahayana teachings, connects Zen with the *Anapanasati* and *Satipatthana Suttas* and many other teachings on attaining *arahhantship* or enlightenment.

Within Zen teachings proper, there are frameworks that help to clarify the process of mindfulness practice. Kapleau (1980) described Yasutani's three essentials of Zen practice as cultivating great faith, great doubt, and great effort. As our practice unfolds, we learn to doubt the face value of our experience. We begin to suspect that there is an intrinsic wellness/goodness in which we can have faith. Because of that faith, we expend great effort to know truly the reality of our experience. These three Zen essentials unfold in the process of mindfulness programs.

The *Prajnaparamita,* Lotus, and Diamond sutras, among many others, offer deep insight into interbeing, loving-kindness, and the ephemeral nature of experience (Conze 1958; Hanh 2009b, 2010; Pine 2001; Tamura 2014). Mahayana sutras however pose a challenge in application to mindfulness approaches simply because of their complex and often tightly woven metaphoric nature. As challenging as it can be for mindfulness program teachers to both grasp and apply the Theravada *Suttas,* the challenge of doing so with the Mahayana/Zen texts can be just as daunting. Nevertheless, a solid acquaintance with the essence of the primary Mahayana/Zen *sutras* is important to providing an overarching perspective of the essence of a mindfulness program.

10.4.3 Zen Koan Principles and Practice

Kabat-Zinn's (2011) connection of *koan* practice and the teacher–participant relationship in mindfulness interventions creates a space for participants to explore their experience without fear of judgment or censure. Understanding Zen *koan* principles helps to encourage this exploration in two ways. First, *koan* study is an intricate process of relationship - building between teacher and student (Loori 2006b) and the face-to-face inquiries lead to letting go of our typical intellectual and philosophical approaches (Yamada 2005). As in the teacher–student relationship in *koan* practice, the mindfulness teacher conveys that every aspect of an experience is legitimate material for inquiry. Unlike the sometimes confrontational or unruly forms in Zen *koan* practice, but in keeping with professional conduct guidelines, the teacher's role of pulling the rug out from under the student takes on a softer aspect of turning the participant towards their intellectual assumptions or experiential state.

Second, Zen *koans* are useful as a device to foster the "don't know" mind (Sahn 1997). As teaching stories or frameworks for inquiring into the nature of our experience, *koans* are a rich source of encouragements to move beyond the mental constructions and directly connect with the experience in the moment. Below are two *koans* that offer insight to typical struggles among participants of a mindfulness program and an overarching model that informs the intention of taking such a program.

Sen-jo's Reality *Koans* are conventionally pithy sketches of dialogue or a scenario through which teachings are transmitted. *Koans* can also come as stories; Caplow and Moon (2013) have compiled twenty-five centuries of narratives by and about women teachers that shine the light on many aspects of our life. The story of Sen-jo and her soul is one; a Chinese folk tale (Aitken 1991; Shibayama 2000; Yamada 2005) about a young woman who decides to leave her parents and an arranged marriage in order to be with the man she loves. Stricken with homesickness and guilt after many years away, she and her husband return only to find her parents confused when she claims to be their daughter. As far as they know, Sen-jo has been in their home all these years, lying in her bed unable to engage with her filial duties or her life. The question is asked: Which is the real Sen-jo?

The question posed by Zen teachers is not about the literal or metaphoric reuniting of Sen-jo with her soul but an inquiry into the idea of dualistic identity (Arnold 2004). Inherent in the question is the implication that the split is real and that resolving the conundrum requires determining which part is truly real and which is fantasy or dream. This overlooks the story material that wraps around the *koan* and it fails to appreciate that the paradox in the story is imposed by our own separation from ourselves (Hori 2006; R. Sasaki quoted in Loori 2006a).

Sen-jo presents us with a direct experience of the delusions that arise when we are asleep to who we are and the joy when we are awake. The components of her story also touch on duty, commitment, an honest desire for a loving relationship, and a wish to be a valued part of community. These themes wrap around the *koan* and inform us of the structure that supports our life. However, the deeper structures of the story are the assumptions and beliefs we hold about who we are and how easily we can be taken apart.

Dukkha arises when we experience ourselves as separated from who we believe we are and from others around us. We attempt to resolve this suffering by various means; in both Buddhist and clinical terms, we engage in denial, obsessions, and mental and physical addictions. We fail to see that the dualism between one self and the other is an illusion, albeit a sometimes helpful illusion. The real question therefore is not which is real Sen-jo but rather how can Sen-jo's experiences and actions become a pilgrimage of identity (Whyte 2001) so she can exist fully and in alignment with each of her roles.

It is typical in clinical mindfulness programs to hear participants speak of their loss of identity. Their experiences with depression and anxiety construct selves of hopelessness and helplessness; injuries that result in loss of mobility and functionality generate beliefs of worthlessness. As painful as the life event can be, *dukkha* is created when the reality of its occurrence and what that means are resisted by clinging to the past, aversion to the present, and confusion about the future. It manifests as the desire to find and reunite with the healthy self. This belief that a split has occurred creates a misperception of life as dualistic: good/bad, pain/no pain, and healthy/ill. It is to this dharma door that the clinician as mindfulness teacher can invite participants to engage in an exploration of impermanence and identity as fluid and ever changing. Similar to the story of Sen-jo, the stories that wrap around the suffering are peeled away; identities as whole, complete, and all the absolute terms are themselves deconstructed. The states of sleep and wakefulness to experience as it unfolds are examined.

Ox Herding The second *koan* that is useful to understand the overarching theme of mindfulness is the story of the ox and its herder. The "taming of the bull" describes our spiritual journey through art and poetry in which the bull or ox is our mind and the herder is the practitioner who seeks to tame that mind. In some renditions, the ox is our Buddha nature not yet realized and in this guise as an unruly ox slowly changes color from black to fully white signifying its transformation. The journey is illustrated in a series of pictures beginning with a sighting of the ox and culminating with returning to one's life having mastered the mind (Loori 2002; Pine 2011). Some sets have 8 or 12 pictures; however, the most common set, attributed to Chinese Zen master Kuo-an Shih-yuan, contains 10 representations of the stages of the path to enlightenment (Kapleau 1980). As Loori (2002) points out the ox-herding pictures form a map of the possible direction that practice can take while still holding a sense of not knowing how that path will unfold. The journey of the ox and its herder also parallels that of the participants in mindfulness programs.

In the first picture, searching for the ox, we become aware that there is a questioning, a wish to know ourselves better or even some aspiration of feeling better than we typically do. Participants in a mindfulness program come with a wide range of suppositions and desires. Pain and suffering has led them to doubt their capacity to manage their life and the ability of any intervention to heal them. The second picture, traces of the ox, depicts our sense that there is something we can do; we may discover meditation, yoga, or some form of practice that provides structure to our life. As we work in this stage, we are also confronted with the reality that there is no quick fix to our *dukkha*. Participants often return after the first week feeling frustrated, dismayed, or even angry that mindfulness practices such as the body scan are not helping. Some do comment that the practices were amazing in transporting them to a blissful state; these are typically "flights into health" and the wise clinician–teacher learns to value the experience, but not become caught in the delusion of cure.

The third picture, seeing the ox, gives us a glimpse of the ox and, although it is stuck deep in the bushes, we have a sense that something solid is present. Participants begin to have glimpses of something unfolding in their practice; there is a sliver of faith building as they get samples of being in their body or noting feelings arise and dissipate. The fourth picture, catching the ox, is a powerful moment of encountering the mind in all its raw unruliness. Most participants report feeling a surge of old thought patterns and doubts as they continue to practice. The dualism they have constructed about mindfulness good/pain bad begins to break down and wisdom arises albeit tentative and inconstant. There is a point in the program where participants either "buy into" the larger possibility of living well or settle for the symptomatic relief they have acquired over the first half of the program.

The fifth picture is the taming of the ox through unrelenting diligence. Old habits are always ready to reassert themselves and, at the same time, we are cultivating trust in our motives and our skills. Compassion arises and with it self-compassion as we learn to befriend ourselves. At this stage of practice, participants begin to feel the confrontational relationship they have with their body and emotions remits, even if only for a while. There are more encouraging encounters with self, other, and the world. Riding the ox home, in the sixth picture, imparts a sense of ease and cooperative connection. The struggle with self and its vicissitudes softens and participants begin to understand how they can be triggered and how to unhook from those types of connections.

The seventh picture shows the ox is gone and the person remains. It points to the teachings of nonself as we realize that there is not absolute mind (ox) that controls or directs us. Instead, who we are emerges out of a myriad of causes and conditions. Participants express a sense of letting go of the ideas and objects that they believed defined them. There is less fear of being controlled by their unruly ox or insight that the ox was really never the problem in the first place. In the eighth picture, all constructs of "self" and "ox" are gone. The seeker and what is sought have transcended their labels. This state comes after lengthy and dedicated practice and may not be evidenced in such a short period of mindfulness training.

The last two pictures represent returning to the source and entering the marketplace. Kuo-an added these two pictures because the truly realized Zen person does not stop at the dropping away of concepts (Kapleau 1980). He saw the highest spiritual development is in our skillful functioning in the quotidian. With deeper and more ardent practice, we are intimate with our experience, embodied, informed by wisdom, live by *sila,* and steadied by practice. We enter into our life with compassion for others and actions that are embedded in that care. This entry into the marketplace is the maturing of our practice. We see our practice as the means to transform *dukkha* but are no longer attached to it in an obsessive way. It becomes simply what we do, moment-by-moment, be it brushing our teeth, fixing a meal, caring for others, or meeting our dying moments. It may be unrealistic to expect participants of an 8-week program to enter these stages given many mature practitioners spend their lives in this process. However, the time limitations of typical mindfulness programs speak strongly to the need for ongoing practice opportunities.

10.5 When Dharma Meets Distress

The teachings in the broader context of *dukkha,* suffering, and the wish to be liberated from it is universal. The path however differs for each individual. Ultimately, it does involve commitment to a process and a willingness to learn how to be different in the face of the realities of life. Dogen, Zen master and founder of the Soto Zen tradition, expressed the essence of how and why we practice as Buddhists: "To study the Buddha Way is to study the self. To study the self is to forget the self. To forget the self is to be actualized by myriad things. When actualized by myriad things, your body and mind as well as the bodies and minds of others drop away. No trace of enlightenment remains, and this no-trace continues endlessly" (Tanahashi 1985). And yet, our intention and trajectory of practice is not that different from the person registering for a mindfulness program. There is a desire to be free of psychological struggles, mental distress, and perhaps even physical pain. In the Buddhist context, however, there is an understanding at the outset that this is a lifetime process demanding tremendous patience and its end point is not relief but liberation. It is understandable that practices which seem to veer away from this lifetime commitment can be seen as "quick fix" ways to lessen suffering without a full transformation.

However, *dukkha* now presents at a scale and intensity that calls for a different approach to transformation and healing. Mental illness and mental distress that arises from physical illness is now a global concern. The statistics are consistent across countries and show a dramatic rise in depression, anxiety, and other psychological disorders (CDC 2011; Marcus et al. 2012). Not only is there an enormous emotional and financial burden on the lives of individuals who suffer from these mental illnesses but also an impact at an economic level (Kazdin and Blase 2011).

The consequences of losing employment because of mental illness and the ensuing stigma also have significant impacts on individuals, their families, and society as a whole (Pescosolido 2013). Turning away from this scope of *dukkha* is inconceivable especially in the face of evidence that suffering benefits from treatments that can be consistent with the fundamental principles of Buddhism.

In order for Buddhist teachings to have the fullest of impact in secular/clinical settings, the principles of what is being transformed and why it needs to be must occupy the foreground of any mindfulness program. While the context of its clinical application is to effect change in presenting symptoms first, the broader and deeper effect of practice on the person must be held close. The balance for the clinician–teacher is to guide the practices so that relief is attained but the larger issue of transforming greed, anger, and delusion are not lost. At the same time, in typical Zen fashion, it is necessary to relinquish investment or hold on the outcome to be a Buddhist-based one.

10.5.1 Upaya in the Treatment Approach and Protocols

The potential for mindfulness-based programs to be beneficial for all those who suffer is significant. However, we must be aware that the people who attend Buddhist venues will not be the same as those who seek psychological assistance and sometimes the two become conflated. In the 35 years since the inception of MBSR, the connection of MBIs to Buddhist thought has become common knowledge. This may be a double-edged sword, attracting those who hope that a spiritual path will take them out of their psychological distress and those who may be willing to explore a path that offers a perspective significantly different from the familiar. At the same time, some participants will be wary of anything that sounds or feels like Buddhist teachings including terminology, ringing of bells, meditation, and yoga movements. Perhaps Buddhist practitioners who attend a program for their own psychological needs will feel a greater discomfort in the secularization of the principles and practices. Each person will require *upaya* or a skillful approach to convey the practices, challenge misunderstanding, and feel reassured that they are being met at their level of understanding and commitment.

Upaya is also necessary in determining the content and form of practices in a mindfulness program. While Buddhist and Western psychology may take differing perspectives of mental disorders and their function (Sharf 2013), the application of mindfulness must be seen as a Buddhist-based intervention in a cultural context (societal, medical, etc.) that has its own criteria for safe and effective protocols. Thus, issues such as diagnostic criteria, medication use, vulnerability to psychosis, and so on need to be considered when selecting practices and forms of interaction.

Regardless of the source of the intervention or the details of its protocols, most individuals coming to a treatment program simply want to get better. Buddhist principles of transforming suffering and Western applications of those principles tend, for the most part, to honor that aspiration. However, there are considerable challenges to accomplishing this process that can arise at many levels. Thus, for the potential secular/clinical teacher, it is important not to confuse a commonality of intention (alleviation of suffering) with a commonality of therapeutic models. Mindfulness in a Buddhist context is not the same as a therapeutic approach with added protocols of meditation or awareness of experience. This means, the onus is on the aspiring teacher to be well informed and educated in the similarities and differences in Buddhist mindfulness practices and their underlying principles as well as the therapeutic model of their own training.

Abbreviations

AN *Anguttara Nikaya;* access to insight, http://www.accesstoinsight.org/index.html

MN *Majjhima Nikaya;* Bodhi (1995)

SN *Samyutta Nikaya;* Bodhi (2000)

Sn *Sutta Nipata;* access to insight, http://www.accesstoinsight.org/index.html

References

Aitken, R. (1991). *The gateless barrier: The wu-men kuan*. Berkeley: North Point Press.

Analayo, B. (2003). *Satipatthana: The direct path to realization*. Birmingham: Windhorse Publications.

Analayo, B. (2013). *Perspectives on Satipatthana*. Cambridge: Windhorse Publications.

Arnold, G. S. (2004). Qian and her soul are separated. *Mountain Record: The Zen Practitioner's Journal, 22*(2), 17–22

Aronson, H. B. (2004). *Buddhist practice on Western ground*. Boston: Shambhala.

Baer, R. A. (2003). Mindfulness training as a clinical intervention: A conceptual and empirical review. *Clinical Psychology: Science and Practice, 10,* 125–143.

Baer, R. A. (Ed.). (2005). *Mindfulness-based treatment approaches*. New York: Academic Press.

Baer, R. A. (2011). Measuring mindfulness. *Contemporary Buddhism, 12*(1), 241–261.

Baumeister, R. F. (2011). Self and identity: A brief overview of what they are, what they do, and how they work. *Annals of the New York Academy of Sciences, 1234*(1), 48–55. doi:10.1111/j.1749-6632.2011.06224.x.

Bodhi, B. (1995). *The middle length discourses of the Buddha: A translation of the Majjhima Nikaya*. Boston: Wisdom Publications.

Bodhi, B. (2000). *The connected discourses of the Buddha: A translation of the Samyutta Nikaya*. Boston: Wisdom Publications.

Bodhi, B. (2005). *In the Buddha's words: An anthology of discourses from the Pali canon*. Boston: Wisdom Publications.

Bodhi, B. (2008). *The Noble Eightfold Path: The way to end suffering*. Onalaska: BPS Pariyatti Editions.

Boulanger, J. L., Hayes, S. C., & Pistorello, J. (2010). Experiential avoidance as a function of contextual concept. In A. M. Kring & D. M. Sloan (Eds.), *Emotion regulation and psychopathology*. New York: The Guilford Press.

Bowen, S., & Kurz, A. (2012). Between-session practice and therapeutic alliance as predictors of mindfulness after mindfulness-based relapse prevention. *Journal of Clinical Psychology, 68,* 236–245.

Buddhadasa, B. (1976). *Anapanasati: Mindfulness of breathing* (B. Nagasena, Trans.). Bangkok: Sublime Life Mission.

Buddhadasa, B. (2010). *The Path of Purification (Visuddhimagga)* (B. Nanamoli, Trans.). Kandy: Buddhist Publication Society.

Caplow, F., & Moon, S. (Eds.). (2013). *The hidden lamp: Stories from twenty-five centuries of awakened wisdom*. Boston: Wisdom Publications.

Carmody, J., & Baer, R. (2008). Relationships between mindfulness practice and leels of mindfulness, medical and psychological symptoms and well-being in a mindfulness-based stress reduction program. *Journal of Behavioral Medicine, 31*, 23–33.

Cayoun, B. A. (2011). *Mindfulness-integrated CBT: Principles and practice*. Chicester: Wiley-Blackwell.

CDC (Centers for Disease Control and Prevention). (2011). Mental illness surveillance among adults in the United States. *MMWR Surveillance Summary*, 60(Suppl. 3), 1–29.

Chodron, P. (2001). *The places that scare you: A guide to fearlessness in difficult times*. Boston: Shambhala Publications.

Coffey, K. A., Hartman, M., & Fredrickson, B. L. (2010). Deconstructing mindfulness and constructing mental health: Understanding mindfulness and its mechanisms of action. *Mindfulness, 1*, 235–253.

Conze, E. (1958). *Buddhist wisdom: The Diamond Sutra and the Heart Sutra*. New York: Vintage Books.

Cowen, S., Chawla, N., & Marlatt, G. A. (2010). *Mindfulness-based relapse prevention for addictive behaviors: A clinician's guide*. New York: The Guilford Press.

Cullen, M. (2011). Mindfulness-based interventions: An emerging phenomenon. *Mindfulness, 2*, 186–193.

Cusens, B., Duggan, G. B., Thorne, K., & Burch, V. (2010). Evaluation of the breathworks mindfulness-based pain management programme: Effects on well-being and multiple measures of mindfulness. *Clinical Psychology & Psychotherapy, 17*(1), 63–78. doi:10.1002/cpp.653.

Davis, J. H., & Thompson, E. (2013). From the five aggregates to phenomenal consciousness: Towards a cross-cultural cognitive science. In S. M. Emmanuel (Ed.), *A companion to Buddhist philosophy* (pp. 585–598). Chichester: Wiley.

Dobkin, P., Hickman, S., & Monshat, K. (2013). Holding the heart of mindfulness-based stress reduction: Balancing fidelity and imagination when adapting MBSR. *Mindfulness*. doi:10.1007/s12671-013-0225-7.

Dunne, J. (2011). Toward an understanding of non-dual mindfulness. *Contemporary Buddhism, 12*(1), 71–88.

Eberth, J., & Sedlmeier, P. (2012). The effects of mindfulness meditation: A meta-analysis. *Mindfulness, 3*, 174–189.

Ekman, P., & Davidson, R. J. (Eds.). (1994). *The nature of emotion: Fundamental questions*. New York: Oxford University Press.

Fairholme, C., Boisseau, C. L., Ellard, K. K., Ehrenreich, J. T., & Barlow, D. H. (2010). Emotions, emotion regulation, and psychological treatment: A unified perspective. In A. M. Kring & D. M. Sloan (Eds.), *Emotion regulation and psychopathology: A transdiagnostic approach to etiology and treatment*. New York: The Guilford Press.

Fjorback, L. O., Arendt, M., Ornbol, E., Fink, P., & Walach, H. (2011). Mindfulness-based stress reduction and mindfulness-based cognitive therapy—A systematic review of randomized controlled trials. *Acta Psychiatrica Scandinavica, 124*, 102–119.

Germer, C. K. (2009). *The mindful path to self-compassion: Freeing yourself from destructive thoughts and emotions*. New York: The Guilford Press.

Germer, C. K., Siegel, R. D., & Fulton, P. R. (2013). *Mindfulness and psychotherapy*. New York: Guilford Press.

Gethin, R. (1992/2001). *The Buddhist path to awakening: A study of the bodhi-pakkhiya dhamma*. Oxford: Oneworld.

Gethin, R. (1998). *The foundations of Buddhism*. Oxford: Oxford University Press.

Gilbert, P. (2005). *Compassion: Conceptualisations, research and use in psychotherapy*: New York: Routledge.

Gilbert, P. (2009). *The compassionate mind: A new approach to life's challenges*. London: Constable & Robinson.
Goldstein, J. (2013). *Mindfulness: A practical guide to awakening*. Louisville: Sounds True.
Gowans, C. (2003). *The philosophy of the Buddha*. New York: Routledge.
Grabovac, A., Lau, M., & Willett, B. (2011). Mechanisms of mindfulness: A Buddhist psychological model. *Mindfulness, 2*(3), 154–166. doi:10.1007/s12671-011-0054-5.
Grossman, P., & Van Dam, N. (2011). Mindfulness, by any other name…: Trials and tribulations of sati in western psychology and science. *Contemporary Buddhism, 12*(1), 219–239.
Gunaratana, B. (2001). *Eight mindful steps to happiness: Walking the Buddha's path*. Somerville: Wisdom Press.
Gunaratana, B. (2012). *The four foundations of mindfulness in plain English*. Boston: Wisdom Publishers.
Hanh, T. N. (1998). *The heart of the Buddha's teaching*. Berkeley: Parallax Press.
Hanh, T. N. (2005). *Interbeing: Fourteen guidelines for engaged Buddhism*. Berkeley: Parallax Press.
Hanh, T. N. (2006). *Transformation and healing: The sutra on the four foundations of mindfulness*. Berkeley: Parallax Press.
Hanh, T. N. (2007). *For a future to be possible: Buddhist ethics for everyday life*. Berkeley: Parallax Press.
Hanh, T. N. (2009a). *Breathe, you are alive! Sutra on the full awareness of breathing*. Berkeley: Parallax Press.
Hanh, T. N. (2009b). *The heart of understanding: Commentaries on the Prajnaparamita Heart Sutra*. Berkeley: Parallax Press.
Hanh, T. N. (2010). *The diamond that cuts through illusion*. Berkeley: Parallax Press.
Hanh, T. N. (2011). *Our appointment with life: Sutra on knowing the better way to live alone*. Berkley: Parallax Press.
Harvey, P. (2000). *An introduction to Buddhist ethics*. Cambridge: Cambridge University Press.
Harvey, P. (2013a). The conditioned co-arising of mental and bodily processes within life and between lives. In S. M. Emmanuel (Ed.), *A companion to Buddhist philosophy*. Chichester: Wiley.
Harvey, P. (2013b). Dukkha, non-self, and the teaching on the four "Noble Truths". In S. M. Emmanuel (Ed.), *A companion to Buddhist philosophy* (pp. 26–25). Chichester: Wiley.
Harvey, P. (2013c). *An introduction to Buddhism: Teachings, history and practices* (2nd ed.). Cambridge: Cambridge University Press.
Hickman, S., Monteiro, L., & Goldstein, A. (2012). *Holding the heart of MBSR: Reflection, collaboration and dialogue on modification or adaptation of the 8-week program*. Paper presented at the Investigating and Integrating Mindfulness in Medicine, Health Care, and Society 10th Annual International Scientific Conference for Clinicians, Researchers and Educators, Norwood, MA.
Hori, V. S. (2006). The steps of koan practice. In J. D. Loori (Ed.), *Sitting with koans*. Somerville: Dharma Communications Press.
Jacobs, A. M., Hopton, J., Davies, D., Wright, N. P., Kelly, O. P., & Turkington, D. (2014). *Treating psychosis: A clinician's guide to integrating acceptance and commitment therapy, compassion-focused therapy, and mindfulness approaches within the cognitive behavioral therapy tradition*. Oakland: New Harbinger Publications.
Kabat-Zinn, J. (2003). Mindfulness-based interventions in context. *Clinical Psychology: Science and Practice, 10,* 144–156.
Kabat-Zinn, J. (2011). Some reflections on the origins of MBSR, skillful means, and the trouble with maps. *Contemporary Buddhism, 12*(1), 281–306.
Kabat-Zinn, J. (2013). *Full catastrophe living: Using the wisdom of your body and mind to face stress, pain, and illness*. New York: Bantam.
Kabat-Zinn, J., Lipworth, L., Birney, R., & Sellers, W. (1987). Four-year follow-up of a mediation-based program for the self-regulation of chronic pain: Treatment outcomes and compliance. *The Clinical Journal of Pain, 2,* 159–173.

Kapleau, P. (1980). *The three pillars of Zen*. New York: Doubleday.
Kazdin, A. E., & Blase, S. L. (2011). Rebooting psychotherapy research and practice to reduce the burden of mental illness. *Perspectives on Psychological Science, 6*(1), 21–37.
Keown, D. (2005). *Buddhist ethics: A very short introduction*. Oxford: Oxford University Press.
Kuyken, W., Byford, S., Taylor, R., Watkins, E., Holden, E., White, K., et al. (2008). Mindfulness-based cognitive therapy to prevent relapse in recurrent depression. *Journal of Consulting and Clinical Psychology, 76*(6), 966–978.
Langer, E. (1990). *Mindfulness*. Cambridge: Perseus Books.
Lazarus, R. S., & Folkman, S. (1984). *Stress, appraisal, and coping*. New York: Springer.
Loori, J. D. (2002). *Riding the ox home: Stages on the path of enlightenment*. Boston: Shambhala.
Loori, J. D. (2006a). Introduction. In J. D. Loori (Ed.), *Sitting with koans*. Somerville: Dharma Communications Press.
Loori, J. D. (Ed.). (2006b). *Sitting with koans*. Boston: Wisdom Publications.
Maex, E. (2011). The Buddhist roots of mindfulness training: A practitioner's view. *Contemporary Buddhism, 12*(1), 165–175.
Marcus, M., Yasamy, M. T., van Ommeren, M., Chisholm, D., & Saxena, S. (2012). Depression: A global public health concern. World Health Organization, Geneva, Switzerland.
Markowitz, F. (2001). Modeling processes in recovery from mental illness: Relationships between symptoms, life satisfaction, and self-concept. *Journal of Health and Social Behavior, 41*(1), 64–79.
McCown, D. (2013). *The ethical space of mindfulness in clinical practice: An exploratory essay*. Philadelphia: Jessica Kingsley Publishers.
McEwen, B. S. (2002). *The end of stress as we know it*. Washington, D.C.: Joseph Henry Press.
McMahan, D. (2008). *The making of Buddhist modernism*. Oxford: Oxford University Press.
Mills, E. (2004). Cultivation of moral concern in Therav¯ada Buddhism: Toward a theory of the relation between tranquility and insight. *Journal of Buddhist Ethics, 11*, 20–45.
Monteiro, L., & Musten, R. F. (2013). *Mindfulness starts here: An 8-week guide to skillful living*. Victoria: Friesen Press.
Monteiro, L., Nuttall, S., & Musten, R. F. (2010). Five skillful habits: An ethics-based mindfulness intervention. *Counselling and Spirituality, 29*(1), 91–103.
Monteiro, L., Musten, R. F., & Compson, J. (2014). Traditional and contemporary mindfulness: Finding the middle path in the tangle of concerns. *Mindfulness*. doi:10.1007/s12671-014-0301-7
Neff, K. (2011). *Self-compassion: Stop beating yourself up and leave insecurity behind*. New York: William Morrow.
Pescosolido, B. A. (2013). The public stigma of mental illness: What do we think, what can we know, what can we prove? *Journal of Health and Social Behavior, 54*(1). doi:10.1177/0022146512471197.
Piet, J., & Hougaard, E. (2011). The effect of mindfulness-based cognitive therapy for prevention of relapse in recurrent major depressive disorder: A systematic review and meta-analysis. *Clinical Psychology Review, 31*(6), 1032–1040.
Pine, R. (2001). *The diamond sutra*. Berkeley: Counterpoint Press.
Pine, R. (2011). *P'u Mindg's oxherding pictures & verses*. New York: Empty Bowl.
Porges, S. (2007). The Polyvagal perspective. *Biological Psychology, 74*(2), 116–143.
Porges, S. (2011). *The Polyvagal Theory: Neurophysiological foundations of emotions, attachment, communication, and self-regulation*. New York: W.W. Norton & Company.
Purser, R., & Loy, D. (2013). Beyond McMindfulness. *Huffington post*. Retrieved from: http://www.huffingtonpost.com/ron-purser/beyond-mcmindfulness_b_3519289.html. Website: http://www.huffingtonpost.com. Accessed 15 July 2013.
Rahula, W. (1978). *Zen and the taming of the bull: Towards a definition of Buddhist thought*. London: Gordon Fraser.
Sahn, S. (1997). *The compass of Zen*. Boston: Shambhala.
Salzberg, S. (2002). *Lovingkindness: The revolutionary art of happiness*. Boston: Shambhala.

Segal, Z. V., Williams, J. M., & Teasdale, J. D. (2012). *Mindfulness based cognitive therapy for the prevention of depression relapse* (2nd edn.). New York: Guilford Press.

Seyle, H. (1974). *Stress without distress*. Toronto: HarperCollins.

Shapiro, S., & Carlson, L. E. (2009a). *The art and science of mindfulness: Integrating mindfulness into psychology and the helping professions*: Washington, DC: American Psychological Association.

Shapiro, S., & Carlson, L. E. (2009b). How is mindfulness helpful? Mechanisms of action *The art and science of mindfulness: Integrating mindfulness into psychology and the helping professions* (pp. 93–104). Washington, DC: American Psychological Association.

Sharf, R. (2013). *Mindfulness or mindlessness: Traditional and modern critiques of "Bare Awareness"*. Paper presented at the conference on Mindfulness in Cultural Context, McGill University, Montreal, QC.

Shibayama, Z. (2000). *The gateless barrier: Zen comments on the Mumokan* (S. Kudo, Trans.). Boston: Shambhala Publications.

Silananda, V. U. (2002). *The four foundations of mindfulness*. Boston: Wisdom Publishers.

Soeng, M. (2006). Zen koan and mental health: The art of not deceiving yourself. In D. K. Nauriyal, M. S. Drummond & Y. B. Lal (Eds.), *Buddhist thought and applied psychological research: Transcending the boundaries*. New York: Routledge.

Tamura, Y. (2014). *Introduction to the Lotus Sutra*. Boston: Wisdom Publications.

Tanahashi, K. (Ed.). (1985). *Moon in a dewdrop: Writings of Zen master Dogen*. New York: North Point Press.

Teasdale, J., Segal, Z. V., Williams, M., Ridgeway, V. A., Soulsby, J. M., & Lau, M. (2000). Prevention of relapse/recurrence in major depression by mindfulness-based cognitive therapy. *Journal of Consulting and Clinical Psychology, 68*, 615–623.

Tekin, Ş. (2011). Self-concept through the diagnostic looking glass: Narratives and mental disorder. *Philosophical Psychology, 24*(3), 357–380. doi:10.1080/09515089.2011.559622.

Thanissaro, B. (2012). *Right mindfulness: Memory and ardency on the Buddhist path*. http://www.holybooks.com/right-mindfulness-memory-ardency-on-the-buddhist-path/. Accessed 3 September 2012.

Thoits, P. A. (2013). Self, identity, stress, and mental health. In C. Aneshensel, J. Phelan & A. Bierman (Eds.), *Handbook of the sociology of mental health* (pp. 357–377). Netherlands: Springer.

Titmuss, C. (2013). The Buddha of mindfulness. The politics of mindfulness. Retrieved from: http://christophertitmuss.org/blog/?p=1454. Website: http://www.christophertitmuss.org. Accessed 22 July 2013

Tuske, J. (2013). The non-self theory and problems inphilosophy of mind. In S. M. Emmanuel (Ed.), *A companion to Buddhist philosophy*. Chicehester: Wiley.

Vøllestad, J., Sivertsen, B., & Nielsen, G. H. (2011). Mindfulness-based stress reduction for patients with anxiety disorders: Evaluation in a randomized controlled trial. *Behaviour Research and Therapy, 49*, 281–288.

Whyte, D. (2001). *Crossing the unknown sea: Work as a pilgrimage of identity*. New York: Riverhead Books.

Williams, J. M., & Kabat-Zinn, J. (2013). *Mindfulness: Diverse perspectives on its meaning, origins and applications*. New York: Routledge.

Wyatt, C., Harper, B., & Weatherhead, S. (2014). The experience of group mindfulness-based interventions for individuals with mental health difficulties: A meta-synthesis. *Psychotherapy Research, 24*(2), 214–228.

Yamada, K. (2005). *The gateless gate: The classic book of Zen koans*. Boston: Wisdom Publications.

Young, S. (2011). Five ways to know yourself. Retrieved from: http://www.shinzen.org/RetreatReading/FiveWays.pdf. Website: http://www.shinzenyoung.org. Accessed 23 September 2014.

Lynette M. Monteiro is a registered psychologist and the director of training at the Ottawa Mindfulness Clinic. She completed an MA on neurobehavioral correlates of human communication disorders and a PhD investigating the efficacy of methylphenidate in the treatment of attention-deficit hyperactivity disorder (ADHD) in preschool-aged children. She is trained in cognitive behavioral therapy (CBT), cognitive processing therapy for veterans and active military personnel, mindfulness-based treatments (mindfulness-based stress reduction (MBSR), mindfulness-based cognitive therapy (MBCT), mindfulness-integrated CBT (MiCBT), mindful self-compassion (MSC)) and Buddhist chaplaincy. Dr. Monteiro's primary treatment interest is with military and first response members experiencing post-traumatic stress disorder (PTSD), and she serves as a personnel selection psychologist for police and military units. As a clinical professor at the University of Ottawa, she is in charge of training PhD clinical psychology candidates in an ethics-based mindfulness intervention. She is coauthor of Mindfulness Starts Here.

Chapter 11
Encountering the Psychological Research Paradigm: How Buddhist Practice Has Fared in the Most Recent Phase of Its Western Migration

Kaisa Puhakka

11.1 Introduction

This chapter examines the adaptations of Buddhist mindfulness practices into protocols that can be studied by the methods of contemporary psychological research and applied in clinical practice in the counseling and health fields. In accordance with the central theme of this book, the question to be explored is whether the power of the Buddha's teachings may have been compromised in the conceptual as well as procedural modifications that have been deemed necessary in these adaptations.

My short answer to this question is "yes," the teachings of the Buddha have been significantly compromised, and their power diluted in most of the research as well as clinical applications thus far. The teachings provide the context for deepening the meditation practice and, likewise, the meditation practice provides a context for the experiential realization of the teachings. Divorcing the practice from the teachings, as has been done in most mindfulness research, therefore significantly limits the power of the practice itself. The reasons why the research paradigm has deemed it necessary to extract the practice out of the context of the teachings are the focus of this chapter. My objective is to show how some of the foundational assumptions of the research paradigm work to rule out of consideration the ontological inquiry that is at the heart of Buddhist mindfulness practice, and also how the specific requirements of the research design that rest upon these assumptions tend to limit research to beginning-level mindfulness practice. Following a brief review of the state of the art of the research and clinical applications of mindfulness meditation, I examine the methodological requirements and their limiting effects in the context of the standard research approach—the randomized controlled trial (RCT) design.

I conclude this chapter by suggesting that, should the deeper aspects of Buddhist practice and its full healing power become of interest to researchers, the pathway

K. Puhakka (✉)
Department of Clinical Psychology, California Institute of Integral Studies, 1453 Mission Street, 5th Floor, 9410 San Francisco, CA, USA
e-mail: kaisap@comcast.net

E. Shonin et al. (eds.), *Buddhist Foundations of Mindfulness*,
Mindfulness in Behavioral Health, DOI 10.1007/978-3-319-18591-0_11

forward would require setting aside some of the paradigmatic assumptions that limit, on a priori basis, what can be studied and how, and returning to a reliance on observation free of a priori assumptions. The possibility of "observation free of a priori assumptions" is denied by the epistemological stance of constructivism, which is widespread among researchers and intellectuals in general today. It is, therefore, important to address how Buddhism meets the challenge of constructivism and how, in so doing, it opens up the horizon of possibilities for psychological research.

Because of the critical focus of this chapter, it is important to acknowledge at the outset that their limitations notwithstanding, the clinical adaptations of mindfulness practice have turned out to be an invaluable contribution to the objective that Buddhism and Western clinical practice share, which is the alleviation of human suffering. These adaptations have given rise to culturally user-friendly techniques that bring relief relatively quickly to large numbers of people without challenging their values, beliefs, or lifestyles. Perhaps the biggest barrier Westerners experience with traditional Buddhist practice is that it requires patience and self-discipline. These are hard to come by especially when one is suffering from relentless physical pain, anxiety, or depression. What is required in terms of patience and self-discipline is less stringent in the clinical adaptations of Buddhist mindfulness and so they are likely to serve the needs of these clinical populations more effectively than would the often more rigorous practices in traditional Buddhism.

It is also important to acknowledge that efforts are currently underway to broaden and deepen the mindfulness training protocols to include central Buddhist principles and values along with the meditation technique (Shonin and Van Gordon 2014; Shonin et al. 2014). I believe that for these efforts to gain momentum and develop further, it will be helpful to have a clear understanding of how and why the research paradigm tends to set a priori limits as to what mindfulness practice can mean and how far or deep it can be taken. In other words, light needs to be shed on the methodological commitments of evidence-supported clinical practice that discourage utilization of the full healing power that is potentially there in Buddhist wisdom and practice. The concern of this chapter is with these a priori limits and the possibility of opening them up to meeting the power of Buddhist practices more adequately.

11.2 Migration of Buddhism Across Cultures

It is always good to remind oneself that Buddhism has been around for over 2500 years and that in the course of this long history it has migrated across great cultural diversity. In the early centuries, the migration took place in Asia, from India to China and other Southeast Asian countries, then to Tibet, and finally to Japan. It is only within the past century or so that Buddhism finally crossed the continental, and perhaps larger cultural, divide from Asia to the West. When chronologically viewed, the Western migration can be thought of as proceeding in three phases, though they could also be thought of as strands insofar as they each have continued to develop alongside one another as somewhat distinct approaches to Buddhism in contemporary Western societies.

11.2.1 *First Phase of Migration to the West: The Scholar–Explorers*

The Western migration began with a few odd scholars and explorers from Europe and America. Some of these became legendary for their daring journeys to difficult-to-access regions of Asia, especially Tibet. Prominent examples include Alexandra David-Neel, Anagarika Govinda, and W. Y. Evans-Wentz. These individuals inspired other young Europeans and Americans to also undertake trips to the East in search of Buddhist teachings. Eventually, Buddhism gained a small foothold in the universities of the USA, Europe, India, and Japan where translations and commentaries of Pali and Sanskrit, later Tibetan, texts were carried out by a handful of linguists, philologists, and philosophers. Rigorous scholarship and fidelity to the texts being translated or commented upon have been of utmost importance in this phase of the Western migration. In contrast with the first explorers, most of these academics took pains to guard their scholarly objectivity by refraining (at least publicly) from engaging in any of the Buddhist practices themselves and from interfacing with the larger public (with some notable exceptions among the more recent scholars, whose writings have been aimed at reaching a larger audience, e.g., Robert Thurman, David Komito, and Jeffrey Hopkins).

The scholarly tradition continues to this day, but remains largely confined to the relative obscurity of an exotic academic specialty. However, the careful translations of and rigorous, sophisticated commentaries on the classic primary texts of all the major Buddhist traditions are the lasting legacy of this tradition.

11.2.2 *Second Phase of Migration to the West: The Awakening of Popular Interest*

It was not until the 1960s that interest in Buddhism was awakened within the general Western public. In contrast to the preceding academic phase, the popular interest in Buddhism was entirely practical, motivated by a search for new values and ways of experience. This was a time of soul searching in the war-weary West, and there was much dissatisfaction and frustration with the established norms of the culture among the younger generation especially in the US (Puhakka 2012). In this climate, Buddhism seemed to hold promise of something new, a transformation at the personal level and methods for achieving it that did not require adherence to particular theological or metaphysical beliefs. Many of the second phase teachers were Asians who have struggled to communicate the message across the cultural and linguistic barriers to their Western students with varying success. Others have been Americans or Europeans who spent years, sometimes decades, in Asia studying with one or more Buddhist masters and then returned to teach in their respective Western countries. Some of the more prominent of these teachers include Chögyam Trungpa, Walpola Rahula, and Shunryu Suzuki.

An interesting feature of this second phase is that, within the past half a century, a variety of Buddhist traditions from several Asian countries became available to Westerners all at once. In the earlier Asian migrations, when Buddhism newly arrived, it was typically represented by one or very few distinct traditions. The simultaneous availability of a vast array of Asian spiritual practices, including Buddhist styles and traditions in contemporary West has both advantages and disadvantages (Walsh 1999). On the one hand, it may encourage superficial "pick-and-choose" kind of spiritual shopping. On the other hand, it may encourage a more flexible approach with less dogmatic adherence to any particular form of belief or practice—thus possibly allowing the essence of Buddhism to shine unencumbered by inessential forms that can occlude it.

With the maturing of both teachers and students, this second phase continues to evolve alongside the more recently emerged third phase. As with any popular adaptations, that of Buddhist practice in America has gone far in accommodating the values, lifestyles, and comfort zones of its new host culture, inevitably becoming diluted in the process. However, there are also many examples of teachers and students, both Western and Asian, who have negotiated the cultural barrier skillfully without compromising the subtlety and depth available in the Buddhist tradition. Their teaching styles tend to be conceptually and doctrinally fluid, capturing what seems to be the timeless essence of Buddhism in a way that resonates with contemporary Westerners. Prominent among these are Jack Kornfield, Thich Nhat Hanh, Stephen Batchelor, Pema Chödrön, and Adhya Shanti, to mention just a few. Most of these individuals spent years if not decades deeply immersed in the study and practice of Buddhism in Asia or in the West, often both. Their deep integration of Buddhist wisdom is often belied by a simple, down-to-earth teaching style aimed at audiences who often have no prior knowledge of Buddhism.

11.2.3 Third Phase of Migration to the West: Empirical Research and Clinical Application of Mindfulness

The third phase of Buddhism's migration to the West began with a new academic interest that started to gain momentum in the 1990s and continues to this day. This time it was psychologists and empirical researchers who took interest in the potential of Buddhist practices to deliver mental and physical health benefits and who wished to explore whether, and how, techniques derived from Buddhism might be incorporated into medical and psychotherapeutic practices. The problem of objectivity that had kept the earlier scholars from engaging in the practical side of Buddhism was still there, but the research methods available for psychologists seemed to promise a solution to this problem.

Despite their common tie to the academia, the third phase has been notably discontinuous with the first, scholarly phase. Most contemporary researchers and clinical practitioners are unfamiliar with the translations of Buddhist texts that have been made available in English by the earlier translators and scholars. The principal concern in the third phase has been with maintaining scientific objectivity, the standards of which are set by the requirements of the research methodology. For the researchers, this has meant that the adaptability of the concepts and techniques of Buddhism to the methodological dictates of empirical research paradigms is more important than scholarly accuracy in how the Buddhist tradition is represented.

The third phase shares with the second phase a concern with the practice side of Buddhism. However, especially researchers (less so counselors and therapists in the field) have felt uneasy with the second phase's embrace of Buddhism as a spiritual practice. To preserve their distance from anything "spiritual," researchers and evidence-supported clinical practitioners have tended to rely on secondary or tertiary sources which present Buddhism in a way that de-emphasizes doctrine and is culturally user friendly to a wider pool of potential research subjects regardless of whether they are interested in Buddhism as a spiritual teaching or approach to life.

11.3 "Essential Buddhism" Amidst Diverse Transmissions

Is the diversity in the transmission styles across cultures a positive, potentially enriching thing, or does it dilute and distort the essential Buddhist teachings? This question begs to be addressed when the concern is with an evaluation of how Buddhism fares through its migrations.

The answers that have been proposed to the above question vary widely. At one extreme is a strict adherence to the texts and teachings attributed to the historical Buddha and his immediate followers, which regards any deviation in style as a distortion of substance—a view somewhat more common among Buddhists in the Theravada tradition. At the other extreme is a broadly inclusive perspective that allows or even calls for a variety of approaches to understanding and practicing the teachings—a viewpoint more commonly held by Buddhists in the Mahayana schools. Then, there are the varieties of positions that fall somewhere between these extremes.

My position leans toward the inclusive end of the spectrum, though I see the question of transmission as being highly complex, potentially involving both distortion and dilution of the original teaching's power and also refinement and enrichment. Which it is depends on how the cultural barriers in the transmission are navigated and this, in turn, depends on awareness of the cultural blinders that might operate on either or both sides of the barrier. By cultural blinders, I mean the often unconscious identifications people have with the worldviews, values, and customs of their ethnic or cultural backgrounds. From the Buddhist viewpoint, such blinders are delusional and inevitably get in the way of understanding the *dharma* (the

Buddha's teachings, or reality as explicated by the teachings). Few today would deny that all humans are subject to cultural blinders—including the Buddha's contemporaries. Inevitably, these blinders were embedded in the language and style of expression of the historical Buddha's own teachings, which were transmitted to subsequent generations by his followers after his passing.

Science, like any other social activity, is embedded in a cultural context in which its methodology is formulated and research carried out. To the extent that researchers are unaware of the foundational assumptions of their methodology, or the cultural context that shape the questions deemed worthy of research, they too are subject to cultural blinders—a point famously made by Kuhn (1970).

Given their inevitable presence, it seems to me that cultural blinders need to be viewed not simply negatively as a hindrance but also as positively as a challenge to be embraced with awareness. When the transmission lacks cultural awareness, the forms of the transmission are likely to confound the teachings with the beliefs and values of the culture, and the latter then become a hindrance that distorts or dilutes the transmission. On the other hand, when there is awareness of the beliefs, values and norms operative in the cultural context of the transmission, these beliefs and values can be skillfully navigated without the transmission getting obscured by them. In reality, transmissions from teachers to students probably tend to fall somewhere on a continuum between these two extremes.

This way of looking at the relationship between culture and Buddhism not only acknowledges distortions and dilutions, but also allows for new openings for communicating. Buddhist teachings uniquely resonate with the recipients of the teachings without compromising their subtlety and depth. Thus, alongside the distortion and dilution of the Buddha's message in popular adaptations across centuries and cultures, arguably some of the later articulations of the teaching and approaches to the practice may have created new openings to their full realization perhaps not available in the original formulations or in the formulations of any single school. If such enrichment occurred in the course of the earlier Asian migrations, it may well also be happening within the current Western migration.

Finally, I address the notion of "essential Buddhism" which has been implicit in the foregoing discussion. If by essential Buddhism is meant that the teachings of Buddhism are not reducible to the forms of the culture within which its transmission takes place, then I affirm such a notion, as I suspect do most people who take up serious study and practice of Buddhism. At the same time, I am aware that any articulation of what this essential Buddhism might be is necessarily context bound. The following characterization of Buddhism is contextualized to my personal understanding as it has been shaped by my journey through scholarly study of the Theravada, early Indian Mahayana, and subsequent Mahayana texts of Tibet, China, and Japan, as well as by decades of practice in both the Theravada and Rinzai Zen traditions.

It is my impression that the Buddha's teachings are most clearly and explicitly stated in the literature of the Pali Canon of the Theravada tradition. The fact that, in this tradition, they are stated from the point of view of the person aspiring to become enlightened no doubt also helps make them more accessible. However, I also believe that significant contributions to the evolution of Buddhism, including new openings to realization of its central message, were made by the Mahayana schools of Madhyamika and Yogacara (Vijnanavada) that flourished in India beginning in the first or second century CE and which became foundational for subsequent traditions of Buddhism in China, Tibet, Japan, and other Asian countries. In these Mahayana schools, the teaching regarding *shunyata* (emptiness, voidness) received greater emphasis than was usually given to them in the Theravada tradition. The teaching regarding emptiness is, in conceptual terms, highly elusive and easily lends itself to misunderstanding, which may have been the reason why it was not prominently featured in the Theravada. Yet, in the Theravada also, it has been acknowledged as the most profound of the Buddha's teachings by the great modern master Buddhadasa (1994) who said of the Buddha regarding the teaching of voidness, "He spoke of no other matter, either directly or indirectly" (p. 27). Furthermore, contributing to the elusiveness of this teaching is the fact that in the Mahayana traditions in which it features prominently, teachings are often conveyed from the standpoint of the enlightened mind as opposed to the standpoint of the person who aspires to enlightenment. This is especially the case in Zen.

To summarize, I consider the essential teachings of Buddhism as consisting of the four noble Truths regarding suffering *(dukkha)* and the teachings regarding impermanence (a*nicca*), no-self (*anatta*), dependent co-arising *(paticca-samuppada),* and emptiness or voidness (s*unnata*, Skr: *shunyata*). In the following pages, technical terms referring to these and other central teachings are spelled in their Pali version, except when the Sanskrit version is more commonly used, the term is spelled in the latter version). These core teachings have been explicated and investigated in direct meditative practice in the Theravada as well as the aforementioned Mahayana traditions. Furthermore, I see these teachings as interrelated, indeed as aspects of one essential teaching much like facets of a diamond. For analytic and didactic purposes, they are typically presented as conceptually distinct with the four noble truths setting the rationale and the path, and the other five central concepts elaborating an understanding through distinct conceptual angles to what deep meditative inquiry reveals as one reality.

It should be noted that the essential Buddhism I have outlined here is rather narrowly construed. It excludes various ideas, which though frequently associated with Buddhist thought and practice, are not present in all of the major traditions of Theravada, Tibetan Buddhism, and Zen. The doctrine of reincarnation and the devotional practices associated with the various Bodhisattvas are examples. The Buddha himself appears to have left unquestioned some of the beliefs current in his culture and society—I imagine (without actually knowing this to be a fact) because he regarded them as being neutral with respect to his teachings. In Mahayana, many indigenous cultural beliefs and practices were considered similarly neutral or even positively facilitating of the transmission of Buddha's teachings. This is especially the case in Tibetan Mahayana, where many of the indigenous beliefs and deities of Tibet were incorporated into the newly arrived Buddhism.

11.4 Buddhist Practices in Psychological Research and Clinical Practice: An Overview

Generally speaking, in all encounters between Buddhism and the new culture into which it enters, some adjustment seems necessary for it to take widespread root in the host culture. But the requirements for cultural acceptability tend to be rather loose and there is usually some give and take of mutual influence, which justifies characterizing the relationship between Buddhism and the host culture as one of "encounter" or "adoption."

This, however, is not the case in the encounter between Buddhism and Western psychology's research tradition. Rather, the host has set clear and strict entry requirements for Buddhism, as it does for anything new to be considered candidate for legitimate subject matter. First and foremost, the candidate must be construable as an object of inquiry amenable to the methodology of empirical research. This methodology sets the standards of scientific objectivity. For researchers, and also for many clinicians, scientific objectivity clearly takes precedence over fidelity to Buddhist doctrine. For this reason, the term "adaptation" in regard to the introduction of Buddhist practices into the domain of research and clinical practice seems appropriate.

The adaptation of Buddhist practices into Western research and clinical practice began in earnest in the 1990s. The adaptation seemed easy and natural, given Buddhism's significant overlap with scientific values and approaches. In particular, an emphasis on inquiry and observation is shared by both traditions. Buddhism also shares with counseling and clinical practice the concern with alleviating suffering. The predominant source for the adaptations of Buddhist techniques has been the Theravada Buddhist tradition. The notable absence of theological or metaphysical beliefs and the emphasis on inquiry and observation in the Theravada especially resonates with Western science. The explicitness and detail with which the nature and sources of suffering, and the steps to liberation from suffering, are articulated in this tradition appeals to scientists who deal in explicit constructs that lend themselves to clear procedures and operational renditions. Furthermore, the analytic language used in explaining the teachings in the Theravada tradition can create the impression that specific techniques can be easily extracted out of the larger context of Buddhist teachings to be studied and applied by themselves.

11.5 Major Adaptations of Buddhist Meditation Techniques

The following look at the various adaptations of Buddhist techniques is by no means meant to present an exhaustive review of the considerable body of research literature that has grown in support of them. The aim is to simply highlight the major adaptations and the issues they have addressed, with references to some illustrative research, and the central concerns of related theoretical and methodological discussions.

11.5.1 Mindfulness-Based Stress Reduction

The introduction of specific Buddhist techniques into Western health practices began with the pioneering work of Kabat-Zinn (1990) who introduced a simple *vipassana* or mindfulness meditation practice to patients suffering from chronic, intractable pain with whom he was working at the Massachusetts University Medical Center. He taught patients to focus their attention on the breath and to use the breath as an anchor to which attention is returned as soon as it veers off to thoughts or emotional reactions. Encouraged by reports of beneficial effects from his patients, Kabat-Zinn standardized his program into an 8-week course of instruction and practice, which allowed his team to assess the program's effectiveness through empirical research. Calling his program mindfulness-based stress reduction (MBSR), Kabat-Zinn also initiated the practice of stripping the descriptions of mindfulness techniques of all Buddhist language and connotations. It should be noted that Kabat-Zinn himself has undertaken years of serious study and immersion in Buddhism, including monastic study in Asia. It is clear from his books addressed to the general public that he knows what he is talking about. His writing is geared for readers with no previous knowledge of Buddhism (and not necessarily much interest in it, either), but he manages to convey the essence of Buddhist wisdom in his clear and deceptively simple style (e.g., Kabat-Zinn 2012). Regarding MBSR, however, Kabat-Zinn has taken pains to present its rationale and technique in a way that is neutral with respect to Buddhist teachings and is amenable to the standards of empirical research. There is by now extensive research literature in support of the beneficial effects of MBSR in easing the suffering of chronic pain patients and also of sufferers of other clinical syndromes such as panic attacks. More recently, Kabat-Zinn developed a standardized 8-week training program for individuals who in turn teach others to become MBSR therapists. These programs are designed for beginners who typically have no previous exposure to *vipassana* meditation or to Buddhism in general.

11.5.2 Mindfulness-Based Cognitive Therapy

Another widely used adaptation of Buddhist meditation is mindfulness-based cognitive therapy (MBCT; Segal et al. 2004; Shapiro et al. 2005; Teasdale et al. 1994), which incorporates Kabat-Zinn's 8-week mindfulness training as a central component. The mindfulness training in MBCT focuses on the patient's negative thinking and ruminative patterns. Unlike traditional cognitive therapy, which addresses the content of these thoughts and teaches patients to substitute positive thoughts for negative ones, MBCT does not attempt to change the content, but the way in which patients relate to their thoughts. The key element in the training is to teach patients to observe their thoughts simply "as thoughts" rather than as a compelling reality. This in turn promotes nonreactive relating to the thoughts and a sense of freedom from them. The important contribution of the mindfulness technique to cognitive-behavioral therapy has been the discovery that negative, ruminative thought patterns can be reduced simply by cultivating nonreactive attention to the goings on in the mind, including these negative patterns. The mindfulness technique has been seen as complementary to the classic cognitive therapy approach and has been found to be, in certain cases, more effective than the latter (Teasdale et al. 1994). In the past two decades, the application of MBCT has expanded from its initial focus on depression relapse prevention to treating other clinical problems such as anxiety, panic, trauma, and addictions (Borkovec et al. 2004; Follette et al. 2004; Marlatt et al. 2004) .

At the present time, MBCT has an established place in the armamentarium of empirically supported cognitive therapies in the USA, as well as in Europe. In England, for example, the National Institute for Clinical Excellence (2009) recommended that MBCT be adopted as part of the standard treatment and management of depression. It is interesting to note that most clinicians in training who are likely to administer standard MBCT programs for their clients may not have practiced mindfulness themselves and have not been required to do so in their clinical training programs. An appeal to having such practice included as part of the clinician training was recently made by Rimes and Wingrove (2011).

11.5.3 Dialectical Behavior Therapy

Among the earliest adaptations of Buddhist mindfulness practice into the general behavioral therapy framework with wide applicability to a variety of emotional and interpersonal problems is dialectical behavior therapy (DBT; Linehan et al. 1991, 2001; Linehan and Schmidt 1995). Linehan drew from her experience as a Zen practitioner as well as her background in cognitive-behavioral therapy to develop a comprehensive treatment program for people suffering from borderline personality disorder. The program consisted of both psychoeducational and meditative components, with the latter being geared toward increasing the person's capacity for self-regulation and tolerance for dysphoric moods. Subsequently, she and her colleagues expanded DBT to treating suicidal patients and patients suffering from addictions and other conditions with impulsivity and self-harming behaviors (Linehan et al. 1999, 2002; Marlatt 1994). Approaches utilizing mindfulness exercises within the DBT framework have also appeared in the self-help literature for coping with various clinical symptoms and for developing distress tolerance and interpersonal effectiveness (Chapman et al. 2011; McKay et al. 2007).

11.5.4 Acceptance and Commitment Therapy

Acceptance and commitment therapy (ACT; Hayes et al. 2001) incorporates mindfulness practice in a broad behaviorist framework. Hayes (2004a, b) characterized ACT as being firmly established in what is called the "third wave" of cognitive-behavioral therapies which generally de-emphasize overt strategies for changing behavior patterns and emphasize more experiential and contextually elaborated processes. Also, ACT is unique among the therapies so far discussed in that it is grounded in a comprehensive program of basic research on language and cognition (Hayes et al. 2004). Acceptance of what is going on moment by moment, attending to its ever widening context without attempting to change anything is at the heart of ACT, and easily recognizable by anyone familiar with Buddhist mindfulness practice. However, Hayes et al. (2004) provide a full account of ACT in terms of contemporary behavior analysis which is expanded from the radical behaviorism of B. F. Skinner and makes no reference to any uniquely Buddhist constructs.

11.6 Central Theoretical and Methodological Concerns

An indication that the research and clinical application around Buddhist meditative techniques has reached a level of maturity is the growing effort in the past decade to develop standardized definitions and operational procedures for key terms and techniques across treatment and research programs. This effort, still very much in its infancy, was started by a gathering of a handful of leading researchers who published their consensus regarding how to define and operationalize mindfulness and related terms (Bishop et al. 2004). The trend of the discussions appears to be in the direction of ever-finer distinctions and operational procedures to pinpoint the empirical basis of the distinctions. The discussions have addressed the multiple meanings of mindfulness; for example, as a mental state, a capacity or disposition, and whether references to subjective events such as awareness, attention, or insight are needed.

Clearly, the objective has been to move away from subjective events in the theoretical discussions and to instead find ways to interpret them either in terms of mechanistic information processing models inspired by computer modeling (Teasdale et al. 1994) or in terms that do not refer to any intervening cognitive processes but to behavior patterns in response to stimuli (Hayes and Wilson 2003; Hayes et al. 2004). The objective in both is to eliminate references to subjective events, but they do it differently. To illustrate, in the cognitive information processing theories, attention is viewed as something that is "deployed" either narrowly or widely, that is, as an inert object analogous to an army unit that is deployed into a battlefield. Hayes et al. (2004) on the other hand, propose that from a behavioral point of view attention "is a way of speaking about patterns of stimulus control" (p. 251). Others, like Bishop et al. (2004) are more willing to stick with terms that refer to subjective events but are closer to how they are understood in Buddhism. For example, they see "mindfulness as a process of gaining *insight* into the nature of one's mind and the adoption of a de-centered perspective ..." (p. 234). The overall objective in all these discussions has been to ground techniques adapted from Buddhism more rigorously in the framework of empirical research and empirically supported clinical theory.

11.7 Two Levels of Inquiry: Psychological and Ontological

Notably absent from the discussions reviewed above has been an interest in researching Buddhist techniques beyond the very beginning-level practice (8 weeks being the standard). One might think this odd, given the prominent emphasis in the Buddhist traditions of rigorous and long-term practices. For example, in Tibetan Buddhist retreats, individuals practice continuous meditation in solitude for as long as 4 years, and in the *sesshin* practice in Zen, individuals engage in continuous meditation practice for 7-day periods at a time. Theravada also includes rigorous, long-term mindfulness practices, and, especially in this tradition, there are systematic and detailed phenomenological accounts of what happens in such practice available, for example, in the classic text of *Visuddhimagga* (Buddhaghosa 1975). There are also modern meditation masters in the Theravada tradition who have provided detailed descriptions of the phases in the cultivation of mindfulness (Mahasi 1985; Pandita 1992). Why has there been so little interest in psychological research and clinical practice to explore the more rigorous practices or the adepts at such practices?

To address this question fully, let us begin by asking: What is it that such rigorous and often long-term Buddhist practice seeks to accomplish? From the viewpoint of those on the journey, the answer could well be "nothing at all" (as it might be in Zen, and also in Tibetan Dzogchen). But such an answer belies a profound shift in the practitioner's orientation to self and world, including the self's striving for liberation or enlightenment. Thus, a profound shift in the understanding of the aims of the practice tends to happen in the course of more rigorous and long-term Buddhist practice. An early indicator of this shift is that the practitioners become less concerned with getting results or feeling better and more interested in gaining insight into the root causes of any and all forms of suffering.

This is a shift from *psychological* to *ontological* inquiry. Psychological inquiry is undertaken from the standpoint of a self and its personal needs and interests, whereas ontological inquiry takes up this very standpoint for observation and experiential analysis in Buddhist practice. Another way to put this is that in psychological inquiry, basic assumptions about the nature of self and world remain intact while in ontological inquiry, these very assumptions are being investigated. Jennings (2010) and others (e.g., Aronson 1998; Engler 2003) have emphasized that the concern of Buddhist teachers is with the inherent and abiding nature of the ontological self, not the personal dramas of the psychological self. As Jennings (2010) noted, it is often difficult for Western students to make the switch from psychological to ontological inquiry. Such a switch is foreclosed, or categorically ruled out, in Western scientific research. Before examining the foundational assumptions of research methodology and how they necessitate such a foreclosure, it may be helpful to consider the psychological–ontological distinction in greater detail, including its roots in the Buddhist traditions.

11.8 The Psychological–Ontological Distinction in Buddhism

This distinction was not explicitly discussed in the Theravada. However, it was implicit in the Buddha's emphasis of the need to investigate his central teachings regarding the (ontological) nature of the self and the world in one's meditative practices so that their true nature as impermanent and lacking in self-existence is realized in direct observation. The shift from psychological to ontological inquiry tends to happen naturally as the practitioners' concern turns from their everyday personal suffering to the generic nature and causes of that suffering.

The first articulation of the psychological–ontological distinction was provided by the Buddhist philosophers of the early Indian Mahayana schools Nagrjuna, Chandrakirti, and Asanga. They distinguished between two orders of reality, that of "relative truth" or "conventional truth" *(samvrtti satya)* and that of "absolute truth" *(paramartha satya)*. (For translations and commentaries regarding *samvrti satya* and *paramartha satya*, see e.g., Kalupahana 2015; Ramaman 1986; Chandrakirti 2004; Puligandla 1975.) The language of these philosophers may sound arcane to contemporary Western ears and a superficial reading of them can easily lend itself to the impression that the distinction is metaphysical or theological, which would certainly be a turnoff to those of a scientific bent of mind. A closer reading of these and other Mahayana texts, however, makes it clear that this distinction grows out of a deep meditative inquiry into the nature and limits of language and conceptual thought and that it refers to an understanding and experience of the same reality from two points of view. The first viewpoint is bound to language and thought, and the various (mostly unconsciously held) beliefs and practices conditioned by one's culture and religion. The second viewpoint is free of such conditions and realizes that the "truths" being held in the former viewpoint are illusory or delusional in that they are true only relative to other things (i.e., the context of beliefs and behavior) that are assumed to be true. This second viewpoint does not reject these relative truths, but simply awakens from what might be thought of as the spell under which they hold a person who takes them to be real (Puhakka 2003).

It is evident from the clinical and research literature that the beneficial effects of mindfulness practice have to do with the taste of liberation from the "spell of reality" which patients experience with the realization that their negative thoughts are "just thoughts" rather than reality. Just 8 weeks of practicing the mindfulness technique can bring about such a realization, as demonstrated by the research literature, which begs the question, why has the research not gone further to study the more comprehensive and long-term practices the benefits of which are well documented in the Buddhist literature?

11.9 Foundational Assumptions: Buddhism and Psychological Research

I believe that the answer to the above question has much to do with the differences in some foundational assumptions between Buddhism and Western psychological research. Buddhism and contemporary psychological research start with a partially overlapping set of such assumptions. They share in common the belief that all truth claims must be grounded in observation. The reliance on observation as the final arbiter of truth is known as the principle of *empiricism* in the Western tradition. When first formulated by the empiricist philosophers Bacon, Hobbes, Locke, Berkeley, and Hume, it was a revolutionary idea that broke out of the Medieval and later Rationalist traditions that had practically ruled out fresh inquiry after Aristotle. Buddhism is unique among spiritual and religious traditions in its whole-hearted embrace of empiricism understood as reliance on direct observation rather than beliefs accepted on the authority of tradition or religious faith.

Empiricism in the Western context, however, became closely associated with two other assumptions, elementism (or atomism) and mechanism. *Elementism* is the notion that what observation yields first and foremost are bits and pieces of sensations or "sense-data" as Berkeley called them, and that these sense-data bear no intrinsic relation to other sense-data, but are discrete, independently existing elements like atoms in empty space. *Mechanism* refers to lawful, predictable processes, such as association, by which complex experience and behavior, including mental states like mindfulness, are constructed out of the sense-data.

While the principle of empiricism is not so much an assumption as a prescription for a method for arriving at truth, elementism and mechanism are assumptions about the nature of what the method reveals. They are accepted a priori rather than established by observation and thus, paradoxically, contradict the principle of empiricism. Nevertheless, these two assumptions were proposed by the same philosophers who proclaimed the principle of empiricism and they are, for many contemporary researchers, synonymous with empiricism itself.

It is important, however, to tease apart these three assumptions and to highlight the a priori nature of elementism and mechanism. While Buddhism embraces the principle of empiricism, it does not accept elementism or mechanism. The core teachings of dependent co-arising *(paticcasamuppada)* counter these assumptions with the notion that all things arise in codependence with other things and hence there are no independently existing elements. The teachings of no-self *(anatta)* and impermanence *(anicca)* further suggest that there are no enduring, self-existent things (including "selves"), but change and impermanence are the very nature of reality.

However, these Buddhist teachings do not have the a priori status, which elementism and mechanism have in psychological research. Most Buddhists regard these teachings as being subject to verification by direct observation, which is undertaken in the practice of mindfulness meditation. This is consistent with the Buddha's admonition for his students to not take any teachings on faith, including his own, but to find out for themselves. As mindfulness practice deepens, the conditional, transient nature of seemingly solid and self-existent entities, such as thoughts and images or even the observing self, becomes evident. The first taste of liberation from the "spell of reality" has much to do with the keen, nonreactive observation that is cultivated in the practice of mindfulness. The reactive patterns to which psychological mechanisms refer are likewise subject to observation in Buddhist meditative practice. Described as mental formations *(samkhara),* these, too eventually dissolve into the ever-changing flow of impermanence.

This leads to another overlapping notion between the two traditions, which is the principle of causation. Buddhism and Western science, including psychological research, both believe that phenomena are related as causes and effects. However, what this means is interpreted differently in the two traditions. If no longer in all of Western science, certainly still in quantitative social science research, causes and effects are interpreted in light of the assumptions of elementism and mechanism, and thus refer to distinct events that are lawfully or predictably connected by the mechanisms of association. The situation is more complex in Buddhism. Initially, the elementistic and mechanistic model of causation works well enough, as there is a convergence of the practitioner's experience with that of the researcher. The teachings in the Theravada tradition are also explained to the beginning practitioner in a language that is compatible with the elementistic–mechanistic model. Thus, for example, dependent co-arising is taught in terms of the series of 12 links that constitute the factors that keep the wheel of *samsara* turning. However, the Buddha taught dependent co-arising in relation to the 12-link formula in four different ways, each from a different link as a starting point to emphasize the interdependence of these factors; that is, that they are each subject to co-arising (Buddhaghosa 1975). As the meditator's practice advances and his understanding of impermanence and of dependent co-arising deepens, seemingly solid structures related as distinct causes and effects begin to dissolve and lose their distinct identities. The one-directional temporal sequence also begins to give way to a simultaneous and two-way and even all-way sense of "interbeing" (to borrow a well-known phrase from *Thich Nhat Hanh*). A contemporary Buddhist practitioner has expressed such a holistic view of dependent co-arising as involving "An overarching awareness that stretches to encompass a metasymmetry of deep, multilayered causality" (Davies 2014, p. 112).

The assumptions of elementism and mechanism, and the notion of causes and effects based on these, usually shape everyday experience and psychological reality and they are also firmly entrenched in the paradigm of psychological research. However, in Buddhist meditative practice, these assumptions are not accepted a priori, but are subjected to observation. They may be deconstructed gradually in the course of the practice, as in Theravada, or at the outset as in many Mahayana schools.

Holding on to the assumptions of elementism and mechanism on a priori basis naturally rules out an inquiry that would deconstruct them. Western research methodology that subscribes to these assumptions cannot, in principle, accommodate their deconstruction in the ontological inquiry, which is at the heart of mindfulness meditation. This foreclosure, of course, is not something that is consciously or explicitly declared. How it happens needs to be uncovered by taking a close look at a typical research design and the specific requirements it imposes upon the subject matter being researched. These requirements are embedded in the foundational assumptions of elementism and mechanism.

11.10 What Can Be Studied and How It Must Be Studied: Requirements Specific to the Research Design

Before turning to the requirements themselves, I will describe the standard research design in some detail for the benefit of readers who may not be familiar with the particulars of psychological research.

11.10.1 RCT: The Gold Standard of Scientific Research

The typical design for research projects is called 'randomized controlled trials (RCT)'. In the RCT design, two or more conditions are administered to volunteer subjects who are suffering from a clinical condition, say depression. One of the conditions administered to the subjects is called treatment, such as an 8-week training in mindfulness. The other condition is called control and may consist of simply continuing usual treatments the subjects may have already been receiving, or some other treatment. The relative effectiveness of the treatment under study is evaluated by "before" and "after" measures of the clinical condition, which are compared for subjects who had received the treatment condition and those who had received the control condition(s). The measures of the clinical condition typically consist of various scales measuring symptoms of depression, sense of well-being, attitudes, and so on. The subjects in the research study are matched in terms of other relevant features such as severity of the symptoms, age, socioeconomic, and educational background, among others. They are then randomly assigned to the treatment and control conditions. To guard against possible researcher bias, those in the research team who administer and score the measures of the clinical condition often are kept in the dark (i.e., blind) as to whether the scores are for the treatment or the control conditions. Further, to ensure comparability across different studies, the administration of the treatment condition needs to be standardized, preferably manualized, procedures that minimizes the effect of variation across different mindfulness training instructors.

Readers familiar with the history of experimental psychology from Pavlov to neo-behaviorism will recognize the stimulus–response (S–R) principle at work in the RCT design, even with the far more sophisticated methodologies that are nowadays used along with greatly expanded cognitive and information processing theories to account for what intervenes between the S (external stimulus) and R (behavioral response). In the RCT design, S refers to the treatment and control conditions, also called independent variables, while the R refers to the clinical conditions or dependent variables.

By widespread consensus, RCT is held as the ideal design for empirical research, its double-blind version being the gold standard, for which reason it is chosen for illustration in this discussion. It should be noted, however, that the same requirements and restrictions also apply to other designs utilized in quantitative research studies on mindfulness.

I now turn to specific requirements of the RCT design and the restrictions they impose on the adaptation of Buddhist practices into the research paradigm. These are the requirements which any event or phenomenon must meet in order to be a legitimate subject for research. They are interrelated, but for purposes of discussion, I am treating them separately in order to examine their specific implications in limiting what can be studied and how when it comes to Buddhist practice. These requirements are: (1) that the phenomenon be quantifiable, (2) that it can be studied with representative samples and standardized sales, and (3) that it be a condition subject to influence by other conditions.

11.10.2 The Quantifiability Requirement

In the RCT design, the clinical as well as treatment and control conditions must be amenable to measurements that are comparable across various subjects and conditions; in other words, they must be quantifiable as variables. This requirement reflects the elementistic assumption discussed earlier, namely that the underlying reality or the phenomena being studied consist of discrete things or events that endure through time and so can be counted. In terms of RCT and other quantitative research designs, the phenomena to be studied are construed either as independent variables (treatment and control conditions) or as dependent variables (clinical outcomes or other measurable responses of the research subjects).

Accordingly, mindfulness has been construed in either of these two ways. For example, when mindfulness is construed as an independent variable as in the above illustration of the RCT design, it refers to the 8-week mindfulness training that is administered as the treatment condition to the research subjects. When mindfulness is construed as a dependent variable, it is construed as the effect or outcome and measured, for example, by scores on a mindfulness scale that has been standardized across a pool of research subjects.

What happens between the independent and dependent variables are not accounted for in this design. The events that intervene between the independent and dependent variables are the research participants' subjective processes as they engage in mindfulness practice. Such processes are either not considered as part of the study, or they may be objects of theorizing in mechanistic information-processing terms, as described earlier. Either way, notions like "awareness," "awakening," or "insight" as a process that is qualitatively changing and evolving in the cultivation of mindfulness have no place in the RCT design. At first glance, it may seem as though these can be included as dependent variables. However, to be treated as dependent variables, they would have to be construed as static, quantifiable responses, such as scores on a mindfulness or self-awareness scale.

From the Buddhist viewpoint, the essential feature of mindfulness practice is the change process over time. This is evident even in the instructions given to beginners, which emphasize not fixating attention, but bringing it into contact with whatever is going on *moment by moment*. It is this activity of attentiveness over time, from one moment to the next, rather than just the instructions given at the outset, that is responsible for the benefits of mindfulness techniques demonstrated by research. Strictly speaking, of course, I have no proof of this statement (nor of its denial, for that matter) in empirical terms. However, common sense suggests that whatever variability occurred between individuals in a given research study had much to do with the constancy and dedication with which the individuals were able to put themselves into actually doing the mindfulness practice.

That the practitioner's engagement in the practice is key to success with mindfulness practice is well recognized in all of the Buddhist practice traditions. The Theravada gives relatively less weight to the role of the teacher, but elaborate preparations and supports are detailed in the eightfold path. These are comprehensive enough to involve all aspects of the practitioner's life. In the Zen and Tibetan traditions, where the teacher–student relationship is more central, the practice lore contains numerous stories about the ingenious and often harsh ways in which the teacher tests the student's readiness for undertaking the practice path on which the teacher would then offer guidance and support. All this suggests that mindfulness practice demands more from its practitioner than, say a casual try of an exotic new dish for culinary pleasure or taking a pill for pain.

Apropos the last remark, it is interesting to note that the logic of the RTC design is the same whether it is applied to the study of effectiveness of drugs or of mindfulness training. The similarity is evident, for example, in Segal et al.'s (2004) characterization of the MBCT training that Ma and Teasdale (2003) had found to result in halving the relapse-recurrence rates in patients as "an 'adequate dose' of MBCT" (p. 59). As I have attempted to show, the logic of the RCT design dictates construing mindfulness in terms of units that are measurable in the manner of drug doses. Qualitative terms that refer to subjective events such as insight or awakening have no place in this logic.

The similarity of RCT designs in drug research and mindfulness research, of course, does not invalidate the research on mindfulness, but it does call attention to substantial limitations on what the research can address regarding mindfulness. The difference between studying psychoactive drugs (or any drugs for that matter) and mindfulness practice is that there is usually just one optimal, measurable dose for the drug being studied, whereas mindfulness is something that can be indefinitely cultivated beyond the first step. From a traditional Buddhist practice viewpoint, this difference is hugely significant. Yet, as suggested above, this difference can be ignored relatively painlessly by the RCT design so long as only the very beginning-level mindfulness practice is being studied. From the viewpoint of the research paradigm and the requirement for quantifiability, this tips the scales in favor of studying just beginning-level meditation practice.

11.10.3 The Requirement of Representative Samples and Standardized Scales for Measurement

Another requirement of the RCT design which also weighs in favor of limiting research to beginning-level mindfulness practice is access to large enough samples of participants to yield robust, statistically significant results that are generalizable to the population to which the results are intended to apply. Large samples are far easier to come by among people who have little or no experience with Buddhist practice than among advanced practitioners. There simply are not very many advanced practitioners to study, much less populations to draw samples from. How is "advanced" defined, anyway? In research studies I have seen where a difference between beginning and advanced practitioners is drawn, the criteria are often rather loose, and as little as 5 years of 1 h of daily sitting practice (by self-report)can make one an advanced practitioner.

In the lore of the Buddhist practice traditions, the criteria are usually not stated in terms of years or months of practice, but rather in terms of how one engages the practice—or one's life—on a moment-by-moment basis. There is a general sense that the cultivation of mindfulness can deepen until the nature of reality and of the self is fully penetrated in enlightenment, which can take decades or a lifetime—or perhaps no time at all, as anecdotes from the Zen sudden enlightenment schools suggest. In any case, there is a clear recognition in the Buddhist practice literature that those who would pursue the path of liberation to its culmination are always few in number. This, however, did not deter efforts to make the path available in the Buddhist practice traditions to those who seek them through teachers and progressively more advanced instructions, nor did it deter efforts to develop practices more suited for laypersons consumed by other demands of life.

The relative scarcity of individuals who would commit themselves to an intensive Buddhist practice as a first priority in their lives has, however, contributed to the absence of study of such individuals in quantitative research paradigms. More regrettably, it has ruled out the study of the actual process of the cultivation of mindfulness and insight beyond the initial sense of freedom from the grip of mental contents. The detailed descriptions of the progress of insight in the Buddhist practice literature imply profound and presumably predictable shifts in the mental states of the practitioners beyond the initial recognition of thoughts "as thoughts" or pain "as sensation." The systematic study of these shifts in the mindfulness practice experience would require a careful phenomenology of the experience of practitioners at various stages of their practice, including adepts at very far reaches of their practice. There have been attempts to develop phenomenologically based criteria for comparing stages in meditation practice (e.g., Walsh 1995). However, such attempts have not been taken up or pursued further in mainstream quantitative research paradigms. Such pursuits fall outside the scope of the RCT design, if for no other reason than that it is practically not easy to identify a group of advanced Buddhist practitioners who could provide data on the development of insight, let alone a population of which they would be a sample.

11.10.4 The Conditionality Requirement

Implicit in the first two requirements is the third which requires that whatever can be studied by the methods of empirical research must be a condition subject to being influenced by other conditions. The conditionality of all that is researchable is implicit in the term "variable" which describes the components in the research design. Accordingly, mental states, including mindfulness states, are "conditional" in that they are subject to influences by various conditions. They are also "conditions" in that they in turn influence other mental states and behaviors.

Buddhism and the paradigm of empirical research are in agreement as to the conditional nature of phenomena, including mental states. But there is a subtle yet profoundly important difference between the two traditions as to what the conditionality requirement is taken to mean regarding reality. In empirical research, the conditionality requirement is taken to be an ontological claim regarding what is and is not real and therefore what can and cannot be investigated. In Buddhism, conditionality is viewed as true relative to the world of phenomena, but not as an ontological claim about the nature of reality itself. According to Buddhism, reality as such can be known; however, nothing can be said about it except that, from the viewpoint of conditioned thought and perception, it is void—a stance elaborated through the teachings of *shunyata* which state that reality as such is devoid (empty) of conceptual determinations and distinctions. This, however, leaves open the possibility of investigating the nature of phenomena and conditionality itself—what I have called ontological inquiry.

An obvious objection to such a possibility from the viewpoint of the research paradigm may be posed as a question: How can a mind that is itself conditioned investigate its own conditions? Scientists would readily grant that conditionality applies to their own minds as much as it does to any empirical research project they may be working on. The conditionality of the latter is evident, for example, in the expectation of results that set the direction and focus of the investigation, including how variables to be studied are set up, and so on. In the paradigm of empirical research, then, the question whether conditionality itself can be investigated raises the specter of infinite regress—(conditional) investigation investigating (conditional) investigation endlessly, or, to put it differently, self investigating self ad infinitum. For the more philosophically minded, this usually clinches the argument against the possibility of an inquiry into conditionality.

How does Buddhism avoid falling into the same infinite regress when it acknowledges that mental states, like all phenomena, are subject to conditions? The Buddhist answer begins by noting that what is being cultivated in mindfulness and other meditative practices is the *activity* of attending, not a static mental state or thing that is subject to conditions. Such a static thing is implied in the research term that refers to attention as something to be "deployed." Again, the significance of this point is easy to ignore when only beginning-level mindfulness practice is considered where the practitioner's attention tends to be largely reactive to needs, desires, fears, and other conditions. The Buddhist answer continues by inviting careful observation of what happens in longer-term cultivation of mindfulness or other practices informed by the Buddha's teachings. With the deepening of practice, attention is gradually, or sometimes suddenly, freed up from the conditions that bind it. This is evident, for example, in the decreased concern of advanced practitioners with achieving results in terms of their personal well-being or enlightenment. One might say that the entire point of the practice is to free up attending to be increasingly present to the moment-by-moment goings on within and without the practitioner. In moments, attention may even be freed from the deep patterns that bind it to the intentional structure of a consciousness divided into subject and object. Unconditioned attention, that is, attention freed from conditions, is capable of seeing into the nature of conditions.

Research is silent on what goes on in the moment when attention is freed from the conditions that bind it. Yet, what goes on in that moment is an actual event; there is nothing metaphysical or mysterious about it. We might say that it is the datum that has been ignored because it does not fit the current paradigm of scientific research. Buddhist practitioners describe this datum as a moment of "awakening." Most people are familiar with awakening in their own immediate experience, for example, when waking up from a dream. That this moment of awakening is usually immediately followed by immersion into another set of conditions called everyday reality can easily obscure the moment of awakening. There are mini-awakenings, such as practitioners of MBCT may experience when they realize that thoughts are "just thoughts." There are greater awakenings along the way that reach to hitherto unconscious identifications and other mental formations, and one wakes up from an entire reactive pattern of thoughts and emotions. And presumably there is a great awakening in which attention is freed from all conditions that would determine it. Such great awakening is called enlightenment or liberation. Nothing mysterious about it, either. The same, however, cannot be said about attempts to identify who is and who is not enlightened.

If this still sounds too strange and mysterious to the researcher, Buddhism has one last argument to offer. It is to invite the researcher to take her own medicine, to set up the experiment on the cushion in the spirit of open-mindedness which is the hallmark of true empiricism, and find out for herself.

11.11 A Path Forward

Were the researcher to follow the above suggestion and take up meditation practice to explore its full depth and range, she would find herself taking up ontological inquiry, not as leap of faith into some new metaphysical or theological belief system, but as a deepening of inquiry that is perfectly consistent with the principle of empiricism as it was originally established by the British empiricist philosophers in the seventeenth and eighteenth centuries. This principle proclaimed the revolutionary idea that truths be accepted not a priori but by verification in experience. By "experience," these philosophers meant direct sensory observation. Our researcher taking up serious Buddhist meditation practice would be returning to the revolutionary spirit inherent in empiricism when embraced without the other a priori assumptions we have discussed in this chapter. Her empiricism would most likely be met with objections from her more conventional colleagues who advocate a research methodology in which empiricism no longer means direct observation, but all sorts of procedures and operations as dictated by the various requirements of the research design, such as the ones reviewed in this chapter. As I have attempted to show, experience and direct sensory observation have indeed taken back seat to a priori methodological dictates which tell the researcher what can and cannot be observed (i.e., only quantifiable data such as scores on scales of measurement) and how they should be interpreted (i.e., through mechanistic information processing models).

It is evident that research bound to these dictates can barely scratch the surface of the powerful healing potential that lies within the Buddhist meditation and wisdom traditions. More than minor revisions in the research paradigm are needed to mine this potential fully in psychological research and clinical practice. At the same time, it behooves one to acknowledge the enormous resistance to any serious reexamination of the paradigm. This resistance operates largely unconsciously as the researchers in the field, usually under pressure to churn out publishable results in short order, seldom find the time or opportunity to reflect deeply on what they are doing. Phenomena that do not fit the established paradigm may not even register on the busy researcher's radar, having been already excluded from consideration by the research design. If they nevertheless manage to register sufficiently to compel questioning of the paradigmatic assumptions, such questioning is not likely to get a sympathetic ear from the established research community.

It is these sorts of considerations about the everyday practice of science that led Kuhn (1970) to opine that new or radically revised paradigms do not have a chance to gain prominence until after the scientists who cling to the established paradigm have passed on. Perhaps I am more optimistic than Kuhn in thinking that the subject matter under discussion here—Buddhist meditative practice—not only challenges the established research paradigm but might also inspire its reexamination. After all, the subject matter is "mindfulness," which may call the researchers to greater mindfulness about what they are doing, perhaps to the kind of deeper inquiry into the conditions and assumptions of their own research that I have called ontological inquiry. This deeper inquiry involves nothing more mysterious than simply returning to the principle of empiricism—to direct, sensory observation.

A shedding of the assumptions of elementism and mechanism while embracing empiricism in an open stance has been done before in the Western philosophy as well as research traditions, for example, by phenomenologists and process philosophers like Henri Bergson and Alfred North Whitehead. A figure known to most psychologists who did this is, of course, William James. When he observed with fresh eyes and a beginner's mind what was present in the immediacy of his experience, no isolated bits of sense data presented themselves to his observation (James 2000, 2013). Rather, around the fringes of what might be thought of as bits of data, there was always something else going on that was noticeable to a discerning observer. He called these subtle goings on "transitional states" and noted that no clear boundaries that distinguished one sense-datum from another were evident in the ongoing stream of consciousness. Because his actual observation did not support the notion that experience was built up from separate bits of sense-data through the mechanism of association, he set this notion aside and called his version of empiricism "radical empiricism."

Why not follow James' example and return to the principle of empiricism pure and simple? Doing so would entail setting aside, for a moment at least, all other assumptions not evident to direct observation and inquire into things afresh. This would seem like an excellent first step toward opening up the established research paradigm for the kind of study of Buddhist meditation that does justice to its full healing power. However, an objection is likely to be raised at this point by researchers and many other contemporary intellectuals that direct observation *not* conditioned by its cultural, linguistic, and psychological context is impossible. This is the epistemological stance of constructivism. But, as an epistemological stance, its categorical denial of the possibility of observation free of conditions, that is, free of contextual influence, is made on a priori basis. While the constructivist claim is consistent with the teaching of dependent co-arising, Buddhism does not accept it on a priori basis, but regards it as subject to observational inquiry. That such an inquiry is enormously challenging is well understood in Buddhism—which is why the cultivation of mindfulness is understood as first and foremost a cultivation—a practice to develop one's capacity for insight into the nature of conditions.

As anyone who has sat on the cushion can attest, sustained direct observation—called bare attention in the mindfulness literature—is not something that people naturally and easily do. But it is a skill that can be developed and fine-tuned. The same practice, viewed in one way, is an ontological inquiry into the conditions of existence. Viewed in another way, it is the cultivation of mindfulness that develops one's capacity for observation that is increasingly free of the conditions that initially shape its content and direction. Thus, one might characterize an important aspect of Buddhist meditative practice as being a gradual or sudden return to the direct observation of pure empiricism.

It is not necessary for the psychological research endeavor to achieve pure empiricism by Buddhist meditative practice or some other way before it takes up the subject of Buddhist practice for research. To start with, it is enough to pay true homage to the spirit of empiricism by giving primacy to phenomena over methodology. The practice of mindfulness techniques as developed in the Buddhist tradition rather than the methodological orthodoxy of established research paradigms would then determine what constitutes data for study. As the study of these techniques and practices progresses, assumptions hitherto accepted unconsciously or on a priori basis might surface for examination and perhaps be set aside. I have no doubt that the inherent openness in such an empiricist stance would naturally lead to methodological innovations to open up the paradigm so it can, if not fully accommodate, at least enter into a dialogue with, an ontological inquiry into any and all assumptions, including methodological ones. Such a dialogue may generate an increasingly transparent and self-modifying approach to methodology that mirrors the subtle shifts of awakening that may happen in the course of Buddhist meditative inquiry.

I believe that nothing less than this kind of open and self-modifying approach is required for research to eventually deliver the full benefits of Buddhist meditation to clinical practice. These benefits would be of an altogether different order than is the alleviation of specific clinical symptoms that has been the concern of most research and clinical practice thus far. The latter kinds of benefits, though immensely valuable for many suffering people, are contingent on ever-changing conditions. The true aim of Buddhist meditation and other practices is liberation from all conditions, what the Dalai Lama calls "unconditional happiness." The benefits of unconditional happiness are immeasurable and understanding what unconditional happiness means, and how it may be realized in practice, would certainly be a worthy undertaking for a research paradigm that is up to the task.

References

Aronson, H. (1998). Review of psychotherapy and Buddhism: Toward an integration by J. Rubin. *Journal of Buddhist Ethics, 5,* 63–73.

Bishop, S. R., Lau, M., Shapiro, S., Carlson, L., Anderson, N. D., Carmody, J., Segal, Z. V., Abbey, S., Speca, M., Velting, D., & Devins, G. (2004). Mindfulness: A proposed operational definition. *Clinical Psychology: Science and Practice, 11*(3), 2310–2241.

Borkovec, T. D., Alcaine, O. M., & Behar, E. (2004). Avoidance theory of worry and generalized anxiety disorder. In R. G. Heimberg, C. I. Turk, & D. S. Mennin (Eds.), *Generalized anxiety disorder: Advances in theory and practice* (pp. 77–108). New York: Guilford.

Buddhadasa, B. (1994). *Heartwood of the Bodhi Tree: The Buddha's teaching on voidness*. Boston: Wisdom.

Buddhaghosa, B. (1975). Viduddhimagga: The path of purification. Kandy: Buddhist Publication Society.

Chandrakirti. (2004). *Introduction to the middle way: Chandrakirti's* Madhyamakavatara *with commentary by Jamgon Mipham*. Boston: Shambhala.

Chapman, A. L., Gratz, K. L., & Tull, M. T. (2011). *The dialectical behavior therapy skills workbook for anxiety: Breaking free from worry, panic, PTSD, and other anxiety symptoms*. Oakland: New Harbinger.

Davies, J. A. (2014). Relational dharma: A modern paradigm of transformation—A liberating model of intersubjectivity. *The Journal of Transpersonal Psychology, 46*(1), 92–121.

Engler, J. (2003). Being somebody and being nobody: A reexamination of the understanding of self in psychoanalysis and Buddhism. In J. Safran (Ed.), *Psychoanalysis and Buddhism*. Boston: Wisdom.

Follette, V. M., Palm. K. M., & Rasmussen Hall, M. L. (2004). Acceptance, mindfulness and trauma. In S. C. Hayes, V. M. Follette, & M. M. Linehan (Eds.), *Mindfulness and acceptance: Expanding the cognitive-behavioral tradition*. New York: Guilford.

Hayes, S. C. (2002). Buddhism and acceptance and commitment therapy. *Cognitive and Behavioral Practice, 9,* 58–66.

Hayes, S. C. (2004a). Acceptance and commitment therapy, relational frame theory, and the third wave of behavioral and cognitive therapies. *Behavior Therapy, 35,* 638–665.

Hayes, S. C. (2004b). Acceptance and commitment therapy and the new behavior therapies: Mindfulness, acceptance, and relationship. In S. C. Hayes, V. M. Follette, & M. M. Linehan (Eds.), *Mindfulness and acceptance: Expanding the cognitive-behavioral tradition*. New York: Guilford.

Hayes, S. C., & Wilson, K. G. (2003). Mindfulness: Method and process. *Clinical Psychology: Science and Practice, 10*(2), 161.

James, W. (2000). *Pragmatism and other writings*. New York: Penguin.
James, W. (2013). *The varieties of religious experience: A study of human nature*. Scotts Valley: CreateSpace Independent Publishing Platform.
Jennings, P. (2010). *Mixing minds: The power of relationship in psychoanalysis and Buddhism*. Somerville: Wisdom.
Kabat-Zinn, J. (1990). *Full catastrophe living*. New York: Dell.
Kabat-Zinn, J. (2012). *Mindfulness for beginners: Reclaiming the present moment—and your life*. Boulder: Sounds True.
Kalupahana, D. (2015). *Mulamadhyamakakarika of Nagarjuna: The philosophy of the middle way*. New Delhi, India: Motilal Banarsidass.
Kuhn, T. (1970). *The structure of scientific revolutions*. Chicago:University of Chicago Press.
Linehan, M. M., & Schmidt, H. (1995). The dialectics of effective treatment of borderline personality disorder. In W. O. O'Donohue & L. Krasner (Eds.), *Theories in behavior therapy: Exploring behavior change* (pp. 553–584). Washington, D.C.: American Psychological Association.
Linehan, M. M., Armstrong, H. E., Suarez, A., Allmon, D., & Heard, H. L. (1991).Cognitive-behavioral treatment of chronically parasuicidal borderline patients. *Archives of General Psychiatry, 48,* 1060–1064.
Linehan, M. M., Schmidt, H., Dimeff, L. A., Craft, J. C., Kanter, J., & Contois, K. A. (1999). Dialectical behavioral therapy for patients with borderline personality disorder and drug-dependence. *American Journal of Addictions, 8,* 279–292.
Linehan, M. M., Cochran, B. N., & Kehrer, C. A. (2001) Dialectical behavior therapy for borderline personality disorder. In D. H. Barlow (Ed.), *Clinical handbook of psychological disorders* (3rd ed., pp. 470–522). New York: Guilford.
Linehan, M. M., Dimeff, L. A., Reynolds, S. K., Contois, K., Shaw-Welch, S., Heagerty, P., et al. (2002). Dialectical behavior therapy versus comprehensive validation plus 12 steps for the treatment of opioid dependent women meeting criteria for borderline personality disorder. *Drug and Alcohol Dependence, 67,* 13–26.
Ma, S. H., & Teasdale, J. D. (2003). Mindfulness-based cognitive therapy for depression: Replication and exploration of differential relapse prevention effects. *Journal of Consulting and Clinical Psychology, 72,* 31–40.
Mahasi, S. (1985). *The progress of insight: A treatise on Buddhist satipatthana meditation*. Kandy: Buddhist Publication Society.
Marlatt, G. A. (1994). Addiction, mindfulness, and acceptance. Content, context, and the types of psychological acceptance. In S. C. Hayes, N. S. Jacobson, V. M. Folllette, & M. J. Dougher (Eds.), *Acceptance and change: Content and context in psychotherapy* (pp. 175–197). Reno: Context.
Marlatt, G. A., Witkiewitz, K, Dillworth, T., Bowen, S. W., Parks, G. A., Macpherson, L. M., Lonczak, H. S., Larimer, M.E., Simpson, T., Blume, A. W., Crutcher, R. (2004). Vipassana meditation as a treatment for alcohol and drug use disorders. In Hayes, S. C., Follette, V. M., and Linehan, M.M. Mindfulness and acceptance: *Expanding te cognitive-behavioral tradition*. New York NY: Guilford (pp. 261–287).
McKay, M., Wood, J., & Brantley, J. (2007). *The dialectical behavior therapy skills workbook: Practical DBT exercises for learning mindfulness, interpersonal effectiveness, emotional regulation, and distress tolerance*. Oakland: New Harbinger.
NICE. (2009). *Depression—The treatment and management of depression in adults: Quick reference guide*. NICE Clinical Guideline CG90. London: National Institute for Clinical Excellence.
Pandita, S. U. (1992). *In this very life*. Boston: Wisdom.
Puhakka, K. (2003). Awakening from the spell of reality: Lessons from Nagarjuna. In S. R. Segall (Ed.), *Encountering Buddhism: Western psychology and Buddhist teachings* (pp. 131–141). Albany: SUNY.
Puhakka, K. (2012). Buddhist wisdom in the west: A 50-year perspective on the contributions of Alan Watts. In P. Columbus & D. Rice (Eds.), *Alan Watts here and now: Contributions to philosophy and psychology*. Albany: SUNY.
Puligandla, R. (1975). *Essentials of Indian philosophy*. Wheaton: Abingdon.

Ramanan, V. K. (1986). *Nagarjuna's philosophy*. Delhi: Motilal Banarsidass.
Rimes, K. A., & Wingrove, J. (2011). Pilot study of mindfulness-based cognitive therapy for trainee clinical psychologists. *Behavioural and Cognitive Psychotherapy, 39,* 235–241.
Segal, Z. V., Williams, J. M.G., & Teasdale, J. D. (2002). Mindfulness-based cognitive therapy for depression. New York: Guilford.
Segal, Z. V., Teasdale, J.D., & Williams, J. M.G. (2004). Mindfulness-based cognitive therapy: Theoretical rationale and empirical status. In S. C. Hayes, V. M. Follette, & M. M. Linehan (Eds.), *Mindfulness and acceptance: Expanding the cognitive-behavioral tradition*. New York: Guilford.
Shapiro, S. L., Astin, J. A., Bishop, S. R., & Cordova, M. (2005) Mindfulness-based stress-reduction for healthcare professionals: Results from a randomized trial. *International Journal of Stress Management, 12,* 164–176.
Shonin, E., & Van Gordon, W. (2014). Manager's experiences of meditation awareness training. *Mindfulness*. doi:10.1007/s12671-014-0334-y.
Shonin, E., Van Gordon, W., Dunn, T. J., Singh, N. N., & Griffiths, M. D. (2014). Meditation awareness training (MAT) for work-related wellbeing and job performance: A randomized controlled trial. *International Journal of Mental Health and Addiction*. doi:10.1007/s 11469-014-9513–2.
Teasdale, J. D., Segal, Z., & Williams, J. M. G. (1994). How does cognitive therapy prevent depressive relapse and why should attentional control (mindfulness) training help? *Behavioural Research and Therapy, 31,* 25–39.
Walsh, R. (1995). Phenomenological mapping: A method for describing and comparing states of consciousness. *The Journal of Transpersonal Psychology, 27,* 1–23.
Walsh, R. (1999). Asian contemplative disciplines: Common practices, clinical applications, and research findings. *The Journal of Transpersonal Psychology, 31,* 83–107.

Part III
Further Buddhist Perspectives on Mindfulness

Chapter 12
Mindfulness and Vigilance in Tsong-kha-pa's Great Treatise on the Stages of the Path to Enlightenment

James B. Apple

12.1 Introduction

This chapter centers upon the theme of mindfulness and vigilance according to Tsong-kha-pa's *Great Treatise on the Stages of the Path to Enlightenment* (Tib. *lam rim chen mo;* hereafter *Great Treatise*). Tsong-kha-pa (1357–1419) was a highly acclaimed Tibetan Buddhist scholar–meditator and founding figure of what became the Gelukpa *(dge lugs pa)* tradition. After briefly introducing the topic of mindfulness and vigilance in the life and works of Tsong-kha-pa, I discuss Tsong-kha-pa's understanding of the nature of mind and mental functions, and then contextualize the place of mindfulness and vigilance within the framework of his exegesis on the meditative process in the *Great Treatise*. The *Great Treatise* is Tsong-kha-pa's masterpiece work that brings together *Mahāyāna* Buddhist moral and mental cultivations into an integrated system of gradual path stages *(lam rim)* that lead to the awakening of Buddhahood.

12.2 Mindfulness and Vigilance in the Life and Works of Tsong-kha-pa

Tsong-kha-pa was a distinguished scholar, monk, philosopher, and meditation master who was one of the most profoundly influential and innovative thinkers in the history of Tibetan Buddhism. Born as the fourth child to an ordinary nomadic family in the Northeast Tibetan province of Amdo, Tsong-kha-pa would later become such a prominent figure in Tibetan Buddhist scholarship that the later Gelukpa *(dge lugs pa)* tradition would call him "the Second Buddha" *(sang rgyas gnyis pa)*.

J. B. Apple (✉)
Department of Classics and Religion, University of Calgary, 2500 University Drive N.W., Calgary, AB T2N 1N4, Canada
e-mail: jbapple@ucalgary.ca

E. Shonin et al. (eds.), *Buddhist Foundations of Mindfulness*,
Mindfulness in Behavioral Health, DOI 10.1007/978-3-319-18591-0_12

Tsong-kha-pa, an erudite and thoroughly trained scholar, was also an accomplished practitioner who blended both theory and practice together, utilizing both the emphasis on monastic discipline and the techniques of Tantric meditation. He is most widely known as the founder of the Ganden-pa *(dga'-ldan pa)* school, which later developed into the present-day Gelukpa *(dge-lugs-pa)* school, of which the 14th Dalai Lama Tenzin Gyatso is affliated (Apple 2004).

Tsong-kha-pa, also known as Jey Rimpochey (Tib. *rje rin-po-che* "precious venerable one"), lived during a unique period of Tibetan Buddhist history that provided the cultural conditions for his meticulous and erudite scholarship. This pivotal point, which Ruegg (2000, p. 5) referred to as the "classical-systematic" period of Tibetan Buddhist doctrinal development, was the cusp between the full assimilation of Indian Buddhism and its systemization, the "high point of Tibetan textual exegesis, philosophical penetration and systematic hermeneutics" (p. 5) during the fourteenth to sixteenth centuries. This was a period of Tibetan Buddhist development in which all the major Indian Buddhist commentaries had been translated into Tibetan, and several generations of indigenous Tibetan interpreters had composed commentaries to Indian Buddhist works. As such, it was a period where it was possible for the first time to examine all Indian Buddhist commentaries in a standardized religious language *(chos skad)* that allowed for new intellectual developments to take place.

The Tibetan scholastic cultural purview that was inherited from India was modeled upon the study, reflection, and exegesis of Indian Buddhist *śāstras*—technical texts composed of stanzas usually accompanied with a commentary (i.e., *Madhyamakāvatāra, Pramāṇavārttika, Abhidharmakośa*). This genre of Buddhist literature had been translated primarily during the second wave *(phyi dar)* of scriptural importation into Tibet several 100 years earlier (tenth to twelfth century). Scholar monks such as Tsong-kha-pa would have memorized such technical treatises and been able to utilize this mnemonic skill in debating and refining subtle hermeneutical points of textual exegesis on a variety of topics within Buddhist scholasticism such as *Abhidharma, Pramāṇa* (epistemology), and Madhyamaka (middle way philosophy).

Tsong-kha-pa was most likely introduced to the basic principles of mindfulness *(smṛti)* and vigilance *(saṃprajanya)* during his initial systematic training in his late teenage years while studying in central Tibet. The late fourteenth century in Tibet was a period where scholars could travel from monastery to monastery to receive teachings in exoteric and esoteric topics from spiritual teachers of diverse lineages. During his late teenage years, Tsong-kha-pa mastered and memorized technical digests of Buddhist scholasticism such as the *Abhisamayālaṃkāra, Abhidharmakośa,* and *Mahāyānasūtrālaṃkara* while studying in central Tibet. In his 20s, he began to write brief texts, preserved in his collected works, such as *The Stairway taken by those of Lucid Intelligence* (*Blo gsal bgrod pa'i them skas;* translated in Apple 2013), a detailed exegesis of Noble beings *(ārya)* based on *Abhidharma* texts, *The Ocean of Eloquence* (*Legs par bshad pa'i rgya mtsho;* translated in Sparham 1993), an examination of the "storehouse, basis-of-all consciousness" (Skt. *ālaya-vijñāna*) in *Yogācāra* literature, and *Notes on the Concentrations and Formless Absorptions* (*bsam gzugs zin bris;* translated in Zahler 2009). These texts provide detailed examinations of topics within *Abhidharma* and *Yogācāra* scholasticism, with the later work discussing his understanding of the preparations for, and actual practice of, the concentrations *(bsam gtan, dhyāna)* and formless absorptions *(gzugs med kyi snoms 'jug, ārūpyasamāpatti)*. This time of formative training in Tsong-kha-pa's life is considered to be the first period of his intellectual development and is referred to as the "*Prajñāpāramitā* study period," a phase which culminates with his writing of the *Golden Garland* (*gser phreng;* translation in Sparham 2008–2013) commentary to the *Abhisamayālaṃkāra* in May or June of 1388. In these works, Tsong-kha-pa only briefly mentions mindfulness and vigilance while discussing the role of these mental qualities within the broader context of path structures and topical exegesis centered around the *Abhidharma, Yogācāra,* and *Abhisamayālaṃkāra.*

After this period of initial intellectual and scholarly development, Tsong-kha-pa entered into a transitional phase lasting almost 10 years where he engaged in meditative retreat, refined his study of exoteric and esoteric Buddhist works, and had a number of visionary encounters with high-level bodhisattvas. During this period, in 1390, Tsong-kha-pa met Lama Umapa Pawo Dorje *(bla-ma dbu-ma-ba dpa'-bo rdo-rje),* who served as an intermediary for Tsong-kha-pa to directly communicate with Mañjuśrī, the tenth-stage bodhisattva of wisdom. According to traditional biographies, during time spent in retreat with Lama Umapa, Tsong-kha-pa was instructed by Mañjuśrī in Madhyamaka philosophy and important points in esoteric tantric practices (Thurman 1982). In 1395, Tsong-kha-pa met Lhodrag drubchen Namkha Gyaltsen (*lho-brag grub-chen nam-mkha' rgyal-mtshan,* 1326–1401) who gave him orally transmitted teachings on the *Bka'-gdams-pa* (hereafter, Kadampa) *Stages of the Path (lam rim)*. Namkha Gyaltsen also served as an intermediary for Tsong-kha-pa to communicate with the bodhisattva Vajrapaṇi who answered a number of Tsong-kha-pa's inquiries. This dialogue is recorded in the *Garland of Supremely Healing Nectars* (*zhu lan sman mchog bdud rtsi'i 'phreng ba,* Thurman 1982), where Tsong-kha-pa asks several questions related to meditation practice. On this topic, Tsong-kha-pa received clarification regarding the faults of laxity and excitement and employing the "watchman of vigilance," key points that contributed to Tsong-kha-pa's initial understanding of serenity *(śamatha, zhi gnas)* and indicated his interest in refining his knowledge of mindfulness and vigilance.

In the spring of the wood-pig year (1395–1396), he reviewed for 6 months the "stages of the path" work of Geshe Drinley *(brin-las-pa)* called the *bstan-rim-chen-mo.* At this time, he gained certainty for the importance of Atiśa's *Bodhipathapradīpa* in understanding the path and made a determination to write a manual based on Atiśa's text. Tsong-kha-pa's period of meditative retreat and study culminated in 1398 when he had a transformative experience of awakening in which he had a direct vision of reality. After this transformative experience, Tsong-kha-pa wrote *The Praise for Dependent Relativity* (*rten 'brel bstod pa;* Gyatso and Woodhouse 2011) which expresses his realization of the profound unity of dependent arising and emptiness. The transformative experience had a great effect upon Tsong-kha-pa as a great amount of his scholastic and cultural activity occurred after the age of 40. As van der Kuijp (1985, p. 47) noted, the year 1398 "...separates the old from the new Tsong-kha-pa. His enormous literary output from that time up to his demise in

1419...set into motion a series of momentous controversies among his contemporaries and immediate successors. These contributed greatly to the further fragmentation of the Sa-skya-pa school and ultimately resulted in the establishment of the more or less autonomous Dga'-ldan-pa doctrinal entity." He gained great renown as the "clarifier" *(gsal-byed-pa)* for his ability to differentiate the purport of Buddhist teachings and his acute analysis displaying refined hermeneutical exegesis on a number of topics and commentaries. In 1401, Tsong-kha-pa gave teachings on the chapter on ethics from Asaṅga's *Bodhisattvabhūmi* (Tatz 1986) as well as the *Gurupañcāśikā* (see Sparham 1999). Tsong-kha-pa's commentary to Asaṅga's *Bodhisattvabhūmi* on the ethics chapter does contain brief comments on mindfulness and vigilance but they are not discussed in an extensive manner.

Tsong-kha-pa and his teacher/colleague Rendawa Shönu Lodrö (*red-mda'-ba gzhon-nu blo-gros,* 1349–1412) then went to Reting *(rwa-greng),* a monastic learning center northeast of Lhasa founded by Atiśa's great Kadampa disciple Dromtönpa Gyalwai Jungné (*'brom-ston-pa rgyal ba'i-'byung gnas*, 1005–1064). The initial time that Tsong-kha-pa spent at Reting was, if we are to follow the traditional biographies (*Rgyal-dbang chos-rje blo-bzang 'phrin-las rnam-rgyal* 2009), the point when he began the initial outlines to his *Great Treatise* as well as when he made an extensive study of, and meditated upon, the principles of meditative serenity (*śamatha, zhi gnas*). It is said that Tsong-kha-pa focused upon the *Mahāyānasūtrālaṃkāra, Madhyāntavibhāga, Abhidharmasamuccaya,* and *Śrāvakabhūmi* for a period of several months and gained a distinctive understanding of the principles of meditative serenity. I think that the traditional biographies are correct that Tsong-kha-pa focused in this manner to gain his perspective on serenity. He cited these texts throughout the section on serenity in the *Great Treatise* and recommended these texts several times for one to study in order to gain a firm understanding of serenity. Although Tsong-kha-pa mentioned, and briefly described, the Kadampa system of achieving serenity through the six powers, four types of attention, and nine mental states (see below), the detailed exegesis that he provided on serenity based on the above mentioned technical digests, along with a few other texts such as Kamalaśīla's *Bhāvanākrama,* marks the distinctive understanding that he provided to the topic of meditative serenity.

Our exegesis and interpretation of Tsong-kha-pa's understanding of mindfulness and vigilance is drawn from the *Byang chub lam rim che ba, The Great Treatise on the Stages of the Path to Enlightenment* (referred to as *Great Treatise* hereafter). This text, completed in 1402, has been referred to as "one of the greatest religious or secular works in the library of our human heritage (Thurman in Cutler and Newland (2000), p. 13) as well as "one of the most renowned works of Buddhist thought and practice to have been composed in Tibet" (Ruegg 2000, p. 17). I have cited throughout this chapter, unless otherwise noted, the English translation of the Lamrim Chenmo Translations Committee's (Cutler, editor-in-chief) *The Great Treatise on the Stages of the Path to Enlightenment,* Volumes I, II, III (Snow Lion, Ithaca: 2000, 2002) and the 1985 Tibetan edition with the title *Byang chub lam rim che ba* published by Tsho Ngön *(mtsho sngon)* People's Press based on the Bya khyung block prints. The translation from Tibetan is followed by brackets that refers to the

Tibetan edition page number and numbers given in parenthesis refers to the English translation of Cutler and Newland.

12.3 Mind and Mental Functions in the Meditative Process of Serenity

For Tsong-kha-pa, the mind (Skt. *citta,* Tib. *sems*) is the fundamental basis of *saṃsāra,* the repeated cycle of rebirth and re-death along with all its sufferings, and *nirvāṇa,* the complete cessation of all suffering. In the context of Tsong-kha-pa's soteriological worldview, what is most important is that one understands the structure of the mind and its accompanying mental processes and then utilize this knowledge as a means for transforming the continuum of one's mental awareness. In broad terms, Tsong-kha-pa outlined in the later portions of the *Great Treatise* two essential trainings of the mind: the cultivation of meditative serenity *(śamatha, zhi gnas)* and then analytical discernment through special insight *(vipaśyanā, lhag mthong)*. In the following brief discussion, I describe the basic presumptions that Tsong-kha-pa has about the mind and mental processes as it relates to his discussion of mindfulness and vigilance in the process of refined mental cultivation.

Tsong-kha-pa considered the mind as an informative awareness endowed with a luminous and pure potential. He understood cognitive knowledge *(rig pa),* mind *(blo),* and conscious awareness *(shes pa)* to be synonyms that refer to mental events, episodes, or states of awareness where a subject *(yul can)* cognizes an object that appears to it (Tsong-kha-pa 1986a). Minds are moments of conscious awareness that are active agents of knowing (Rinbochay and Napper 1980) that arise together with facets or functionary processes *(caitta, sems byung),* some of which are classified as virtuous, variable, or afflictive. Tsong-kha-pa also assumed that the mind in its natural state is luminous *(gsal ba)* and pure *(rnam dag)*. It is luminous because it is free of conceptualization with respect to the object that appears to it (Wallace 1998). Impure mental afflictions such as ignorance and attachment are considered adventitious *(glo bur ba)* to the mind. The mind's luminous and pure nature did not mean for Tsong-kha-pa that the mind has always primordially been free from mental afflictions. Rather, due to the mind's lack of having a substantial existence *(rdzas pa)* or intrinsic essence *(rang bzhin med pa),* luminosity and purity signify the potential to be free from negative mental afflictions, such as malice and hatred. The mind has the potential to be reconditioned and reoriented, purified of negativities, due to the fact that mental afflictions lack intrinsic essence (Tsong-kha-pa 1986b, pp. 339–340).

Tibetan Buddhist scholars like Tsong-kha-pa view the mind as consisting of a series of individual moments of conscious awareness that relate to their objects rather than being merely a reservoir of information or an apparatus of a mechanical brain that produces thoughts and ideas (Dreyfus 2002; Rinbochay and Napper 1980). This sequential flow of causally interrelated moments of awareness constitutes a mental continuum *(santāna, rgyud)*. The mental states that comprise such a stream of awareness may apprehend real or imaginary things as their objects of cognition *(shes bya)*. Tsong-kha-pa posits many different types of mind or consciousness (*blo rig*[*s*]) based on the general understanding of mind as "that which is clear and cognizes." He classified multiple types of awareness or consciousness (*blo rig*[*s*]) such as sense awareness, mental awareness, gross minds, subtle minds, and very subtle minds. A sevenfold scheme of awarenesses drawn from the Indian Buddhist epistemological tradition was posited in relation to distinguishing valid *(tshad ma)* from nonvalid *(tshad min)* modes of cognition and awareness. Tsong-kha-pa also posited various types of awareness in relation to their mode of activity. In terms of how they engage their objects, minds may be categorized into either conceptual *(rtog pa)* or nonconceptual minds *(rtog med)*. Awareness may be classified into either sense awareness *(dbang shes)* or mental awareness *(yid shes)* from the standpoint of the objects which dominate.

This later classification is important to note, as Tsong-kha-pa in his discussion of the cultivation of meditative serenity emphasized that mental awareness should be directed inward when placing attention on an object of meditation (*dmigs pa; Great Treatise,* vol. 3, p. 44). This is because, for Tsong-kha-pa, objects of meditation are only to be perceived and focused upon by mental awareness rather than the five spheres of sensory objects and their awarenesses. This means that the techniques of mindfulness and vigilance consists of perceptions of purely mental awarenesses that focus on inner objects of meditation and internal symptoms of agitation and slackness (Wallace 1998).

Another important classification that Tsong-kha-pa presumed in his discussion of the meditation process is the analysis of awareness in terms of primary minds *(citta, sems)* and mental facets, factors, or functions *(caitta, sems byung)*. Mind and mental functions arise at the same time and are essentially identical. However, they may be defined separately from each other, with the mind being an awareness of the mere nature of an object, while a mental factor or function is an awareness which is defined in terms of its aspectual function (Apple and Dunne 2001). From the beginnings of the classical-systematic period of Tibetan Buddhist scholasticism, of which Tsong-kha-pa was a major figure, the study of mind and mental functions was based largely on the *Abhidharmasamuccaya* (Rahula 2001). This treatise lists 51 mental functions, including five omnipresent mental functions *(kun 'gro lnga, pañcasarvatraga)*, 5 mental functions for a determined object *(yul nges pa, pratiniyataviṣaya)*, 11 virtuous mental functions *(dge ba, kuśala)*, six fundamental afflictions *(rtsa nyon drug, ṣaḍmūlakleśa)*, 20 secondary afflictions *(nye nyon, upakleśa)*, and four variable mental functions *(gzhan 'gyur bzhi, caturanyathābhava)*. Related to this typology, Tsong-kha-pa described the ways in which virtuous and accurate mental factors or states may be identified and cultivated, while non-virtuous and erroneous mental states, once identified and understood, may be replaced and discarded.

In his discussion of the meditative process that employs mindfulness and vigilance, Tsong-kha-pa only emphasized a few of these mental functions in his descriptive exegesis. Mindfulness itself is included among the five mental functions for a determined object in Asaṅga's *Abhidharmasamuccaya* (Rahula 2001). In general, mindfulness is the mind's "not forgetting" of an object of meditation and has the function of non-distraction. Tsong-kha-pa understood that any achievement of concentration is necessarily accomplished through this distinctive state. Vigilance is a refined introspective awareness that arises with the presence of mindfulness. It is considered an aspect of discernment *(shes rab, prajñā)* and functions to provide watch over the cultivation of mindfulness as will be discussed below.

Among the five omnipresent mental functions, Tsong-kha-pa mentioned intention *(sems pa, cetanā)* and attention *(yid la byed pa, manaskāra)* in his discussion of meditative serenity. Intention is a mental function that makes the mind be drawn or incited toward an object. This mental function is discussed toward the end of Tsong-kha-pa's exegesis on mindfulness and vigilance as it will help drive awareness to rid itself of the negative mental states of laxity and excitation. Tsong-kha-pa described intention with the analogy of how iron is helplessly drawn to a magnet, as the mind helplessly becomes involved with an object due to this mental function. Another omnipresent mental function, attention, directs the mind toward a distinctive object of meditation. Concentration *(ting nge 'dzin, samādhi)* is mentioned throughout Tsong-kha-pa's discussion and is considered to be a power related to mental function of pliancy *(shin tu sbyangs pa, praśrabdhi),* one of the 11 virtuous mental functions.

Tsong-kha-pa placed attention on excitement or agitation *(rgod pa, auddhatya)* and laxity *(bying ba, laya)* among the mental processes related to the afflictions. Excitement, listed among the 20 secondary afflictions, is a derivative of attachment, and it is a mental function that engages with craving and is drawn to previously experienced desirable qualities. In the discussion of mindfulness in the *Great Treatise,* Tsong-kha-pa made a distinction between laxity *(bying ba, laya)* and lethargy. Lethargy or sluggishness *(rmugs pa, styāna)* is an unsuitable mental function in which physical and mental heaviness becomes associated with delusion. Mental afflictions increase in dependence upon this mental function. Laxity, for Tsong-kha-pa, was caused by lethargy, and it is a slackness of awareness that lacks vivid clarity. The understanding of these mental states infuses Tsong-kha-pa's discussion of the path in the *Great Treatise* and is presumed in his exegesis of mindfulness and vigilance.

12.4 Tsong-kha-pa's *Great Treatise*: An Encyclopedic Manual of Mahāyāna Buddhist Mental Cultivation

The *Great Treatise on the Stages of the Path* is an encyclopedic manual of detailed instructions that outlines practices for bodhisattvas (Tib. *byang chub sems pa*) who follow the Mahāyāna Buddhist path to Omniscient Buddhahood. The *Great Treatise* instructions are set out in sections which are further divided into subsections and individual rubrics, with each division providing reasoned discourse supported by scriptural citations to guide the practitioner through a series of mental cultivations that lead to awakening (Ruegg 2000). In this manner, the analytical procedures, reasoned discourses, and scriptural quotations discussed in the *Great Treatise* are not primarily understood as polemical rhetoric against former commentators or partisan diatribes against opponent groups, but, rather, may be read as an internal dialogue that leads the practitioner gradually through a series of cultivations aimed at profound mental transformation. Tsong-kha-pa's *Great Treatise* embodies a series of spiritual exercises utilizing reasoned discourse to bring about a transformation of the person from the mental afflictions *(nyon mongs)* and karmic propensities such that they are able to achieve long-lasting peace beyond suffering *(mya ngan las 'das pa)* and ultimately, through achieving complete Buddhahood, accomplish the welfare of others. The exercises in this instance consist of a combination of meditative stabilizing procedures *('jog sgom)* and analytical meditative realizations *(dpyad sgom)* that familiarize and condition the mind *(goms)* with wholesome qualities and cognitive insight. The aim of such practices is to produce within the mental continuum wholesome qualities such as faith, love, and compassion.

As the *Great Treatise* outlines in detail the path to full Buddhahood *(rdzogs pa'i sangs rgyas)* it is considered an all-inclusive guide to training. In fact, the *Great Treatise* is not part of the official philosophical curriculum in Gelukpa *(dge-lugs-pa)*-based monastic institutions, but rather is often utilized for contemplation in meditative retreat by both lay and monastic practitioners (Napper 2001). Each section describes the necessary meditative cultivations for proceeding in a gradual manner. The first section of the text outlines how to rely upon a spiritual teacher *(bla ma),* an individual who Tibetan Buddhists regard as absolutely necessary for a being's spiritual development and who is considered the root of the path *(lam gyi rtsa ba)*. After this section, the rest of the work presents various stages of training one's mind. These instructions include coming to understand the rare and precious opportunity that human rebirths provide for reaching Buddhahood and then the way in which one develops that opportunity into the occasion for full awakening for the benefit of all sentient beings. The manner of actualizing the precious human rebirth for Buddhahood is encapsulated within a schema outlining three types of spiritual capacity: training the mind in the stages of the path in common with individuals of small capacity (*skyes bu chung*), training in the stages of the path in common with individuals of moderate spiritual capacity *(skyes bu 'bring),* and training in the stages of the individual of great capacity *(skyes bu chen po)*.

Training the mind in the stages of the path for individuals of small capacity *(skyes bu chung)* motivates a practitioner away from the concerns of the present life and encourages the cultivation of spiritual practices that are thought to result in the higher rebirth as humans or gods in future lives. These exercises include contemplating death and impermanence *('chi ba mi rtag pa),* the sufferings of the lower realms of existence *(ngan 'gro' sdug bsngal),* taking refuge in the three jewels of Buddha, Dharma, and Sangha, and developing conviction in the karmic principles of cause and effect.

Training in the stages of the path for individuals of moderate spiritual capacity *(skyes bu 'bring)* focuses on disenchantment with cyclic existence, and striving for their own liberation from cyclic existence. These cultivations focus on the four truths of the Noble One, the Buddha. That is, the inherent suffering in cyclic existence *(saṃsāra),* of how cyclic existence is perpetuated, the nature of its cessation, and training in the actualization of the truth of the path that leads to cessation. The truth of the path is subsumed under the three trainings *(bslab pa gsum)* of morality *(tshul khrims),* concentration *(ting nge 'dzin),* and wisdom *(shes rab).*

The trainings on the stages of the path for individuals of great spiritual vision or capacity *(skyes bu chen po)* are for those who strive for omniscient and compassionate Buddhahood, "in order to extinguish all the sufferings of all living beings" (*Great Treatise,* 131 [87]). The text elaborately details the altruistic aspiration for awakening *(byang chub sems skyed, bodhicittodpāda),* which is considered the gateway *('jug sgo)* to the Mahāyāna path of bodhisattvas. After instructions for developing this unique aspiration, the *Great Treatise* then describes the purifying trainings for bodhisattvas who have generated that mind.

The cultivation of the altruistic aspiration for awakening entails both training for the welfare of others and developing one's own mental continuum with awakened qualities. Training for other's welfare includes such practices as generating universal equanimity, love, and compassion for all beings and cultivating the exchange of one's self with others *(bdag gzhan mnyam brje).* The practices that develop awakened qualities within one's own mental continuum consist in the training of the six perfections *(phar phyin drug).* That is, the trainings in generosity *(sbyin pa, dāna*), ethical discipline *(tshul khrims, śīla),* patient forbearance *(bzod pa, kṣānti),* energy *(brtson 'grus, vīrya),* concentration *(bsam gtan, dhyāna),* and insight or wisdom *(shes rab, prajñā).* The later two perfections, concentration and insight, are treated in long and extensive sections of the *Great Treatise.* Tsong-kha-pa discussed the perfection of concentration in an extensive manner under the heading of how to cultivate meditative serenity *(zhi gnas),* the essence of concentration.

12.5 Mindfulness and Vigilance in Tsong-kha-pa's Great Treatise

In Tsong-kha-pa 's *Great Treatise,* mindfulness and vigilance are discussed in the context of developing and achieving meditative serenity *(śamatha, zhi gnas).* Meditative serenity (*Great Treatise,* p. 11–103 [468–563]) and insight (*Great Treatise,* pp. 107–359 [564–805]; *vipaśyanā, lhag mthong*) are part of the training in the last two of the six perfections of the Mahāyāna path as serenity is a practice within the perfection of meditative stabilization *(dhyāna, sam gtan),* and insight is a practice within the perfection of wisdom (*prajñā, shes rab*). Tsong-kha-pa considered meditative serenity and insight to be the root of all meditative concentrations *(samādhi, ting nge 'dzin)* found within Mahāyāna and Hīnayāna pathways.

Tsong-kha-pa (*Great Treatise,* p. 47 [504], pp. 89–90 [549], p. 107 [564]) described meditative serenity as having three features consisting of (1) non-discursiveness *(mi rtogs pa),* (2) clarity *(gsal ba)* that is free from laxity, and (3) having a distinctive benefit of delight *(dga' ba)* and bliss *(bde ba).* Meditative serenity consists of an undistracted mind that has mental one pointedness (*Great Treatise,* p. 47 [504]) consisting of no discursive thought at all. Tsong-kha-pa briefly described the complementary aspect of meditation to serenity, insight, as "the wisdom that properly distinguishes the meaning of an object of knowledge" (*shes bya'i don yang dag par rab tu 'byed pa'i shes rab*; *Great Treatise,* p. 19 [474.19]). The section on insight (*Great Treatise,* pp. 107–359 [564–805]) is around two and half times longer than the discussion of serenity and is often considered a separate work known as "Special Insight" (*lhag mthong chen mo*; Jinpa 2002). In the section on insight, Tsong-kha-pa delineated in detail a number of topics that refined his understanding of insight such as identifying the object of negation (Lopez 2001), the relationship between dependent arising and emptiness (Napper 1989), the distinction between "Prāsaṅgika" and "Svātantrika" types of Mādhyamikas (Dreyfus and McClintock 2002), and the uniting of insight and serenity among other topics.

For our purposes here, insight, in brief, consists of the proper examination and detailed analysis that distinguishes the exact particulars of an object. Insight therefore necessarily requires analysis (*Great Treatise,* pp. 327–350 [769–795]. Insight distinguishes the diversity *(ji lta ba)* of conventional things and cognizes their real ultimate nature *(ji snyed pa),* which, for Tsong-kha-pa, is emptiness *(śūnyatā, stong pa nyid),* the lack of intrinsic existence or essence in persons (*Great Treatise,* pp. 289–308 [730–752) and objects (*Great Treatise,* pp. 309–325 [752–769). Ascertainment based on insight eradicates afflictions that perpetuates beings suffering and rebirth.

Serenity and insight must both be cultivated as neither one alone achieves sustained cognitive ascertainment and transformation (*Great Treatise,* pp. 19–23 [476–480]). For Tsong-kha-pa, although insight provides knowledge which is not derived from serenity, non-discursive serenity nevertheless provides insight with a quality of steadiness that is more powerful than insight alone, and this enables a discerning consciousness to analyze selflessness without distraction (*Great Treatise,* pp. 21–22 [477–478]). Tsong-kha-pa, based on the analysis of a number of technical digests by Asaṅga, Bhāviveka, Kamalaśīla, and Śāntideva among others, strongly emphasized that the sequence in which one newly develops serenity and insight for the first time is based on achieving serenity first followed by cultivating insight. This sequence leads to a special type of mental pliancy that is able to be maintained in insight (*Great Treatise,* pp. 23–26 [481–483]). Meditators with more experience may alternate the sequence of practice in cultivating serenity and insight.

Tsong-kha-pa discussed how to train in meditative serenity *(zhi gnas la bslab tshul)* in three broad sections with multiple divisions and subdivisions. He first briefly outlined (1) the preconditions for meditative serenity (*zhi gnas kyi tshogs; Great Treatise,* pp. 28–30 [484–486]), discusses (2) how to cultivate serenity *(zhi gnas sgom pa'i tshul)* based on the preconditions (*Great Treatise,* pp. 30–79 [486–537]), and then the (3) measure of the successful cultivation of serenity (*Great Treatise,* pp. 79–90 [536–550]). The preconditions for meditative serenity include such things as dwelling in a quiet and amendable area, having little desires, cultivating contentment, and having pure ethical discipline. The section on how to cultivate serenity consists of instructions on the actual practice *(dngos gzhi)* of meditation that leads to serenity. At this point, Tsong-kha-pa provided an exegesis on the correct bodily posture for meditation *(lus kyi spyod lam)* and the meditative process *(bsgom pa'i rim)* itself. He outlined the contours of the meditative process as follows:

> the "stages of the path" tradition indicates that you achieve serenity by means of the eight antidotes which eliminate the five faults listed in Maitreya's *Separation of the Middle from the Extremes* (*Madhyānta-vibhāga*). Personal instructions passed down from Geshe Lak-sor-wa (dGe-bshes Lag-sor-ba) explain that in addition to that you have to achieve serenity through the six powers, the four types of attention, and the nine mental states which Asaṅga's *Śrāvakabhūmi* explains. (*Great Treatise*, pp. 31–32 [487]).

The structure of the meditative process that Tsong-kha-pa follows is based on a combination of two systems of practice that developed within the Kadampa stages of the path tradition. This tradition consists of the system of the five faults and eight antidotes, based on Maitreya's *Separation of the Middle from the Extremes (Madhyānta-vibhāga),* and the system of powers, attentions, and nine mental states from Asaṅga's *Śrāvakabhūmi* and Maitreya's *Mahāyāna-sūtrālaṃkāra.* Tsong-kha-pa identified Geshe Lak-sor-wa (eleventh century), a Kadampa master who was a direct disciple of Atiśa's student Nag-tsho lo-tsā-ba Tshul-khrims rgyal-ba (b. 1011), as the scholar who combined these two systems for the first time. Tsong-kha-pa then cited the stages of the path commentary of the prominent Kadampa master Sha-ra-ba Yon-tan-grags (1070–1141) to briefly outline and authorize his exegesis of this system and the classical texts that serve as its source. The *Great Treatise* states,

> The methods of the nine mental states are included in the four attentions, and the six faults and the eight applications which are their antidotes are the method [for achieving] all concentrations. This is agreed upon in all teachings about the techniques for meditative stabilization—including those in most *sūtras,* Maitreya's *Ornament for the Mahāyāna Sūtras* and *Separation of the Middle from the Extremes,* Asaṅga's texts on the levels (i.e. *Yogacārabhūmi*) and Kamalaśīla's three *Stages of Meditation.* Those who first have the preconditions for concentration will definitely attain concentration if they use these methods to work at it. (*Great Treatise*, p. 32 [487])

The following table (see Table 12.1) outlines the relationship of the nine mental states, six forces, the four types of attention as factors for achieving meditative serenity. As the details of this system have been explained in other studies on Gelukpa *(dge lugs pa)* meditation practice (Hopkins 1983; Wallace 1998; Zahler 2009), I reference it here to illustrate the place of mindfulness and vigilance within the broader structures of Tsong-kha-pa 's system of developing meditative serenity.

Within the division on the meditative process, Tsong-kha-pa outlined what he termed "the method of developing flawless concentration *(ting nge 'dzin skyon med skyed pa'i tshul)*" followed by an overview of the stages in which the (nine) mental states develop *(sems gnas skye ba'i rim pa).* The subdivision on developing flawless concentration describes the varied objects of meditation *(dmigs pa)* and how to focus the mind on an object of meditation. Objects of meditation include universal objects (*khyab pa'i dmigs pa; Great Treatise,* pp. 35–36 [490–492]), objects for purifying behavior (*spyad pa rnam par sbyong ba'i dmigs pa; Great Treatise,* p. 36 [492]), objects of meditation for the skilful (*mkhas pa'i dmigs pa; Great Treatise,* pp. 36–37 [492–493]), and objects for purifying afflictions (*nyon mongs pa rnam par sbyong ba'i dmigs pa; Great Treatise,* pp. 37–39 [493–496]). Tsong-kha-pa stated that a meditator should focus on an object that appeals to them based on the varied dispositions of the meditator (*Great Treatise,* p. 42 [499]). In the context of the Kadampa stages of the path tradition that Tsong-kha-pa followed, focusing on the bodily form of the Buddha is considered the most beneficial object for developing concentration (Wallace 1998).

After outlining and describing the objects of meditation, Tsong-kha-pa detailed the manner in which one focuses the mind *(sems ji ltar gtod pa'i tshul)* on the object of meditation in order to achieve a concentration of meditative serenity (*zhi gnas kyi ting nge 'dzin;Great Treatise,* pp. 15–16 [503]). He specified that this concentration has two special features: an intense mental clarity *(gsal cha)* and non-discursive stability *(mi rtog pa'i gnas cha)* that single pointedly stays on the object of meditation (*Great Treatise,* p. 47 [504]). Tsong-kha-pa noted that there are two major flaws which obstruct intense clarity and non-discursive stability. He explained that,

> Since the development of this sort of vivid clarity is blocked as long as there is laxity, while one-pointed non-discursiveness is blocked as long as there is excitement, laxity and excitement are the chief obstacles to achieving genuine concentration. So if you do not understand how to identify accurately the subtle and coarse forms of laxity and excitement, or if you do not know how to correctly sustain a concentration which stops these once you have identified them, then it will be impossible for you to develop serenity, not to mention insight. Hence, those who diligently seek concentration should master these techniques. (*Great Treatise,* p. 48 [505])

At this point, Tsong-kha-pa provided his initial explanation of the techniques of mindfulness and vigilance. He then outlined the role that mindfulness plays within the context of developing serenity, more clearly identified the flaws of laxity and excitement, and then discussed the application of vigilance. The *Great Treatise* begins its exegesis on mindfulness and vigilance with the following statement:

> Here, concentration refers to your attention remaining one-pointedly on an object of meditation; in addition it must stay with the object continuously. Two things are needed for this: (1) a technique in which your attention (*sems*) is not distracted from whatever it had as its original object of meditation, and (2) an accurate awareness (*ji lta ba bzhin shes pa*) of whether you are distracted and whether you are becoming distracted. The former is mindfulness; the latter is vigilance. (*Great Treatise,* p. 48 [505])

Mindfulness and vigilance are two aspects of focusing the mind on an object of meditation while developing a sustained concentration of serenity. According to Tsong-kha-pa , mindfulness centers on the meditative object, and vigilance closely monitors the very awareness that one places on that object. Tsong-kha-pa (*Great Treatise*, p. 61 [518]) stressed that it is very important to distinguish mindfulness from vigilance for if one jumbles these awarenesses together it will lead to a jumbled state of concentration. With these points in mind, Tsong-kha-pa provided a detailed exegesis on the definition and implementation of mindfulness in the context of meditation.

12.6 Mindfulness in the *Great Treatise*

In the *Great Treatise,* mindfulness *(dran pa)* is the foundation of cultivating concentration and primarily signifies to not forget the object of meditation and become distracted while one is meditating. The idea is that one apprehends an object of meditation with one's attention and stabilizes the attention on the object without analyzing anything anew. Tsong-kha-pa based his discussion of mindfulness on Asaṅga's *Abhidharmasamuccaya* and noted that it has three features. The *Great Treatise* explains:

> ...mindfulness has three features. (1) Its observed object is "a familiar object," since mindfulness does not occur with regard to a previously unfamiliar object. In this case, the image of a previously ascertained object of meditation appears. (2) Its subjective aspect or manner of apprehension is your mind's not forgetting the object, as indicated by the phrase "your mind is not forgetful." In this case, it is your mind's non-forgetfulness of the object of meditation….(3) Its function is to keep your attention from wandering from the object of meditation. (*Great Treatise,* p. 49 [506])

A critical point in the technique of mindfulness for Tsong-kha-pa centered on properly understanding mindfulness as the "non-forgetfulness of the object of meditation" *(dmigs rten ma brjed pa)*. This entails being continuously mindful of the object of meditation with one's attention fixated without any diversion. As he clarified,

> What does non-forgetfulness mean? It is not mentioned in reference to merely being able to remember what your guru taught you about the object of meditation, thinking or saying "The object of meditation is like this" when you cast your mind to it or when someone asks you about it. Rather, it refers to how your attention is fixed on the object of meditation and brings it to mind clearly without even the slightest distraction. If you are distracted, you lose your mindfulness to the extent that you are distracted. Therefore, after you have set your attention on the object of meditation in the manner explained above, you think, "In this way, I have fixed my attention on the object of meditation." Then, without new examination, you sustain the force of that awareness in unbroken continuity. (*Great Treatise,* p. 49 [506])

Maintaining a state of sustained attention to the object of meditation is the most critical point in the technique of developing mindfulness. Tsong-kha-pa, citing Bhāviveka's *Madhyamakahṛdaya* and Kamalaśīla's *Bhāvanakrama,* utilized the traditional analogy of the mind being like an elephant which is bound with the rope of mindfulness to a pillar that represents the object of meditation. While the rope of mindfulness binds the wild elephant of the mind to the pillar, the iron hook of vigilance controls lapses in attention. This analogy demonstrates how mindfulness fixes in a sustained manner one's attention on an object of meditation, while vigilance intervenes to restrain any backsliding from sustained attention. Tsong-kha-pa then specified,

> Mindfulness directly and continually fastens your attention to the object of meditation. However, indirectly vigilance also focuses your attention on the object of meditation, for you depend on noticing actual or incipient laxity and excitement with vigilance, and then stabilize your attention on the primary object without falling under their influence…[therefore,]…both mindfulness and vigilance focus your mind on the object of meditation. (*Great Treatise,* p. 50, [507])

On this account, mindfulness and vigilance are two complementary facets of focusing the mind on an object of meditation in the process of developing serenity. While mindfulness is the technique of direct focus on the object, vigilance does so in an indirect manner while monitoring one's attention. In addition to understanding that mindfulness is a direct focused attention on an object of meditation, Tsong-kha-pa asserted that mindfulness must ascertain its meditative object with a sense of certitude in order to have potent clarity. Otherwise, one may develop a casual level of mindfulness that is clear, but lacks the vivid intensity of certain knowledge *(nges shes)* that is bereft of subtle laxity.

12.7 Excitement and Laxity: The Two Great Flaws that Hinder Meditative Serenity

As mentioned above, Tsong-kha-pa described excitement and laxity as the two major flaws that inhibit the development and perdurance of the concentration of meditative serenity. The two main antidotes to excitement and laxity are mindfulness and vigilance. Tsong-kha-pa defined excitement and laxity in detail before providing more precise instructions on the application of vigilance in relation to mindfulness.

Tsong-kha-pa based his definition of excitement on Asaṅga's *Abhidharmasamuccaya.* As with the definition of mindfulness, he specified three aspects to this definition noting excitement's object, subjective aspect, and its function:

> (1) Its object is an attractive and pleasant one. (2) Its subjective aspect is that your mind is unquiet and scattered outward. As it is a derivative of attachment, it engages its object with a sense of craving. (3) Its function is to impede stabilization of your mind on its object. (*Great Treatise,* p. 58 [514])

Tsong-kha-pa explained that excitement is when an inwardly fixed state of attention becomes helplessly distracted toward sensory objects. Tsong-kha-pa identified excitement as derived from attachment *('dod chags, rāga)*. Tsong-kha-pa's placing of excitement in relation to attachment was based on his study of *Abhidharma.* As mentioned above, during the period of Tibetan Buddhist scholasticism when Tsong-kha-pa was a major figure, the study of mind and mental functions was based largely on the *Abhidharmasamuccaya.* This treatise lists 51 mental functions, of which there are 6 fundamental afflictions *(rtsa nyon drug, ṣaḍmūlakleśa)* and 20 secondary afflictions *(nye nyon, upakleśa)*. As attachment is one of the six fundamental afflictions, Tsong-kha-pa was stating that excitement is derived from this mental affliction rather than the mental function of distraction *(rnam par g.yeng ba, vikṣepa),* which is one of the 20 secondary afflictions.

Tsong-kha-pa noted that while it is easy to recognize excitement, laxity is hard to comprehend since it is not clearly identified in the authoritative classic texts (*Great Treatise,* p. 60 [516]). He considered a proper understanding of laxity a major point for practicing flawless concentration. In this regard, he emphasized that there is a distinction between laxity *(bying ba)* and lethargy *(rmugs pa)* that is not often recognized (*Great Treatise,* p. 58 [515]). Based on Kamalaśīla's *Intermediate Bhāvanakrama,* Tsong-kha-pa understood lethargy to be *a cause of* laxity. Lethargy, based on the *Abhidharmasamuccya* and *Abhidharmakośabhāṣya,* is a derivative of delusion and consists of a heaviness and unserviceability of mind and body. On the other hand, laxity

> means that your mind's way of apprehending the object of meditation is slack, and it does not apprehend the object with much vividness or firmness. So even if it is limpid, if your mind's way of apprehending the object is not highly vivid, then laxity has set in…. Laxity may be virtuous or ethically neutral, whereas lethargy is either a nonvirtuous or ethically neutral mental obstruction, and it is invariably a derivative of delusion. (*Great Treatise*, p. 59 [616])

In this way, Tsong-kha-pa emphasized that his understanding of laxity accords with the explanation given in Kamalaśīla's *Intermediate Bhāvanakrama* and that one should be attentive with a subtle awareness that recognizes this understanding. This is because one may mistakenly think that one's mind has flawless concentration by merely having a limpid clarity that is devoid of a darkened and cloudy mental awareness. Along with this mistaken presumption, one may think that "good relaxation is good meditation" (*glod pa rab la sgom rab; Great Treatise*, p. 51 [508]). However, such a limpid mental state lacks the vividness that concentration requires. As the limpid quality of a relaxed mind is not sufficient, a degree of intensifying or tightening *(grims cha)* is necessary to properly apprehend the object of meditation. A balance between relaxation and intensity must be found. As Tsong-kha-pa stated,

> Thus, if you use an intense cognition that is too tight, you may have clarity, but excitement will predominate so that it will be hard to develop stability.... If you sustain your meditation after becoming greatly relaxed, then you may have stability, but laxity will predominate so that there is no vivid intensity. It is very hard to find the right balance of tension so as to be neither too taut nor too relaxed, and for this reason it is hard to develop a concentration free from laxity and excitement. (*Great Treatise*, p. 51 [508–509])

In addition to the issue of finding the right balance between relaxing and tightening one's attention, another matter in question is how to sustain mindfulness while in a state of concentration. How does one maintain a sustained and powerful state of mindfulness while concentrating? Does one stop concentrating and then examine one's mind? Does one think about how the object of meditation is being apprehended during concentration? Tsong-kha-pa addressed these points in the *Great Treatise* when he stated that,

> It is not that you stop your concentration and then look at your mind. Rather, while maintaining your state of concentration, you just look to see whether your attention is staying where it was previously set on the primary object of meditation and, if it is not, whether there is laxity or excitement. After you have settled into concentration, you monitor this at moderate intervals, neither too often nor too seldom. If you do this while the intensity and force of the previous awareness are not quite gone, it takes place within the perspective of this awareness. This has the purpose of both enabling long-lasting, intense stability, and letting you quickly recognize laxity and excitement. Accordingly, this is how you sustain your mindfulness, for a necessary cause of powerful and continuous mindfulness is sustaining your meditation by repeatedly reminding yourself, at intervals, of the intended object of meditation. (*Great Treatise*, p. 53 [511])
>
> Therefore, you maintain mindfulness to stop forgetfulness wherein you stray from the object of meditation. Hence, non-forgetfulness of the object of meditation—wherein forgetfulness is stopped—is when you "mentally express" the object of meditation; you bring the object of meditation to mind again and again. For example, when you are anxious about forgetting something you know, it will be hard to forget if you recall it again and again. Thus, you have to remind yourself of the object of meditation at moderate intervals in order to develop strong mindfulness. (*Great Treatise*, p. 54 [512])

Mindfulness is applied while concentrating in order to prevent distraction away from the object of meditation as well as to not backslide into completely forgetting the meditative object. Strong mindfulness with vivid intensity is maintained by recollecting the object of meditation at brief intervals during concentration. For Tsong-kha-pa, through monitoring at brief intervals, mindfulness is sustained and the ability to quickly identify the presence of either laxity or excitement is enhanced. However, a sustained mindfulness that understands laxity or excitement is not sufficient to develop a level of concentration that is free of subtle flaws. Vigilance is necessary to reach a level of concentration where even subtle flaws of laxity or excitement are removed in order that one may reach a state of flawless meditation.

12.8 Vigilance in the *Great Treatise*

Vigilance *(saṃprajanya, shes bzhin)* is closely related to a state of discernment and intelligence *(saṃprajñā)* that knows accurately. Its emphasis is traditionally upon "the immediate awareness and assessment of the position, activity, and so on of the body, the mind, and one's situation" (Crosby and Skilton 1995, p. 31). Although it is not found among the 51 mental functions listed in Asaṅga's *Abhidharmasamuccaya,* non-vigilance is listed among the 20 secondary mental afflictions where it is defined as an "intelligence filled with defilements" (Rahula 2001, p. 17). As previously mentioned, vigilance closely monitors the very awareness that one places on an object of meditation. Based on Śāntideva's *Bodhicaryāvatāra* (5.33a–c; 5.108), vigilance for Tsong-kha-pa was an exact awareness *(ji lta ba bzhin shes pa)* that arises based on mindfulness and is able to detect laxity and excitement even at the point when they are about to occur. Tsong-kha-pa explained,

> It is not enough just to have an understanding of laxity and excitement; you have to be able to develop vigilance that accurately detects whether laxity or excitement is present during meditation. Moreover, by gradually developing powerful vigilance, not only must you develop vigilance that recognizes laxity and excitement as soon as they occur, you must also develop a vigilance that recognizes them when they are on the verge of occurring, before they have actually arisen. (*Great Treatise,* p. 60 [517])

In this way, vigilance is a precise awareness that is able to detect even an inclination toward laxity or excitement (Wallace 1998). One is not able to be sure that one's meditative session is free of laxity and excitement until one develops a potent level of vigilance that recognizes when subtle laxity and excitement are about to take place.

In Tsong-kha-pa's understanding, vigilance is able to detect laxity and excitement at a subtle level that is more refined than coarse laxity and excitement. This indicates the distinctive focal awareness that vigilance has apart from mindfulness. Although Tsong-kha-pa intermittently mentioned subtle laxity and excitement, he did not specifically address how subtle levels are different than coarse levels of laxity and excitement. Wallace (1998, p. 171) provided an informative summary of the distinction between subtle and coarse levels of laxity and excitement in Tsong-kha-pa's stages of the path writings:

> While excitation is a problem from the beginning of the training in quiescence [i.e., *meditative serenity*], laxity arises only when the attention is stable. When coarse laxity is present, the clarity of the mind is poor; but when just subtle laxity remains, it is only the potency, or full intensity, of clarity, that is absent. When the mind comes under the sway of coarse excitation during meditation, the meditative object is forgotten altogether while the attention is distracted elsewhere; but in the case of subtle excitation, although the attention is chiefly fixed on the meditative object, there is still peripheral distraction, indicating that the mind is not completely focused on its chosen object. (*brackets added*)

In order to cultivate the type of vigilance that Tsong-kha-pa advocated, one must develop a sustained level of mindfulness that avoids distraction and does not forget the object of meditation. This is because the development of continual mindfulness is the most important cause of vigilance. As Tsong-kha-pa asserted, a sustained and continual level of mindfulness prevents a prolonged occurrence of laxity and excitement which enables these two flaws to be readily recognized when they do occur. Tsong-kha-pa (*Great Treatise,* p. 61 [518]) followed Sthiramati's *Madhyāntavibhāgaṭikā* in understanding that vigilance appears when mindfulness is fully present. In this regard, Tsong-kha-pa offered the following instructions to maintain vigilance,

> Focus your mind on a visualized image of the body of a deity, etc., or focus on a subjective aspect such as the quality of experience being simply luminous and aware. Then, while you stay mindful as explained above, hold your attention on the object while continuously monitoring whether it is scattering elsewhere. Know that this is critical for the maintenance of vigilance…. Thus, with this method you develop vigilance that notices laxity and excitement when they are on the verge of arising, while with the method for maintaining mindfulness you prevent forgetfulness in which attention is distracted and slips away. (*Great Treatise*, p. 61 [518])

Sustained mindfulness holds one's attention on an object of meditation, while vigilance, developed as a result of that mindfulness, monitors the very awareness that one places on that object. Through maintaining mindfulness, vigilance is able to recognize the occurrence of subtle laxity and excitement. However, as Tsong-kha-pa noted, if one does not make an effort to stop laxity and excitement as soon as they occur, the failure to apply a remedy to these two flaws will become a major obstacle to concentration. Tsong-kha-pa therefore advocated the cultivation of intention *(sems pa, cetanā)* as a remedy that counteracts the failure to engage in eliminating laxity and excitement, stating,

> For example, iron filings are compelled to move under the influence of a magnet. Similarly, the mental process of intention moves and stimulates your mind toward virtue, nonvirtue, or the ethically neutral. So it here refers to an intention that applies your mind to the elimination of laxity or excitement when one of them occurs. (*Great Treatise*, p. 62 [519])

Tsong-kha-pa then discussed remedies for mental laxity through applying the mental process or function of intention by expanding the mind upon the object of meditation. This includes reflecting upon good qualities like the Three Jewels, light, or a beautiful image of the Buddha (*Great Treatise,* pp. 63–64 [520–521]). He also discussed remedies that are applied to excitement by bringing attention to disillusioning things that cause the mind to be drawn inward. This includes bringing objects like impermanence to the mind. Tsong-kha-pa gave a summary of the meditative process of developing flawless meditation by emphasizing how vigilance contributes to the vivid intensity necessary for concentration. He stated,

> In summary, withdraw your mind from scattering and excitement, inwardly fixing it upon the object of meditation, and seek stability. Each time stability occurs, take great precautions against laxity and bring forth a vivid intensity. You will achieve flawless concentration by alternating between these two. Do not expect to attain stability by means of mere limpidity, which lacks the vividness that goes along with an intense way of apprehending the object. (*Great Treatise*, p. 67 [525])

In concluding the section on counteragents to laxity and excitement, Tsong-kha-pa explained that one needs to utilize the application of equanimity when laxity and excitement are absent. Tsong-kha-pa explained,

> Through meditation, turning your attention inward when your mind is excited and stimulating your mind when it is lax, you gain confidence that laxity and excitement will not occur during each suitable meditation session. At this point you are still extremely wary of laxity and excitement, just as at the outset. Sustaining this is the problem. Your mind will become distracted, so at that time you must know to relax,.... This entails relaxing the effort, but not sacrificing the intensity of the way you apprehend your object. Therefore, this cultivation of equanimity is not to be done every time laxity and excitement are absent, but once you have reduced the force of laxity and excitement; for when you have not done so, there is no equanimity. (*Great Treatise*, p. 68 [526–527])

After discussing the practice of mindfulness and vigilance as techniques to counter the flaws of laxity and excitement in the cultivation of meditative serenity, Tsong-kha-pa then went through the attainment of serenity by the nine stages in which the mental states develop (*Great Treatise*, pp. 73–79 [529–536]), including a brief explanation of six forces and four states of attention (see Table 12.1). Tsong-kha-pa concluded the chapters on meditative serenity with a discussion on how one measures the successful cultivation of serenity (*Great Treatise*, pp. 79–90 [536–550]).

Table 12.1 Stages of meditative serenity (read from bottom to top)

Nine mental states	Six forces	Four attentions
9. Balanced placement	Acquaintance	Spontaneous focus
8. One-pointed attention	Enthusiasm (7, 8)	Uninterrupted focus
7. Complete pacification		Intermittent focus
6. Pacification	Vigilance (5, 6)	
5. Taming		
4. Close placement	Mindfulness (3, 4)	
3. Patched placement		
2. Continuous placement	Reflection	Tight focus (1, 2)
1. Mental placement	Hearing	

12.9 Conclusion

Tsong-kha-pa understood mindfulness and vigilance to be essential components to cultivating the concentration of meditative serenity. In Tsong-kha-pa's exegesis, mindfulness is a non-distracted focal attention on a meditative object, while vigilance closely monitors the very awareness that one places on that object. Mindfulness and vigilance are abilities that contribute to the intense clarity and non-discursive stability found in the concentration of meditative serenity. Mindfulness and vigilance are developed with effort and application until the advanced level of the ninth mental state (see Table 12.1). In the ninth mental state, a continual stream of mindfulness and vigilance is maintained without effort enabling the concentration of meditative serenity to be focused for long periods of time without being interrupted (*Great Treatise*, p. 76 [533]).

Mindfulness is considered to be the non-forgetfulness of the object of meditation that is not distracted by the flaws of laxity and excitement. Mindfulness from this standpoint is the retention of information in an active mode of apprehension. The active mode of mindfulness contributes to the overall goal of attaining meditative serenity through retaining a focused attention on an object of meditation. In this goal-directed context, mindfulness is an ability related to memory and may be developed in the practice of meditation. Vigilance is a discerning awareness that complements mindfulness and detects subtle levels of laxity and excitement, flaws which hinder meditative serenity. In this way, mindfulness for Tsong-kha-pa was not "the present-centered non-judgemental awareness of an object but the paying close attention to an object" (Dreyfus 2011, p. 47). Mindfulness is not limited to being present-centered as it retains information on an object of meditation through awarenesses related to memory. Sustained mindfulness contributes to the ability to develop vigilance. Mindfulness, coupled with vigilance, is not nonjudgmental as the flawed mental state of excitement as well as the mind's flawed non-vivid mode of apprehension embodied in the state of laxity must be recognized and removed. Flawed mental states and modes of apprehension are therefore evaluated and discarded within goal-directed processes contributing to meditative stability.

Vigilance is an active introspective awareness that monitors mindfulness and is a mental function that can accompany a primary mental awareness. Vigilance observes and monitors mindfulness and is traditionally described as playing the role of a watchman or spy (Hopkins 1983; Rinbochay and Napper 1980). Vigilance is *not* considered by Tibetan scholars like Tsong-kha-pa to be the same as reflexive awareness or self-awareness *(svasaṃvedana, rang rig)*. Self-awareness, as found in discourses of Tibetan Buddhist thought, specifically refers to a consciousness that apprehends, in a simultaneous non-dualistic manner, the knowing of consciousness itself rather than the consciousness that derives from an external sensory object while hearing, thinking, and so forth (Buswell and Lopez 2014). Tsong-kha-pa considered Buddhist thinkers who advocate this type of awareness, usually affiliated with Yogācāra trends of Mahāyāna Buddhist thought, to be "absolutizing consciousness" (Jinpa 2002, p. 127). In Tsong-kha-pa's view, reflexive awareness was counter to the radically nonessentialist and dependently designated nature of consciousness that is promoted within the Madhyamaka teachings that he followed.

I shall not explore the complexities of Tsong-kha-pa's arguments and outright rejection of this concept here (See, for example, Tsong-kha-pa 2009, pp. 351–367). Rather, vigilance, in brief, is different from reflexive awareness; in that it is a mental function that one seeks to cultivate as a part of the training of one's awareness. Reflexive awareness, on the other hand, is considered to function throughout all stages of mental operations and is not referred to as a technique for developing awareness in meditation (Hopkins 1983; Rinbochay and Napper 1980). Moreover, as Hopkins (1983, p. 377) pointed out, reflexive awareness "does not involve analysis as whether the mind is wandering or remaining with its object." How vigilance functions as an introspective awareness that monitors mindfulness relates to Tsong-kha-pa's Madhyamaka understanding of perception. He posited two types of perception: (1) the sensory awareness that directly cognizes form and so forth, and (2) a mental awareness that cognizes objects by the force or experience of sensory awareness. This entails that mental awarenesses do not directly cognize sensory objects, but rather, they recollect them (Tsong-kha-pa 2009, p. 362). However, inner experiences such as laxity and excitement are, as mentioned above, detected by mental awareness. For Tsong-kha-pa, vigilance actually perceives an immediate previous moment of awareness. This understanding enabled Tsong-kha-pa to maintain a sequential flow of dependently interrelated moments of awareness without need of positing an extra layer of simultaneous awareness like reflexive awareness.

In sum, in Tsong-kha-pa's theory and practice of meditative serenity, mindfulness centers on the meditative object and vigilance closely monitors the very awareness that one places on that object. Coupled with the mental application of intention and equanimity, mindfulness and vigilance enable a practitioner to check, and subsequently immobilize the flaws of laxity and excitement, which hinder the clarity and vividness that the concentration of meditative serenity requires.

References

Apple, J. (2004). Tsong-kha-pa blo-bzang grag-pa. In P. G. Jestice (Eds.), *Holy people of the world a cross-cultural encyclopedia*. Santa Barbara, Calif.: ABC-CLIO.

Apple, J. (2013). *A Stairway taken by the Lucid: Tsong kha pa's study of noble beings New Delhi: Aditya Prakashan.*

Apple, J., & Dunne, J. D. (trans). (2001) *The necklace of clear understanding: An elucidation of the system of mind and mental states by Tshe-mchog-gling yongs-'dzin, Dka'-chen Ye-shes rgyal-mtshan* (Foundation for the Preservation of Mahāyāna Buddhism).

Buswell, R. E., & Lopez, D. S. (2014). Svasaṃvedana. In R. E. Buswell & D. S. Lopez (Eds.), *The Princeton dictionary of Buddhism*. Princeton: Princeton University Press.

Crosby, K., & Skilton, A. (1995). The *Bodhicaryāvatāra*. Oxford/New York: Oxford University Press.

Cutler, J. W. C., & Newland, G. (Eds.). (2000, 2002). *The great treatise on the stages of the path to enlightenment* (Vols. 1–3). Ithaca: Snow Lion.

Dreyfus, G. (2002). Is compassion an emotion? A cross-cultural exploration of mental typologies. In R. J. Davidson, A. Harrington (Eds.), *Visions of compassion: Western scientists and Tibetan Buddhists examine human nature*. New York: Oxford University Press

Dreyfus, G. (2011). Is mindfulness present-centred and non-judgmental? A discussion of the cognitive dimensions of mindufulness. *Contemporary Buddhism, 12*(1), 41–54.

Dreyfus, G. B. J., & McClintock, S. L. (2002). *The Svātantrika-Prāsaṅgika distinction: What difference does a difference make?* Boston: Wisdom.

Gyatso, L., (blo-bzang rgya-mtsho) & Graham Woodhouse. (2011). *Tsongkhapa's praise for dependent relativity*. Boston: Wisdom.

Hopkins, J. (1983). *Meditation on emptiness*. London: Wisdom.

Jinpa, T. (2002). *Self, reality and reason in Tibetan philosophy: Tsongkhapa's quest for the middle way*. London: RoutledgeCurzon.

Lopez, D. (2001). Painting the target: On the Identification of the object of negation (*dgag bya*). In G. Newland (Ed.), *Changing minds: Contributions to the study of Buddhism and tibet in honor of Jeffrey Hopkins* (pp. 63–81). Ithaca: Snow Lion.

Napper, E. (1989). *Dependent-arising and Emptiness: a Tibetan Buddhist Interpretation of Madhyamika philosophy emphasizing the compatibility of emptiness and conventional phenomena*. London: Wisdom.

Napper, E. (2001). Ethics as the basis of a tantric tradition: Tsong kha pa and the founding of the dGe lugs Order in Tibet. In G. Newland (Ed.), *Changing minds: Contributions to the study of Buddhism and Tibet in honor of Jeffrey Hopkins* (pp. 63–81). Ithaca: Snow Lion.

Rahula, W. (2001). *Abhidharmasamuccaya. The compendium of the higher teaching (Philosophy) by Asaṅga*. (Translated by Sarah Boin-Webb). Fremont: Asian Humanities.

Rgyal-dbang chos-rje blo-bzang 'phrin-las rnam-rgyal. (2009). *'Jam mgon chos kyi rgyal po tsong kha pa chen po'i rnam thar thub bstan mdzes pa'i rgyan gcig ngo mtshar nor bu'i phreng ba dang mdzad rnam zhal thang*.

Rinbochay, L., & Napper, E. (1980). *Mind in Tibetan Buddhism: Oral commentary on Ge-shay Jam-bel-sam-pel's presentation of awareness and knowledge, composite of all the important points, opener of the eye of new intelligence*. London: Rider.

Ruegg, D. S. (2000). *Studies in Indian and Tibetan Madhyamaka thought*. Part 1. Wien: Arbeitskreis für Tibetische und Buddhistische Studien, Universität Wien.

Sparham, G. (1993). *Ocean of eloquence: Tsong-kha-pa's commentary on the Yogācāra doctrine of mind*. Albany: SUNY.

Sparham, G. (1999). *The fulfillment of all hopes: Guru devotion in Tibetan Buddhism*. Boston: Wisdom.

Sparham, G. (2008–2013). *Golden garland of eloquence*. Four volumes. Fremont: Jain.

Tatz, M. (1986). *Asanga's chapter on ethics with the commentary of Tsong-Kha-Pa, the basic path to awakening, the complete Bodhisattva*. Lewiston: Edwin Mellen.

Thurman, R. A. F. (1982). Revised 2006. *The life and teachings of Tsong Khapa*. Dharmsala: Library of Tibetan Works and Archives.

Tsong-kha-pa blo-bzang grags-pa, 1357–1419. (1985). *Lam rim chen mo. mNyam med Tsong-kha-pa chen pos mdzad pa'i byang chub lam rim che ba*. Kokonor, Tibet: mTsho ngon mi rigs dpe skrun khang. Translated by the Lamrim Translation Committee. See Cutler (2000, 2002).

Tsong-kha-pa blo-bzang grags-pa, 1357–1419. (1986a). *Sde bdun la 'jug pa'i sgo don gnyer yid kyi mun sel*. Kokonor, Tibet: mTsho ngon mi rigs dpe skrun khang.

Tsong-kha-pa blo-bzang grags-pa, 1357–1419. (1986b). *Shes rab kyi pha rol tu phyin pa'i man ngag gi bstan bcos mngon par rtogs pa'i rgyan 'grel pa dang bcas pa'i rgya cher bshad pa legs bshad gser phreng zhes bya ba bzhugs so (=Legs bshad gser phreng)*. Kokonor, Tibet: mTsho ngon mi rigs dpe skrun khang. Also Collected Works, 1977, Volumes 26+27, gSung 'bum lHa sa edition, v. tsa and tsha. See Sparham, 2008–2012.

Tsong-kha-pa blo-bzang grags-pa, 1357–1419. (2009). *Dbu ma dgongs pa rab gsal*. Lhasa: Ser gtsug nang bstan dpe rnying 'tshol bsdu phyogs sgrig khang.

Van der Kuijp, L. W. J. (1985). Apropos of a recent contribution to the history of central way philosophy in Tibet: Tsong Khapa's speech of gold. *Berliner Indologische Studien, 1*, 47–74.

Wallace, B. A. (1998). *The bridge of quiescence: Experiencing Tibetan Buddhist meditation.* Chicago: Open Court.
Zahler, L. (2009). *Study and practice of meditation: Tibetan interpretations of the concentrations and formless absorptions*. Ithaca: Snow Lion.

James B. Apple is an associate professor of Buddhist studies at the University of Calgary. He received his doctorate in Buddhist studies from the University of Wisconsin-Madison. He has published over 30 articles focusing upon the critical analysis of *Mahāyāna sūtras* and topics within Indian and Tibetan Buddhist forms of Buddhism. His most recent books include *A Stairway taken by the Lucid: Tsong kha pa's Study of Noble Beings* (2013) and *Stairway to Nirvāṇa* (2008).

Chapter 13
Mindfulness in Similes in Early Buddhist Literature

Tse-fu Kuan

13.1 Introduction

The term "mindfulness" is translated from *sati* in Pali or *smṛti* in Sanskrit. This Indic word originally meant memory, but as Bodhi (2011, p. 22) noted "the Buddha assigned the word a new meaning consonant with his own system of psychology and meditation". Different people have translated this word in various ways (cf. Kuan 2008, p. 1; Gethin 2011, pp. 263–264). The word "mindfulness" has become the most popular English translation of this Indic word or even "the only possible English translation of *sati*" (Gethin 2011, p. 265). However, what the term "mindfulness" means in the context of Buddhism is still an issue to be settled. This chapter is an attempt to unfold the meaning of mindfulness through investigation of several similes in early Buddhist literature.

By early Buddhist literature, I am here referring to the *sūtras/suttas* that were transmitted by early Buddhist schools and thence have come down to us. Among these early schools, only the Theravādins, dating back approximately to the third century BCE, survive until today, and so their corpus of *suttas* in the five *Nikāyas* is the only complete collection of early Buddhist discourses to survive intact. Therefore, the Pali *suttas* are taken as the primary sources of this study. The Chinese *Āgamas,* equivalent to the *Nikāyas,* were translated in the fourth and fifth centuries CE from Prakrit and Sanskrit originals transmitted by other schools. I refer to some *sūtras* in the *Āgamas* when their Pali counterparts are not clear or when comparison between the Pali and Chinese versions is useful.

T.-f. Kuan (✉)
College of General Studies, Yuan Ze University, 135 Yuan-Tung Road, Chung-Li District, Taoyuan City 320, Taiwan

E. Shonin et al. (eds.), *Buddhist Foundations of Mindfulness,*
Mindfulness in Behavioral Health, DOI 10.1007/978-3-319-18591-0_13

The Buddha liked using similes to explain his doctrine. In many *suttas,* he is recorded as saying, "I have given this simile in order to convey a meaning" (e.g. It 114, MN I 117–118, 155, II 260). The Buddha's disciples also often made up similes to preach and elucidate the Buddha's teaching. Many *suttas* record that they said, "I shall give you a simile, for some wise people here understand the meaning of a statement by means of a simile" (e.g. DN II 324, MN I 523, SN II 114). The Buddha and his disciples gave hundreds of similes as found in the *Nikāyas*. In line with this literary style, the Buddha's teaching on mindfulness is accompanied by or even embedded in quite a few similes. It is essential to scrutinize those similes in order to penetrate the meanings and implications in the discourses on mindfulness.

Mindfulness plays an extremely important part in Buddhism. Conze (1962, p. 51) pointed out:

> If one were asked what distinguishes Buddhism from all other systems of thought, one would have to answer that it is the Dharma-theory and the stress laid on mindfulness. Mindfulness is not only the seventh of the steps of the holy eightfold path, the third of the five virtues, and the first of the seven limbs of enlightenment. On occasions it is almost equated with Buddhism itself.

Basically speaking, Buddhism refers to the Buddha's teaching. What did he teach? Gethin (1998, p. 59) answered, "The early sūtras present the Buddha's teaching as the solution to a problem. This problem is the fundamental problem of life. In Sanskrit and Pali the problem is termed *duḥkha/dukkha,* which can be approximately translated as 'suffering'". Then, he suggested that the basic orientation of Buddhism has its classic formulation by way of "four noble truths". Likewise, Rahula (2000, p. 16) said:

> The heart of the Buddha's teaching lies in the Four Noble Truths (*Cattāri Ariyasaccāni*) which he expounded in his very first sermon .... In this sermon, as we have it in the original texts, these four Truths are given briefly. But there are innumerable places in the early Buddhist scriptures where they are explained again and again, with greater detail and in different ways.

The Buddha's teaching on mindfulness at many places in early Buddhist literature represents alternative ways of expounding the Four Noble Truths and fits into this classic formulation of Buddhism. In this chapter, my discussion of mindfulness is occasionally related in the context of the Four Noble Truths in the hope of elucidating mindfulness from a more comprehensive perspective. The Four Noble Truths are (see DN II 305–313, SN V 414 ff. and passim):

1. *Dukkha* generally rendered as "suffering"
2. The origin of *dukkha (dukkha-samudaya)*
3. The cessation of *dukkha (dukkha-nirodha)*
4. The way leading to the cessation of *dukkha (dukkha-nirodha-gāminī paṭipadā)*

The translation "Four Noble Truths" is problematic. Harvey (2009) critiqued this standard translation and convincingly argued that the four referents (see above) of the Four Noble Truths cannot be "noble truths", and suggested that the four are "true realities for the spiritually ennobled" (cf. also Cousins 2001, p. 38). Later on Harvey

(2013, p. 13, etc.) modified his rendering and called them "the Four True Realities for the Noble Ones", which I adopt for my discussion in this chapter.

13.2 Prevention

In the *Dukkhadhamma Sutta* of the *Saḷāyatana Saṃyutta* in the *Saṃyutta Nikāya,* the Buddha gave an instruction on how a monk should behave in daily life (translation based on Bodhi 2000, p. 1249):

> And how, monks, has a monk comprehended a mode of conduct and way of living in such a way that as he conducts himself thus and as he lives thus, evil unwholesome states of covetousness and dejection do not flow in upon him? Suppose a man should enter a thorny forest. There would be thorns in front of him, thorns behind him, thorns to his left, thorns to his right, thorns below him, and thorns above him. He would go forward, being mindful (*sato* in CS and BJT, agreeing with 正念 at T II 314a; Ee has *yato*, which must be wrong), he would go back, being mindful, thinking: 'May no thorn [prick] me!' So too, monks, whatever in the world has an agreeable and pleasing nature is called a thorn in the Noble Discipline. (SN IV 189)

At the beginning of this *sutta,* its title *dukkhadhamma (dukkha states)* is explained by virtue of the five aggregates, that is, material form, feeling, perception, volitional formations and consciousness (MN IV 188). This *sutta* has a Chinese parallel, namely *sūtra* 1173 of the *Saṃyukta Āgama* (T 99), which is widely ascribed to the Mūlasarvāstivāda tradition (Lü 1963, p. 242; Enomoto 1984a, p. 1071, b, p. 99; Mizuno 1996, pp. 373–375; Hiraoka 2003; Oberlies 2003, p. 64.). Different from the Pali *sutta,* this Chinese *sūtra* begins with an exposition relating to *dukkhadhamma* (苦法, **duḥkha-dharma*) in terms of the Four True Realities for the Noble Ones (T II 314a). It is difficult to tell which version is authentic and the possibility cannot be ruled out that there is a third version in another school, but it has been lost. A viable way to find out the meaning of *dukkha/duḥkha* in this text is to examine the simile. Both Pali and Chinese versions of the simile are largely identical. In this simile, the thorn is apparently used as a metaphor for *dukkha* at the end of the simile: "whatever in the world has an agreeable and pleasing nature is called a thorn in the Noble Discipline". Why does the Buddha regard anything agreeable and pleasing as a thorn? The answer is implied in the ensuing passage. The Buddha said that having understood the above discourse, one should understand restraint and non-restraint. His explanation of non-restraint *(asaṃvara)* is as follows (restraint *(saṃvara)* is explained in the converse way):

> On seeing a visible form with the eye, a monk is intent on it in the case of an agreeable visible form, and is upset at it in the case of a disagreeable visible form. He dwells without having established mindfulness of his sentient organism (*kāyasati*)…[and so on through all the six senses]. (SN IV 189)

Corresponding roughly to the above Pali passages, the Chinese version reads:

> How does a sharp thorn hurt the Noble Dharma and Discipline? That is, the agreeable and lovely visible form. Thus a sharp thorn hurts the Noble Dharma and Discipline. How does

> the agreeable and lovely visible form hurt the Noble Dharma and Discipline? That is, the five cords of sensual desire: When the eye cognizes a visible form, desire arises and sensual pleasure is nourished; when the ear cognizes a sound...the nose cognizes an odor...the tongue cognizes a taste...the body cognizes a touch, desire arises and sensual pleasure is nourished. Thus the agreeable and lovely visible form hurts the Noble Dharma and Discipline. Thus a learned noble disciple conducts and lives in such a way that he prevents and foresees so that unwholesome states of covetousness and dejection concerning the world do not flow into his mind. (T II 314b)

As mentioned above, the thorn is apparently used as a metaphor for *dukkha,* and the thorn refers to "whatever in the world has an agreeable and pleasing nature". Contrary to our common sense, agreeable and pleasing things are regarded as *dukkha* or suffering. The reason is as follows: Agreeable and pleasing things are cognized by one's senses, five senses in the Chinese version, but six (five senses plus *manas,* the mind organ) in the Pali. When such cognition occurs, sensual pleasure is nourished, and one is intent on such pleasing objects cognized by one's senses. On the other hand, when disagreeable things are cognized by one's senses, one is upset at such objects. Therefore, "evil unwholesome states of covetousness and dejection flow in upon him" in the words of the Pali *sutta* quoted above, or "unwholesome states of covetousness and dejection concerning the world flow into his mind" in the words of the Chinese *sutta. Dukkha* (First True Reality for the Noble Ones) is this very situation in which one falls under the sway of evil unwholesome states and remains a prey to covetousness and dejection. The "origin of *dukkha*" (Second True Reality for the Noble Ones) in this context is non-restraint of the senses according to the Pali *sutta* or failure to foresee and prevent the danger that happens when one's senses contact their objects according to the Chinese version.

This simile implies that "the way leading to the cessation of *dukkha*" (Fourth True Reality for the Noble Ones) includes the constant practice of mindfulness in every movement so as to protect oneself from evil unwholesome states of covetousness and dejection, which result from contact with agreeable objects and disagreeable objects as well. In this discourse, mindfulness is employed in a sense similar to "vigilance" as described in cognitive psychology. As Sternberg (2009, p. 142) stated:

> Vigilance refers to a person's ability to attend to a field of stimulation over a prolonged period, during which the person seeks to detect the appearance of a particular target stimulus of interest. When being vigilant, the individual watchfully waits to detect a signal stimulus that may appear at an unknown time.

A person is endowed with sense organs, through which he is always exposed to various kinds of stimulus. A monk's daily life is compared to entering a thorny forest. In such a forest or a field of stimulation, he has to be mindful or attentive all the time, for the sake of being able to detect the appearance of a particular target stimulus of interest, that is, agreeable objects and disagreeable objects. To put in the words of Anālayo (2013, p. 22), mindfulness makes him aware as soon as something manifests through the senses that could disturb his mental equipoise. When he is able to detect agreeable objects, which are compared to thorns, as soon as they appear, he can avoid being hurt by them in such a way that his mind is not infatuated nor entangled with them, thereby set free from covetousness and dejection. This escape from the emotional agitation amounts to the "cessation of *dukkha*" (Third True Reality for the Noble Ones), which is comparable to the prevention of being pricked by thorns.

This type of mindfulness is particularly emphasized with reference to coming into contact with enticing or distracting objects. In the *Janapada Sutta* of the *Satipaṭṭhāna Saṃyutta* in the *Saṃyutta Nikāya,* the Buddha made the following simile: Suppose a great crowd were to assemble to see the most beautiful girl of the country singing and dancing. A man would be ordered to carry around a bowl of oil full to the brim between the crowd and the girl, and he would be killed if he spilt even a little oil. The Buddha explained that "the bowl of oil full to the brim" represents *kāyagatā sati* (SN V 170), which is rendered as "mindfulness directed to the body" by Bodhi (2000, p. 1649). This Pali expression *kāyagatā sati* should not be construed as mindfulness directed to the physical body, because *kāya* here refers not to the physical body alone, but to "an individual that is able to perceive through his senses" as Kuan (2008, pp. 99–103) demonstrated. The term *kāyagatā sati* is synonymous with *kāyasati* (mindfulness of one's sentient organism) that appears in the *Dukkhadhamma Sutta* quoted above (see Kuan 2008, pp. 43–44).

Moreover, Kuan (2008, pp. 131–132) also showed that *kāyagatā sati* and the four *satipaṭṭhānas* (establishments or foundations of mindfulness), that is, mindfulness of the body, of feelings, of mental states and of *dhammas,* are just different expressions of the same practice based on different schemes of classification of phenomena. In this connection, it is noteworthy that the Chinese counterpart of this Pali *sutta,* namely *sūtra* 623 of the *Saṃyukta Āgama,* has a passage not found in the Pali version. Following the simile of the oil bowl, this passage states that the Buddha exhorts the monks to dwell in the establishment of mindfulness of the body (身念處), which is apparently equivalent to *kāyagatā sati* in the Pali version. This is immediately explained as contemplation of the body, of feelings, of mental states and of *dhammas,* to wit the four establishments of mindfulness (T II 174c). We do not know whether this passage is a later interpolation into the Mūlasarvāstivāda version preserved in Chinese or the Pali version omits it from the original (or earlier) version. In any case, it is certain that what is meant in this discourse is not mindfulness of the physical body alone, but is mindfulness in a much more comprehensive sense.

This simile of the oil bowl is analogous to that of the thorny forest in the *Dukkhadhamma Sutta.* In both cases, one has to be mindful of every bodily and mental movement one makes at every moment in order to avoid *dukkha,* which refers either to death (the result of being distracted by the girl) or to being hurt by thorns (covetousness and dejection resulting from contact with sense objects). Both are related to the restraint of the senses. The implication is that if a person fully recognizes the nature of suffering inherent in the agreeable objects (and also disagreeable objects) perceived by his senses, and if he really wants to escape from suffering, then he will naturally be determined to maintain his mindfulness by guarding his senses all the time.

13.3 Healing

While a person is in contact with incoming sensory data, his mindfulness can have an introspective function with regard to his own mind. This function serves as a remedial measure when the above preventive mindfulness fails to act and he gets hurt. Owing to the non-restraint of his senses in contact with agreeable and disagreeable objects, evil unwholesome states of covetousness and dejection arise in his mind. Then, he should be able to resume the faculty of mindfulness so as to notice and recognize these states and get rid of them in time. In the *Sunakkhatta Sutta* of the *Majjhima Nikāya,* the Buddha provided a simile that describes this function of mindfulness (translation based on Ñāṇamoli and Bodhi 2001, p. 866):

> Suppose, Sunakkhatta, a man were wounded by an arrow thickly smeared with poison (*visa*).... A surgeon would cut around the opening of the wound with a knife, then he would probe for the arrow with a probe, then he would pull out the arrow and would expel the poisonous humour without leaving a trace of it behind. (MN II 259)

As the Buddha explained later, the "wound" is a designation for the six internal bases, that is, the six senses. "Poisonous humour" *(visa-dosa)* and "arrow" stand for ignorance and craving, respectively. "Probe" is a designation for mindfulness (MN II 260). It should be noted that the Buddha regarded both ignorance and craving as the cause of *dukkha* or suffering. Ignorance *(avijjā)* is the first link in the dependent origination *(paṭiccasamuppāda)* formula explaining the cycle of rebirth, that is, explaining the arising of *dukkha* (MN III 63 and passim). On the other hand, according to the standard exposition of the Four True Realities for the Noble Ones, the second True Reality is defined, thus "This is the True Realities for the Noble Ones concerning the origin of *dukkha*: it is this craving (*taṇhā*) which leads to rebirth ..." (SN V 421 and passim). As Rahula (2000, pp. 29 and 54) reminded us, neither craving nor ignorance should be taken as the first cause for "everything is relative and interdependent". The following remark by Gombrich (1988, pp. 65–66) may help to clarify the relationship between ignorance and craving:

> [T]wo rival analyses of life's problems were already on offer. I have dubbed them the intellectualist—which locates the nub of the problem in our lack of true understanding—and the emotionalist—which blames our lack of self-control. The Buddha wonderfully combined the two. You cannot see things straight because you are blinded by passion, and you allow your emotions to run you because you do not see things as they are.

Therefore, it is reasonable to see the origin of *dukkha* as both ignorance and craving. The two factors are interconnected, and neither of them overrides the other.

Again, we find in this simile that mindfulness functions in the context of the six senses, but here instead of a preventive, it serves as an antidote to the unwholesome states that have invaded an individual. This kind of mindfulness has a healing function. Just like a surgeon uses a probe, a practitioner uses mindfulness to search the unwholesome states that have invaded his mind. The Pali word for probe, *esanī,* is cognate with the noun *esanā,* which means "seeking, search" (DOP I 552). This probe-like mindfulness may be compared to "search" as described in cognitive psychology. Sternberg (2009, p. 145) defines it thus, "Search refers to a scan of the environment for particular features—actively looking for something when you are not sure where it will appear". Without the probe-like mindfulness, a person is unable to locate the unwholesome states in his mind even if he seems to be aware of their existence. It is only when the probe-like mindfulness finds out craving and ignorance (which are compared to an arrow and poison) that he is able to get rid of the *dukkha* that already assailed him.

In this connection, it should be noted that search associated with this simile and vigilance associated with the simile of a thorny forest are among the four main functions of attention as classified by cognitive psychologists (Sternberg 2009, p. 141). Mindfulness in Buddhism has a certain affinity to attention in psychology. As Nyanaponika Thera (1962, p. 30) observed, "Mindfulness, in its specific aspect of bare attention …. When attending to the sixfold sense impressions, *attention or mindfulness* is kept to a bare registering of the facts observed" (italics added). In the opinion of this Theravāda monk, mindfulness has an aspect of attention and can even be paraphrased as attention. But mindfulness *(sati)* in Buddhism is by no means coterminous with attention in psychology. Kuan (2012, pp. 43–47) has discussed the relationship between the two concepts.

13.4 Binding

13.4.1 A Pillar for Binding Six Animals

The *Chapāṇa Sutta* in the *Saḷāyatana Saṃyutta* of the *Saṃyutta Nikāya* has the same exposition of restraint and non-restraint as that in the *Dukkhadhamma Sutta* cited above "On seeing a visible form with the eye, a monk is not intent on it …. He dwells with *kāyasati* established" (SN IV 199–200). After this exposition, the text gives a further explanation with the following simile (abridged):

> Suppose a man would catch six animals with different domains and bind them to a firm post or pillar. Each animal would pull in the direction of its own domain. The snake would pull [and think]: 'Let me enter an anthill.' The crocodile would pull [and think]: 'Let me enter the water.' The bird would pull [and think]: 'Let me fly in the sky.' The dog would pull [and think]: 'Let me enter a village.' The jackal would pull [and think]: 'Let me enter a charnel ground.' The monkey would pull [and think]: 'Let me enter a forest.' In the end they would be tired and stay near the post or pillar. So too, for a monk whose *kāyagatā sati* is developed, the eye does not pull in the direction of agreeable forms, nor are disagreeable forms repulsive. The same applies to the other five senses. Thus there is restraint. A firm post or pillar is a designation for *kāyagatā sati*. (SN IV 200)

This passage appears to be a supplementary explanation for restraint and non-restraint as expounded earlier, and *kāyasati* in the earlier exposition of restraint and non-restraint is rephrased as *kāyagatā sati* in this supplementary explanation.

It is obvious that the six animals stand for the six senses, each of which has its own domain. Each of the six senses has a habitual tendency to indulge in agreeable things and to be repelled by disagreeable things in its domain. It is this propensity that brings *dukkha* to sentient beings as discussed above. Therefore, this habitual tendency can be seen as the origin of *dukkha,* that is, the Second True Reality for the Noble Ones. In order to end *dukkha,* it is essential to stop this unwholesome tendency, the origin of *dukkha.* The way to stop this tendency, that is, the Fourth True Reality, is described in this *sutta* as *kāyagatā sati*, "mindfulness directed to one's sentient organism". This practice of mindfulness is compared to a firm post or pillar. Just as the six animals are trained to be detached from their domains by means of binding them to a firm pillar, the six senses are restrained by the persevering practice of mindfulness. According to this text, mindfulness directed to one's sentient organism functions as a pillar that restrains the six senses and thus seems to be somewhat repressive. On the contrary, however, this practice of mindfulness liberates the individual by freeing his mind from its habitual and compulsive unwholesome reactions to the sense objects, reactions including covetousness and dejection.

13.4.2 A Post for Binding an Elephant

The *Dantabhūmi Sutta* of the *Majjhima Nikāya* (MN 125) contains a basic structure of discourse that is similar to those found in several other *suttas* such as MN 27 and MN 51. This structure is composed of a standard gradual path proceeding from morality *(sīla),* concentration *(samādhi),* wisdom *(paññā)* to liberation *(vimutti).* The *sutta* begins with a prince's visit to the novice Aciravata. After a futile conversation with the prince, the novice reported this to the Buddha. Thereupon, the Buddha gave him two similes that could have helped him convince the prince. Then, the Buddha related a long simile of taming a forest elephant for explaining how to train a monk. It is in this context that the gradual path formula is introduced. After a description of the stage of training in morality *(sīla),* the Buddha expounded the preliminaries to the four attainments of concentration *(samādhi)* called the four *jhāna*s. These preliminaries are guarding the doors of the sense faculties, being moderate in eating, being devoted to vigilance, mindfulness and full awareness, starting meditation in a sitting posture and abandoning the five hindrances (MN III 134–135). Following these preliminaries, the four establishments of mindfulness *(satipaṭṭhāna)* are integrated into this gradual path as follows:

A. Having abandoned these five hindrances, defilements of the mind and weakeners of wisdom, he dwells contemplating the body as a body, ardent, fully aware, possessed of mindfulness, in order to remove covetousness and dejection concerning the world ... feelings ... mind .... He dwells contemplating *dhammas* as *dhammas,* ardent, fully aware, possessed of mindfulness, in order to remove covetousness and dejection concerning the world. (It is difficult to translate *dhammas*. Here *dhammas* can cover virtually whatever phenomena become the objects of consciousness, which are contemplated from the Buddhist perspective. See Kuan 2008, pp. 126–128.)

B. Just as the elephant tamer plants a large post in the earth and binds the forest elephant to it by the neck in order to subdue his forest habits, to subdue his forest memories and thoughts, to subdue his forest distress, fatigue and fever, to make him delight in the village, and to inculcate in him habits congenial to human beings, so these four *satipaṭṭhānas* are the bindings for the mind of the noble disciple in order to subdue his habits based on the household life, to subdue his memories and thoughts based on the household life, to subdue his distress, fatigue and fever based on the household life, and in order that he may attain the method and realize Nirvana.
C. Then, the Tathāgata disciplines him further: "Come, monk, dwell contemplating the body as a body, but do not think thoughts (*vitakka*) connected with the body; dwell contemplating feelings as feelings, but do not think thoughts connected with feelings; dwell contemplating mind as mind, but do not think thoughts connected with mind; dwell contemplating *dhammas* as *dhammas,* but do not think thoughts connected with *dhammas*".
D. With the stilling of *vitakka* and *vicāra,* he enters and dwells in the second *jhāna,* which has internal tranquility and singleness of mind, without *vitakka* and *vicāra,* with joy and pleasure born of concentration … the third *jhāna* … the fourth *jhāna.*
E. When his mind is thus concentrated, purified … and attains imperturbability, he directs his mind to knowledge of the recollection of past lives … to knowledge of the death and rebirth of beings … to knowledge of the destruction of the taints …. His mind is liberated from the taint of sensual desire, from the taint of becoming, from the taint of ignorance (MN III 136).

Bodhi remarked that, in paragraph A, the four establishments of mindfulness are expounded in the place usually reserved for the four *jhāna*s (Ñāṇamoli and Bodhi 2001, p. 1338 note 1176). In my opinion, paragraphs A and B correspond closely to the first *jhāna,* while paragraph C is related with the practice leading from the first to the second *jhāna.* The expression "having abandoned these five hindrances, defilements of the mind and weakeners of wisdom" in paragraph A is a standard account preceding the usual *jhāna* formula (e.g. MN I 181, 270) and marks the moment of entering the first *jhāna.* Paragraph B shows that just as the post binding the elephant tames him and makes him delight in the village, away from the forest, so the four *satipaṭṭhānas* make one enjoy being away from the household life. This is related to one of the first *jhāna*'s characteristics: joy and pleasure born of seclusion *(vivekajaṃ pīti-sukhaṃ)*—being secluded from sensual pleasures and secluded from unwholesome states (*vivicc' eva kāmehi vivicca akusalehi dhammehi*).

Anālayo (2006, pp. 15–16) contended that this positioning of the four *satipaṭṭhānas* after a removal of the five hindrances is unexpected, "since, according to the Pāli and Chinese versions of the *Satipaṭṭhāna Sutta,* awareness of the presence of the five hindrances is an integral part of *satipaṭṭhāna* practice". In fact, there are two Chinese versions of the *Satipaṭṭhāna Sutta.* The version in the *Madhyama Āgama,* just like the Pali version, includes introspection of the five hindrances in its exposition of the fourth *satipaṭṭhāna,* contemplation of *dhammas.* The other Chinese version in the *Ekottarika Āgama,* however, makes no mention of the five hindrances; instead, its exposition of the fourth *satipaṭṭhāna* contains only the seven enlightenment factors and the four *jhāna*s.

This fact casts a doubt on the authenticity of introspection of the five hindrances as found in the Pali and *Madhyama Āgama* versions. Moreover, Bronkhorst (1985, p. 312) argued that the passage on introspection of the five hindrances is a later addition since it does not appear in the Chinese *Ekottarika Āgama.* With references to some other scholars, he assumed that this *Ekottarika Āgama* belongs to the Mahāsāṃghikas, which "may have emerged as a separate sect around 116 or 137 years after the death of the Buddha …, long before the other sects whose collections of Sūtras have been preserved. This would make it at least conceivable that the Sūtras of the Mahāsāṅghikas should preserve some early features where the texts of the other sects show in common a further development". Kuan (2013b) demonstrated that the Chinese *Ekottarika Āgama* is most probably affiliated with the Mahāsāṃghikas. While the Pali canon belongs to the Theravāda still thriving today and the Chinese *Madhyama Āgama* belongs to the extinct Sārvāstivāda (Lü 1963, p. 242; Kumoi 1963, p. 248; Mayeda 1964, pp. 643–644; Enomoto 1984a, p. 1071; Thich Minh Chau 1991, pp. 18–27; Anālayo 2012b, pp. 516–521), both schools descended from the Sthaviras, opposed to the Mahāsāṃghikas at the first schism, according to the sources of various schools (e.g. Dīp V 16–47 of the Theravāda; *Bu zhiyi lun* 部執異論 T XLIX 20a–21b of the Sarvāstivāda; **Śāriputraparipṛcchā* 舍利弗問經 T XXIV 900b–c of the Mahāsāṃghika). This may explain why the *Ekottarika Āgama* version of the *Satipaṭṭhāna Sutta* differs so much from the other two versions and reinforces the possibility that the section on the five hindrances did not exist in the pre-sectarian (or original) *Satipaṭṭhāna Sutta.* Therefore, there is no problem with practising the four establishments of mindfulness after abandoning the five hindrances from the textual perspective. From the doctrinal point of view, as Kuan (2008, pp. 65–80) elucidated, the four establishments of mindfulness can be practised in the context of concentrative *(samādhi)* meditation in order to achieve the four *jhāna*s and even higher meditative attainments, all of which can be called "absorption". Bronkhorst (2012, pp. 193–194) also points out that the four establishments of mindfulness play a role in attaining "absorption" by referring to a passage in MN 118 (III 85–86).

Paragraph C is problematic. My translation is based on Ee. Anālayo (2006, p. 13 note 32) pointed out that while the Siamese edition agrees with Ee, the Burmese and Ceylonese editions read in all four cases of contemplation: "Do not think thoughts connected with sensual desire" *(mā ca kāmūpasaṃhitaṃ vitakkaṃ vitakkesi)*. Bodhi also mentioned the variant readings, and on the basis of two editions (Burmese-script Buddhasāsana Samiti edition of the *Majjhima Nikāya,* BBS and Sinhala-script Buddha Jayanti Tripitaka Series edition of the *Majjhima Nikāya,* SBJ) rather than Ee he translated: "Come, bhikkhu, abide contemplating the body as a body, but do not think thoughts of sensual desire. Abide contemplating feelings as feelings … mind as mind … mind-objects as mind-objects, but do not think thoughts of sensual desire" (Ñāṇamoli and Bodhi 2001, p. 995 and 1338 note 1177). The Chinese counterpart of this *sutta* in the *Madhyama Āgama* (MĀ 198) reads, "You should contemplate the internal body as a body, but do not think thoughts connected with sensual desire … contemplate feelings … mind … *dhammas* (法) as *dhammas*, but do not think thoughts connected with non-*dhamma* (非法, **adhamma*)" (T I 758b). This Chinese version agrees partly with the Burmese and Ceylonese editions of the Pali version in that both versions contain the instruction "do not think thoughts connected with sensual desire". However, this instruction applies to all four cases of contemplation or *satipaṭṭhāna* in the Pali version, whereas it applies only to the case of contemplating the body in MĀ 198. In the case of contemplating *dhammas*, the instruction is "do not think thoughts connected with non-*dhamma*". The omissions in the text seem to suggest that in the other two cases, namely contemplation of feelings and contemplation of mind, there could be instructions other than "do not think thoughts connected with sensual desire" and "do not think thoughts connected with non-*dhamma*", but we just do not know what they are. MĀ 144 (T I 652b) has a passage almost identical to the passage quoted from MĀ 198 above, but this passage is not found in the Pali counterpart of MĀ 144, that is, MN 107 (III 1–7). It is very likely that this is an abridged stock formula created by the *Sārvāstivādins,* and they interpolated this formula into several *sūtras* in their *Āgamas,* among which only the *Madhyama Āgama* survives intact until today, and so this formula is now found only in the above two *sūtras,* MĀ 144 and MĀ 198 (by searching CBETA). As Kuan (2013a, pp. 65–68) illustrated, such interpolations are not uncommon in early Buddhist literature.

Which version of the instruction in paragraph C could be original or the earliest? The possibility of the Chinese version can be ruled out as discussed above. We are left with the following two options:

1. The reading in the Burmese and Ceylonese editions "do not think thoughts connected with sensual desire" may lead to a contradiction. In paragraph A, a monk has abandoned the five hindrances, one of which is sensual desire. If a monk has abandoned sensual desire, it is redundant to instruct him: "Do not think thoughts connected with sensual desire".
2. The reading in Ee and the Siamese edition "do not think thoughts connected with the body, feelings, mind and *dhammas*" in paragraph C, when juxtaposed with paragraph D, gives coherence to this *sutta* passage. If a monk follows this instruction and does not think *(vitakketi)* thoughts *(vitakka)* connected with the body, feelings, mind and *dhammas,* he virtually stops his thoughts in general. This seems to indicate one of the second *jhāna*'s characteristics, namely "without *vitakka* and *vicāra*" *(avitakkaṃ avicāraṃ)* as stated in paragraph D. According to PED 620 s.v. *vitakka,* the two terms *vitakka* and *vicāra* "denote one & the same thing: just thought, thinking, only in an emphatic way". Stuart-Fox (1989, pp. 86, 89–92) also argued, "the term *vicāra* was used only to reinforce the meaning of *vitakka*" and he showed that several passages distinguishing between these two terms in the Pali *Nikāyas* are interpolations, to judge from their Chinese counterparts. If we read with Ee and the Siamese edition "do not think thoughts (*vitakka*) connected with the body, feelings, mind and *dhammas*", then paragraph C represents a function of mindfulness suggested by Kuan (2008,

p. 69), that is, to stop the mind proceeding from *saññā* (simple cognition) to *vitakka* (thought) and the ensuing cognitive proliferation *(papañca)*.

Paragraph D describes the second *jhāna* up to the fourth *jhāna*. Paragraph E begins with a standard account of developing the three knowledges subsequent to the attainment of the fourth *jhāna*. As Bucknell and Stuart-Fox (1986, p. 170, 178) demonstrated, the three knowledges *(ñāṇa)* can be identified with wisdom *(paññā)*, the last stage of the three trainings *(sikkhā)* that are usually considered to constitute the Buddhist practice or "path". The three trainings refer to morality, concentration and wisdom (see e.g. Vism I. 8–10, p. 5. Cf. DN I 206–208, AN I 229 ff., MN I 301). The third knowledge, that is, knowledge of the destruction of the taints *(āsava)*, marks the achievement and commencement of liberation, hence the ensuing description: "… His mind is liberated from the taint of sensual desire, from the taint of becoming, from the taint of ignorance …". The taint of sensual desire and the taint of ignorance correspond, respectively, to the emotionalist and intellectualist causes of *dukkha* mentioned above. Liberation from these two taints signifies the eradication of the origin of *dukkha* or the abandoning of the Second True Reality for the Noble Ones (see SN V 422. Cf. Harvey 2009, p. 198). The term "becoming" *(bhava)* means rebirth or continuing existence (Bucknell and Stuart-Fox 1986, p. 88; Buswell and Lopez 2014, p. 69), so liberation from the taint of becoming denotes the end of the round of rebirths. Liberation from the above three taints indicates the realization of Nirvana or the cessation of *dukkha (dukkha-nirodha)*, the Third True Reality for the Noble Ones. The gradual path covering the three trainings delineated in this *sutta* is the way leading to the cessation of *dukkha*: the Fourth True Reality for the Noble Ones.

13.4.3 Constrained or Tamed?

The above two similes, that is, a pillar for binding six animals and a post for binding an elephant, appear to depict the practice of mindfulness as rather grudging and constrained. Rather, this may imply that the practice of mindfulness requires painstaking efforts. According to the *Ariyapariyesanā Sutta* (MN I 168), shortly after his attainment of Nirvana, that is, Awakening, the Buddha described the Dharma, or Truth, that he had just realized as "going against the stream *(paṭisotagāmin)*". Human nature is prone to negligence. People tend to be distracted by objects that may arouse unwholesome mental responses and to stray from the wholesome objects that they should be aware of. In his *Visuddhimagga*, the great exegete Buddhaghosa explained mindfulness thus, "Because of its being firmly set in the object of awareness, it should be seen as like a post" (Vism XIV.141, p. 393; translation by Gethin 2011, p. 272). This explanation presumably alludes to the *sutta* passages as those cited above. The way mindfulness trains the mind of a practitioner is comparable to how a post planted in the earth is employed to bind the animals and thereby tame them. In the last simile, the person who tames the elephant stands for the Buddha, who tames his disciples with the training in mindfulness. In this connection, it is worth noting that one of the Buddha's epithets is "unsurpassed leader of persons to be tamed" (*anuttaro purisadammasārathi,* e.g. MN I 179, 344).

13.5 Altruism

13.5.1 Loving-Kindness

The development of loving-kindness as a practice of mindfulness is unusual for its altruistic aspect, which seems to be lacking in the foregoing types of mindfulness. The well-known *Metta Sutta* in the *Sutta-nipāta* describes the development of loving-kindness *(mettā)* as a practice of mindfulness *(sati)*. This *sutta* contains ten verses. The following is from the first verse and the seventh to ninth verses (Sn 143, 149–151):

> 143. This is what should be done by one who is skilful at the good in order to attain[1] the peaceful state …
> 149. Just as a mother would protect her own son, her only son, with her life, so one should develop the immeasurable mind towards all beings. 150. One should develop the immeasurable mind of loving-kindness towards the whole world[2]—upwards, downwards and across, without obstruction, without hatred, without hostility. 151. Standing, walking, sitting, or lying down, as long as one is free from drowsiness, one should practise this mindfulness (*sati*).

The simile in this *sutta* compares the practitioner to a mother of only one son and all beings to her only son. But the implication is even more complicated. This practice of mindfulness entails imagination. It would be easier for a woman who has only one son to arouse this essential imagination on the basis of her real experience. For

[1] Here the absolutive *abhisamecca* should be rendered as "in order to attain" rather than "having attained" as Norman (1992, p. 16) translated. See Gombrich (1998, p. 15) and Kuan (2008, p. 115).

[2] I translate "so one should develop the immeasurable mind towards all beings. 150. One should develop the immeasurable mind of loving-kindness towards the whole world" from "*evam pi sabbabhūtesu mānasam bhāvaye aparimāṇaṃ*. 150. *Mettañ ca sabbalokasmiṃ mānasam bhāvaye aparimāṇaṃ*" (Sn 149–150, p. 26). Norman (1992, p. 17) translated this passage as, "so one should cultivate an unbounded mind towards all beings, 150. and loving-kindness towards all the world. One should cultivate an unbounded mind". This translation treats *Mettañ ca sabbalokasmiṃ* in verse 150 as a continuation of the sentence in verse 149. But the editors of the *Sutta-nipāta*, D. Andersen and H. Smith, saw this phrase as the beginning of a sentence and thus capitalized *Mettañ;* in contrast, they used the lower case for words that do not stand at the beginning of a sentence. It is more plausible to read this passage in the way Andersen and Smith understood it. "*Mettañ ca sabbalokasmiṃ mānasam bhāvaye aparimāṇaṃ*" in verse 150 should be taken to mean that *mettañ* (loving-kindness) qualifies *mānasam aparimāṇaṃ* (immeasurable mind) since all the three words are in the accusative, and they serve as the object of the verb *bhāvaye* (should develop). Gombrich (1998, p. 14 note 12) also regarded *mettañ* as adjectival and took *mettaṃ mānasaṃ* to mean "friendly thought". At another place, Gombrich (1998, p. 15) translated *mettaṃ mānasam aparimāṇaṃ* as "loving thoughts, boundless", which is similar to my translation: "immeasurable mind of loving-kindness".

most people, however, they have to first imagine that they are a mother of just one son and how much they love him and endeavour to protect him. Then, they have to develop the "constructive imagination" in such a way that they love all beings as much as they love their only son, who exists in fantasy rather than in reality. Such "constructive imagination", an idea put forward by Hamilton (1996, p. 61), is regarded as a form of mindfulness by Kuan (2008, p. 53). In this *sutta,* the expression "immeasurable mind" *(mānasam aparimāṇaṃ)* indicates the extent to which the practitioner of this mindfulness should expand his capacity for developing such constructive imagination, or deliberately conceptualizing the spiritually wholesome and beneficial quality "without limit", namely loving-kindness towards "all sentient beings", the thought of whom apparently arises in him through visualization or something like that.

The "peaceful state" *(santaṃ padaṃ)* at the beginning of this *sutta* refers to Nirvana as demonstrated by Kuan (2008, p. 116). Accordingly, this *sutta* articulates that the ultimate goal, Nirvana, is built on altruistic attitudes towards all beings. This idea is somewhat similar to the idea that characterizes Mahāyāna Buddhism, as Williams and Tribe (2000, p. 102) outlined:

> [T]hose superior people whose motivation is the very highest take as their goal freedom from suffering for all, that is, perfect Buddhahood, motivated by the wish to attain the greatest possibility to benefit others. These are followers of the Great, the Supreme, Path—the Mahāyāna.

Therefore, a Mahāyāna practitioner's supreme liberation from suffering or *dukkha* is based on his kind wish to benefit all others to the extent that his liberation is inseparable from all sentient beings. However, as Gombrich (1998, pp. 26–27) comments, the Theravāda tradition is so conservative that wherever the words loving-kindness *(mettā)* and compassion *(karuṇā)* are mentioned in the texts, the reference is to thought not to acts of kindness—other than preaching. He points out that the Theravādin *Abhidhamma,* for example, the *Dhammasaṅgaṇi,* defines loving-kindness *(mettā)* negatively as absence of hatred *(adosa)* and considers it to be a component of every morally wholesome *(kusala)* thought (Dhs §1056), and therefore not necessarily directed at any object; "loving-kindness" is thus rendered somewhat bloodless.

While the *Metta Sutta* designates "developing the immeasurable mind of loving-kindness towards the whole world" as a practice of mindfulness, this practice is apparently meant to be a meditative exercise. It takes all the beings in the world as the basis or object *(ārammaṇa)* of meditation. The practitioner pays intensive attention to the suffering *(dukkha)* and happiness *(sukha)* of living beings, developing empathy for their situations, which may involve imaginative empathy based on personal experiences. According to Buddhaghosa's exposition in his *Visuddhimagga,* the practitioner should first pervade himself with loving-kindness, and then he should be mindful *(anussaritvā < anu-sati)* of the amiable words, admirable virtues and so on of a dear and revered teacher or his equivalent and so forth, thereby developing loving-kindness thus, "May this good person be happy and free from suffering". The *Visuddhimagga* says that such a practitioner attains absorption *(appanā),* which denotes that this mindfulness practice of loving-kindness is aimed at meditative attainments. In the same way, loving-kindness is next developed towards a very dear friend, a neutral person and a hostile person (Vism IX. 8–12, pp. 245–246). This exposition is apparently intended to cover all categories of sentient beings.

The *Visuddhimagga* argued that loving-kindness should first be developed towards oneself because if one develops loving-kindness thus, "May I be happy", thinking, "Just as I desire happiness and dislike suffering, as I want to live and not to die, so do other beings", making himself the example, then the wish for other beings' welfare and happiness arises in him (Vism IX. 10, pp. 245–246). In support of this argument, the *Visuddhimagga* invoked a verse spoken by the Buddha (translated by Bodhi 2000, p. 171):

> Having traversed all quarters with the mind,
> One finds none anywhere dearer than oneself
> Likewise, each person holds himself most dear
> Hence, one who loves himself should not harm others (SN I 75 and Ud 47)

It is true that if a person does not recognize the very fact that he loves himself, he is unlikely to realize that other beings also love themselves, and thus unlikely to love others in the way they love themselves. The last line of the verse may imply a more positive sense: "One who loves himself should love others". This axiom underlies the practice of mindfulness that is developing the immeasurable mind of loving-kindness towards all beings. A similar but more sophisticated principle is exemplified by the following simile in a discourse on mindfulness.

13.5.2 Acrobatics

In the *Sedaka Sutta* of the *Satipaṭṭhāna Saṃyutta* in the *Saṃyutta Nikāya,* the Buddha gave a simile of an acrobat and his apprentice Medakathālikā as follows (abridged):

> The apprentice Medakathālikā climbed up a bamboo pole and stood on the teacher's shoulders. The acrobat told his apprentice: 'You protect me and I will protect you. Thus protected by one another, we will display our skills, collect our fee, and get down safely from the bamboo pole.' Then the apprentice said: 'That is not the way. You protect yourself and I will protect myself. Thus each self-protected, we will display our skills, collect our fee, and get down safely from the bamboo pole.' (SN V 168–169; translation based on Bodhi (2000, p. 1648))

Explaining this simile, the Buddha said:

> Just as the apprentice Medakathālikā said to the teacher: 'I will protect myself', thus should the establishment of mindfulness (*satipaṭṭhāna*) be practised. 'I will protect others', thus should the establishment of mindfulness be practised. One who protects himself protects others. One who protects others protects himself. And, monks, how does one who protects himself protect others? By practising, developing and cultivation. Thus one who protects himself protects others. And, monks, how does one who protects others protect himself? By forbearance, harmlessness, loving-kindness (*mettatā*) and sympathy (*anudayatā*). (SN V 169)

The Buddha surely approved of what the apprentice said. Did he disapprove of what the teacher said? The answer is negative since the Buddha said, “I will protect others” just as the teacher said, “I will protect you”, and he also asserted, “One who protects others protects himself”. On the whole, the stress is admittedly laid on self-protection, which is seen as providing the foundation for protecting others. Meanwhile, the Buddha could not have derogated the importance of protecting one another. This *sutta* is cited in the *Bhaiṣajya-vastu of the Mūlasarvāstivāda Vinaya* (根本說一切有部毘奈耶藥事, T 1448). This version of the *sutta* shows disapproval of the acrobat teacher’s idea and the Buddha stated, “If one intends to protect others, then one cannot protect himself” (T XXIV 32b). This expression, not found in the SN and SĀ versions, is most likely to be an interpolation as the *Mūlasarvāstivāda Vinaya* is a rather late composition, probably between the fourth and seventh centuries CE (Kuan 2013b, p. 615).

The Buddha said, “How does one who protects himself protect others? By practising, developing and cultivation”. His answer to the question he himself raised is not clear. This is the Pali version transmitted by the Theravāda tradition. Let us look at the Chinese version in the *Saṃyukta Āgama* (T 99) of the Mūlasarvāstivāda tradition. The above statement by the Buddha is parallel to the following in the Chinese version: “The mind itself approaches, develops and realizes protection. Thus one who protects himself protects others” (SĀ 619 at T II 173b). This is my tentative rendering from the Chinese translation of the *Saṃyukta Āgama*. Anālayo’s (2012a, p. 2) rendering is “Becoming familiar with one’s own mind, developing it, protecting it accordingly and attaining realization—this is called ‘protecting oneself protects others’”. This ancient Chinese translation is very obscure. de Jong (1981, p. 108) cogently argued that the *Saṃyukta Āgama* was translated from Sanskrit. Below is my attempt to reconstruct the Sanskrit original of part of the foregoing passage.

The Pali “By practising, developing and cultivation” is *āsevanāya, bhāvanāya* and *bahulīkammena*. We can assume that the Sanskrit original of the foregoing passage extant in Chinese translation corresponds in some way to the Pali. The Chinese rendering 親近, “to approach”, is likely to be translated from a Sanskrit word with the root *√sev* (SJD 1502 s.v. *Sev*: 親近), which is probably equivalent to the Pali *āsevanāya* (instrumental of *āsevanā,* derived from *ā-√sev*), “by practising”. The Chinese rendering 修習, “to develop”, is a standard translation of *bhāvanā* (SJD 956 s.v. *bhāvanā* 修習), which is exactly identical to the Pali *bhāvanāya* (instrumental of *bhāvanā*). The Chinese rendering 隨護 is apparently translated from *anurakṣaṇa* or *anurakṣaṇā* (SJD 65 s.v. *anurakṣaṇa* [neuter] and *anurakṣaṇā* [feminine]: 護, 隨護). Both words can simply mean 護, “to protect”, while 隨 is a typical rendering of the prefix *anu* and hence meaningless. They are equivalent to *anurakkhaṇa* and *anurakkhaṇā* in Pali, which also mean “protection, guarding” (PED 41; DOP I 132). Neither of these two words nor their cognate, however, appears in the Pali passage quoted above. The Chinese rendering 作證, “to realize” or “to witness”, is usually translated from words derived from *sākṣāt-√kṛ* (SJD 1456 s.v. *sākṣāt-√kṛ*: 作證). It has no counterpart (such as *sacchikaroti*) in the Pali passage quoted above. This verb seems to have 隨護, “to protect”, as its object, so I translate “realizes protection". Accordingly, the Chinese (originally Sanskrit) *Saṃyukta Āgama* probably says, "The mind itself practises, develops and realizes protection. Thus one who protects himself protects others". This seems to convey a more complete sense than does the Pali: "By practising, developing and cultivation. Thus one who protects himself protects others". The Chinese version makes it clear that it is the mind that needs practice and development, which are aimed to realize mental protection rather than physical protection [alone].

One's mental practice or self-protection as a means to protect others is related to the Buddha's statement quoted above: "'I will protect myself', thus should the establishment of mindfulness (*satipaṭṭhāna*) be practised". Therefore, one's mental practice as self-protection actually refers to mindfulness. This practice of mindfulness is primarily meant to protect oneself and can be considered to be self-restraint as the simile of a thorny forest indicates above. It is evident that self-restraint, in turn, also protects others.

The Buddha said, "How does one who protects others protect himself? By forbearance, harmlessness, loving-kindness *(mettatā)* and sympathy (*anudayatā*)". This is connected with the Buddha's statement in the same *sutta:* "'I will protect others', thus should the establishment of mindfulness be practised". Accordingly, mindfulness is associated with forbearance, harmlessness, loving-kindness and sympathy, and is thus applied to some ethical attitudes with regard to interpersonal relations. The practice of mindfulness helps one develop beneficial and wholesome attitudes towards others and can thus protect others. This practice leads to positive reciprocal interactions between oneself and others, so it also conduces to protection of oneself. Such reciprocal relationship can extend infinitely to all beings. In a similar vein, Salzberg (2011, p. 178) described loving-kindness as "an inner knowing that all our lives are inextricably interconnected".

Acknowledgments Professor Peter Harvey and the editors of this book read an earlier draft of this chapter and provided valuable suggestions, for which I am very grateful. I would also like to thank Ven. Anālayo for directing me to useful sources and Professor Richard Gombrich and Mr. L. S. Cousins for their helpful advice.

Abbreviations

AN	Aṅguttara Nikāya
BJT	Buddha Jayanti Tripitaka Series (electronic version)
CBETA	*CBETA Chinese Electronic Tripiṭaka Collection,* Version 2014. Taipei: Chinese Buddhist Electronic Text Association
CS	*Chaṭṭha Saṅgāyana Tipiṭaka,* Version 4.0 (digital version). Igatpuri: Vipassana Research Institute
Dhs	Dhammasaṅgaṇi
Dīp	*The Dīpavaṃsa: an ancient Buddhist historical record,* ed. and tr. by Hermann Oldenberg. London: Williams and Norgate, 1879
DN	Dīgha Nikāya
DOP I	*A dictionary of Pāli,* Part I, ed. Margaret Cone. Oxford: Pali Text Society, 2001

Ee	European edition, that is, Pali Text Society edition
It	Itivuttaka
MĀ	Madhyama Āgama 中阿含經 Zhong ahanjing
MN	Majjhima Nikāya
SĀ	Saṃyukta Āgama 雜阿含經 Za ahanjing
SJD	漢訳対照梵和大辞典 (A Sanskrit-Japanese dictionary with equivalents in Chinese translation), ed. Unrai Wogihara 荻原雲来, revised edition. Tokyo: 講談社, 1986
SN	Saṃyutta Nikāya
Sn	Sutta-nipāta (by verse)
T	*Taishō Shinshū Daizōkyō* 大正新脩大藏經, ed. Takakusu Junjirō 高楠順次郎, Watanabe Kaigyoku 渡邊海旭 and Ono Genmyo 小野玄妙, Tokyo: Taishō Issaikyō Kankōkai, 1924–1934. (Cited from CBETA)
Vism	Visuddhimagga of Buddhaghosācariya, ed. Henry Clarke Warren, reprint. Delhi: Motilal Banarsidass Publishers, 1989. (First published 1950 Cambridge, Massachusetts: Harvard University Press)
Ud	Udāna

References to Pali texts are to the Pali Text Society editions, unless otherwise noted.

References

Anālayo, B. (2006). The Chinese version of the Dantabhūmi Sutta. *Buddhist Studies Review, 23*(1), 5–19.

Anālayo, B. (2012a). Protecting oneself and others through mindfulness: The acrobat simile in the Saṃyukta-āgama. *Sri Lanka International Journal of Buddhist Studies, 2,* 1–23.

Anālayo, B. (2012b). *Madhyama-āgama studies*. Taipei: Dharma Drum.

Anālayo, B. (2013). *Perspectives on satipaṭṭhāna*. Cambridge: Windhorse.

Bodhi, B. (2000). *The connected discourses of the Buddha*. Oxford: Pali Text Society.

Bodhi, B. (2011). What does mindfulness really mean? A canonical perspective. *Contemporary Buddhism, 12*(1), 19–39.

Bronkhorst, J. (1985). Dharma and Abhidharma. *Bulletin of the School of Oriental and African Studies, 48*(2), 305–320.

Bronkhorst, J. (2012). *Absorption: Human nature and Buddhist liberation*. Paris: UniversityMedia.

Bucknell, R. S., & Stuart-Fox, M. (1986). *The twilight language: Explorations in Buddhist meditation and symbolism*. London: Curzon.

Buswell, R. E., Jr., & Lopez, D. S., Jr. (2014). *The Princeton dictionary of Buddhism*. Princeton: Princeton University Press.

Conze, E. (1962). *Buddhist thought in India: Three phases of Buddhist philosophy*. London: George Allen & Unwin Ltd.

Cousins, L. S. (2001). *Pain and its ending: The four noble truths in the Theravāda Buddhist Canon*. *Journal of Buddhist Ethics, 8,* 36–41.

de Jong, J. W. (1981). Fa-hsien and Buddhist texts in Ceylon. *Journal of the Pali Text Society, 9,* 105–115.

Enomoto, F. 榎本文雄. (1984a). 說一切有部系アーガマの展開——『中阿含』と『雜阿含』をめぐって——(The Development of the Āgamas of the Sarvāstivāda Lineage: Concerning the Madhyama Āgama and the Saṃyukta Āgama). 印度學佛教學研究 *Journal of Indian and Buddhist Studies, 32*(2), 1073–1070.

Enomoto, F. 榎本文雄. (1984b). 阿含經典の成立 (Formation of the Āgama Texts). 東洋學術研究 *Journal of the Oriental Studies, 23*(1), 93–108.
Gethin, R. (1998). *The foundations of Buddhism*. Oxford: Oxford University Press.
Gethin, R. (2011). On some definitions of mindfulness. *Contemporary Buddhism, 12*(1), 263–279.
Gombrich, R. (1988). *Theravada Buddhism: A social history from ancient Benares to modern Colombo*. London: Routledge & Kegan Paul Ltd.
Gombrich, R. (1998). *Kindness and compassion as means to nirvana in early Buddhism*. Amsterdam: Royal Netherlands Academy of Arts and Sciences.
Hamilton, S. (1996). *Identity and experience: The constitution of the human being according to early Buddhism*. London: Luzac Oriental.
Harvey, P. (2009). The Four Ariya-saccas as 'true realities for the spiritually ennobled'—the painful, its origin, its cessation, and the way going to this—rather than 'Noble Truths' concerning these. *Buddhist Studies Review, 26*(2), 197–227.
Harvey, P. (2013). The Saṅgha of Noble Sāvakas, with particular reference to their trainee member, the person 'practising for the realization of the stream-entry-fruit'. *Buddhist Studies Review, 30*(1), 3–70.
Hiraoka, S. 平岡聡. (2003). 『雜阿含經』と說一切有部の律藏 (The Saṃyukta Āgama and the Vinaya of the Sarvāstivāda). 印度學佛教學研究 *Journal of Indian and Buddhist Studies, 51*(2), 818–813.
Kuan, T.-f. (2008). *Mindfulness in early Buddhism: New approaches through psychology and textual analysis of Pali, Chinese and Sanskrit sources*. London: Routledge.
Kuan, T.-f. (2012). Cognitive operations in Buddhist meditation: Interface with western psychology. *Contemporary Buddhism, 13*(1), 35–60.
Kuan, T.-f. (2013a). The Pavāraṇā Sutta and "liberation in both ways" as against "liberation by wisdom". *Bulletin of the School of Oriental and African Studies, 76*(1), 49–73.
Kuan, T.-f. (2013b). Legends and transcendence: Sectarian affiliations of the Ekottarika Āgama in Chinese translation. *Journal of the American Oriental Society, 133*(4), 607–634.
Kumoi, S. (1963). Āgama (2). In G. P. Malalasekera (Ed.), *Encyclopaedia of Buddhism* (Vol. I, fasc. 2, pp. 244–248). Government of Ceylon.
Lü, C. (1963). Āgama (1). In G. P. Malalasekera (Ed.), *Encyclopaedia of Buddhism* (Vol. I, fasc. 2, pp. 244–248). Government of Ceylon.
Mayeda, E. 前田惠學. (1964). *A history of the formation of original Buddhist texts* 原始佛教聖典の成立史研究. Tokyo: Sankibo-Busshorin.
Mizuno, K. 水野弘元. (1996). 仏教文献研究 *(A study of Buddhist literature)*. Tokyo: 春秋社.
Ñāṇamoli, B., & Bodhi, B. (2001). *The middle length discourses of the Buddha,* revised edition. Oxford: Pali Text Society.
Norman, K. R. (1992). *The group of discourses (Sutta-nipāta)* (Vol. II). Oxford: Pali Text Society.
Nyanaponika, T. (1962). *The heart of Buddhist meditation: A handbook of mental training based on the Buddhist way of mindfulness*. London: Rider & Company.
Oberlies, T. (2003). Ein bibliographischer Überblick über die kanonischen Texte der Śrāvakayāna-Schulen des Buddhismus. *Wiener Zeitschrift für die Kunde Südasiens, 47,* 37–84.
Rahula, W. (2000). *What the Buddha taught*. Oxford: Oneworld.
Salzberg, S. (2011). Mindfulness and loving-kindness. *Contemporary Buddhism, 12*(1), 177–182.
Sternberg, R. J. (2009). *Cognitive psychology* (5th ed.). Belmont: Wadsworth Cengage Learning.
Stuart-Fox, M. (1989). Jhāna and Buddhist scholasticism. *Journal of the International Association of Buddhist Studies, 12*(2), 79–110.
Thich Minh Chau, B. (1991). *The Chinese Madhyama Āgama and the Pāli Majjhima Nikāya*. Delhi: Motilal Banarsidass.
Williams, P., & Tribe, A. (2000). *Buddhist thought: A complete introduction to the Indian tradition*. London: Routledge.

Tse-fu Kuan is an associate professor in the College of General Studies at Yuan Ze University in Taiwan. He received his doctoral degree in Oriental studies from the University of Oxford. His primary research interests include early Indian Buddhism and comparative studies of Buddhist texts in Pali, Sanskrit and Chinese. He is an editor of the *Journal of the Oxford Centre for Buddhist Studies*.

Chapter 14
Types of Mindfulness, Orders of Conditionality, and Stages of the Spiritual Path

Tim Lomas and Jnanavaca

14.1 Introduction

The concept of mindfulness has found a hugely receptive audience within Western psychology over recent years. In the wake of Kabat-Zinn's (1982) pioneering mindfulness-based stress reduction (MBSR) programme, the number of academic papers focusing on mindfulness has grown exponentially, with over 500 studies published on it in 2012 alone (Shonin et al. 2013). However, as much as this interest is to be welcomed, it is worth reflecting critically on what *type* of mindfulness is being explored in such work. Mindfulness has tended to be conceptualised and operationalised in contemporary academia in using cognitive theories of attention and awareness (Bishop et al. 2004). Such theories can be seen as modern constructs, generated by a culture of thought that, influenced by emergent technologies, views the mind mechanistically in terms of computer metaphors (Crowther-Heyck 1999). That said, it is not necessarily the case that constructs such as attention are completely out of tune with the spirit of the original Buddhist teachings. For instance, the *Amitayus jhana sutta,* which provides instructions for a meditation on the sun, states, "[C]ause your mind to be firmly fixed on it so as to have an unwavering perception by the exclusive application of your mind" (part II, verse 9). Thus, conceptualising mindfulness using constructs such as attention is not necessarily inappropriate; however, it may nevertheless be somewhat limiting.

In particular, having been generally operationalised in this cognitive way, mindfulness has become largely decontextualised from its Buddhist origins. Although Buddhist teachings informed the construction of initiatives like the MBSR programme, this influence has tended to remain largely implicit, with many people

T. Lomas (✉)
School of Psychology, The University of East London, Stratford Campus, Water Lane, London E15 4LZ, UK
e-mail: t.lomas@uel.ac.uk

Jnanavaca
London Buddhist Centre, 51 Roman Road, Bethnal Green, London E2 OHU, UK

E. Shonin et al. (eds.), *Buddhist Foundations of Mindfulness,*
Mindfulness in Behavioral Health, DOI 10.1007/978-3-319-18591-0_14

engaging with mindfulness in a secular way, without reference to Buddhism (Shapiro 1994). One may indeed argue that this decontextualisation was necessary in order for mindfulness to find a receptive audience in secular Western societies. King (1999) suggested that it is exactly the ease with which meditation *can* be shorn of its religious connections and presented as a relaxation tool, for example, that has enabled it to take root and flourish in such societies. However, now that mindfulness has achieved critical and popular acceptance, we would argue that the time has come to *re*contextualise it, which indeed is the spirit of this book as a whole. Even in its limited, decontextualised way, mindfulness as currently operationalised within Western academia has had a powerful, transformative effect across diverse fields, from medicine (Fortney and Taylor 2010) to education (Erricker and Erricker 2001). However, in Buddhist teachings, the concept of mindfulness is just one part of a much wider nexus of thought and practice, which have much farther-reaching implications in terms of wellbeing and psychological development. Considered in this original context, the potential for mindfulness to generate beneficial outcomes is thus perhaps far greater.

This chapter is an attempt at recontextualisation, informed and influenced by the contemporary Buddhist teacher Sangharakshita, whose perspective and location within Buddhism is briefly outlined below.[1] Buddhism comprises such a vast,

[1] Throughout its long and illustrious history, numerous traditions have emerged and developed within Buddhism; in broad brush strokes, we can paint a picture involving the early Therevadan schools; the later Mahayahan movement; followed still later by the Vajrayanan (Tantric) efflorescence; moreover, even within these different traditions can be found diverse schools of thought. As such, any presentation and interpretation of Buddhism is necessarily partial, drawing only on select sources while ignoring other equally interesting or worthy sources. The authors here have taken their interpretation of Buddhism from one of the foremost contemporary Buddhist teachers, Urgyen Sangharakshita, who has been central to the efforts to transmit and interpret Buddhism to the "West" (Subhuti 1994). Sangharakshita was born in London in 1925, originally named Dennis Lingwood. After being posted to India during the Second World War, he stayed on to pursue his interest in Buddhism, studying under numerous revered Buddhist masters (including Dhardo Rimpoche, teacher of the Dalai Lama; recounted in Sangharakshita 1997). He was ordained within the Therevadan tradition in 1950, whereupon he received the honorific "dharma name" Urgyen Sangharakshita, a Pali term meaning "Protector of the Sangha". He returned to England in 1964, and after leading the English Sangha Trust for 2 years, founded the Western Buddhist Order (WBO) in 1967, a monastic order, encompassed by the wider Friends of the Western Buddhist Order (FWBO). In 2010, the movement changed its name to the Triratna Buddhist Order/Community; this change, eschewing the word "Western", was partly to reflect the dissemination and migration of the movement across the world (e.g. India is currently the country with the largest number of members). "Triratna" is a Sanskrit term which means the "three jewels"—referring to the tripartite model of Buddha (teacher), Dharma (teachings), and Sangha (community)—to which members are said to turn for refuge (i.e. commit to) at their ordination.The emergent Triratna movement is considered one of the main forms that Buddhism has taken as it has been transmitted to the West, with around 80 centres/groups in the UK alone (Bluck 2006). The movement is innovative in that it does not exclusively situate itself within any of the dominant Asian Buddhist traditions (a fact that has perturbed some traditionalists within the wider Buddhist community who value the "authority of lineage and Asian precedent"; Vishvapani 2001, para. 60). Rather, Sangharakshita has sought to select practical and doctrinal elements from across various traditions, with the aim of presenting a "core of common material" constituting the "essence" of Buddhism which, divested of anachronistic cultural accretions, may be "relevant" to the "West" (Subhuti 1994). His attitude to the ca-

diverse collection of teachings that any one presentation is necessarily partial—all we can do to mitigate this partiality is to reflexively acknowledge how we have arrived at our particular exegesis and interpretation. Here, we shall identify and draw together three threads that can be found within the canonical literature and its supporting commentaries. The chapter is in two parts: The first part introduces the threads themselves and the second part will trace the links and associations between the threads. The first thread concerns the origins of the English term mindfulness, and the idea that in traditional Buddhist teachings there are different *types* of mindfulness, captured by various Pali terms that each have specific nuances and inflections. (All terms will be written in the text in Pali, and will generally be defined on first usage.) Here we focus on three particular Pali words, reflecting on their meanings and implications: *sati* (perhaps best defined as awareness infused with a spirit of recollection), *appamada* (awareness infused with an ethos of ethical care), and *sampajañña* (awareness infused with a sense of spiritual progress). The second thread concerns a central Buddhist teaching, *paṭiccasamuppāda*, the law of dependent origination (i.e. all things arise dependent on conditions). One interpretation of this law holds that conditionality operates at a number of different orders of existence, from the causality of physical laws (e.g. the law of gravity) to the kind of causality that explains the evolution of enlightened consciousness in human history. The third thread is the widespread notion (not limited to Buddhism) that a person's psychological development unfolds through a series of identifiable stages; here we focus on one particular Buddhist stage-wise model that elucidates five broad stages of the spiritual path.

Moreover, we not only present these threads but in the second part of the chapter seek to weave them together by articulating commonalities among them. We do this by identifying three key phases of practice, each outlined in a section. The first section focuses on the first type of mindfulness, *sati*. Here, we weave in the second thread by arguing that *sati* is associated primarily with the recognition of the three lowest orders of causality—physical, biological, and psychological. Here we also

---

nonical texts is encapsulated thus: "Some of the discussions and classifications of the Abhidharma are very helpful, but others are less so. We must therefore study it with the analytic and critical spirit of the Abhidharma itself…. If we were to swallow everything indiscriminately … we would probably get intellectual, spiritual, or aesthetic indigestion" (Sangharakshita 1998, p. 17). The two central meditation practices taught within the movement are: the mindfulness of breathing, which is a canonical Therevadan teaching, as recommended in the *Anapanasati sutta* (sutra on mindfulness of breathing) for example (Roth 2006); and the *metta bhavana,* which likewise has roots in the Therevadan tradition, such as the *Karaniya mettā sutta* from the *Khuddakapatha* (Blackburn 1999). For practitioners who are more experienced (e.g. ordained), the movement also promotes more advanced practices including the "Six Element" practice, a meditation on the insubstantiality of self which also has origins in traditional Therevadan Buddhism (e.g. the *Bahudhàtuka sutta*); and the Sadhana practice, a deity visualisation meditation associated with the Tibetan Vajra tradition (Nyima and Gyaltsap 2013). In addition to these, the movement has developed pujas based on various teachings, such as the "Heart Sutra" (*Prajñāpāramitā sutta*), a classic Mahayanan teaching (Conze 2001); and a "sevenfold puja" based on the *Bodhicaryavatara* ("Way of the Bodhisattva") by the eighth-century teacher Śāntideva (2002), which features within the Mayahanan and Vajrayanan traditions (Batchelor 1987).

weave in the third thread by suggesting that *sati* is linked to embarkation on the spiritual path, that is, to the first stage of psycho-spiritual development. The second phase centres on the second type of mindfulness, *appamada*. Here we weave in the second thread by suggesting that *appamada* is linked to the recognition of a fourth type of causality, namely karmic causality. We furthermore weave in the third thread by arguing that *appamada* is connected to the fulfilment of the first stage of psycho-spiritual development and to progression through the second stage of development. Finally, the third section of the chapter addresses the third type of mindfulness, *sampajañña*. Here we weave in the second thread by proposing that *sampajañña* is associated with the recognition of a final type of causality, dharmic causality. We further weave in the third thread by arguing that *sampajañña* is connected to the third, fourth, and fifth stages of psycho-spiritual development.

14.2 Part 1: The Three Threads

In part 1, we outline the three threads in turn: types of mindfulness, orders of causality, and stages of psycho-spiritual development. In each case, we identify the original Buddhist teachings that are the source of these threads, as well as point out the particular contemporary slant—influenced by Sangharakshita—that we bring to these teachings.

14.2.1 Thread 1: Types of Mindfulness

Our first thread concerns the concept of mindfulness itself, and the notion that there may be different types of mindfulness. Recent years have witnessed an emergent debate in the psychological literature around the term mindfulness—around what it means— and how well it serves as an English translation of concepts found in the original Buddhist texts (McCown et al. 2010). This debate raises interesting questions pertaining to exegesis and hermeneutics (i.e. how we access and interpret original texts), and to translation and discursive equivalence (i.e. how we retain the original meanings in the English terms we use). The crux of the issue is this: In the Buddhist texts, there are a number of conceptually similar Pali/Sanskrit terms, relating to awareness and attention, each with subtly different nuances and meanings embedded within them. However, by historical accident, only one of these terms has been highlighted and translated into English, namely *sati*. Moreover, the English word chosen for this translation, mindfulness, arguably does not capture the nuances of the original term. Consequently, not only is mindfulness perhaps an inadequate translation of the original Pali term *sati,* but the exclusive focus on this word in the psychological literature means that the significance of the other Pali/Sanskrit terms relating to awareness in Buddhist teachings is also being overlooked.

So, where did the term mindfulness come from? As Gethin (2011) elucidates, the word was first used by the great Buddhist scholar, T. W. Rhys Davids, in 1881, as a translation of *sati*. Within the Brahmanical tradition of ancient India, the word *sati* had connotations of "remembrance" and "recollection" (Peacock 2014). Within a Buddhist context, however, it did not refer to historical or chronological memory per se, but to a state in which one recollects or remembers the activity that "one is engaged in, in the present moment" (Peacock 2014, p. 6). This meaning of *sati* is to an extent evident in the pre-eminent contemporary definition of mindfulness formulated by Kabat-Zinn (2003, p. 145), who explicitly cited the term *sati* as the origin of his formulation, as "the awareness that arises through paying attention on purpose, in the present moment, and nonjudgmentally to the unfolding of experience moment by moment". However, it is interesting to consider the process through which mindfulness was selected as an appropriate translation of *sati*. As Gethin (2011) noted, Rhys Davids appeared to have some uncertainty over the choice of this English word. In Rhys Davids, (1881) translation of the *Mahaparinibbana sutta,* mindfulness was rendered as "mental activity" (p. 9) and simply "thought" (p. 63), but it was only with Rhys Davids, (1910) translation of the *Mahasatipatthana sutta* that he settled on the term mindfulness. Indeed, as others have pointed out, *sati* is a very difficult word to translate (Bodhi 2011). For example, Shapiro et al. (2006) suggested that the term is too cognitive and cerebral, and overlooks qualities of emotional warmth present in the original, and thus a better translation might be "heart-mindfulness". Moreover, the word mindfulness is semantically confusing—while one can appreciate the value of a word that is the antonym of being mindless, the notion of a full mind arguably misses the mark.

Aside from the adequacy of the term mindfulness as a translation for *sati,* a perhaps more significant issue is the number of Buddhist concepts linked to *sati* that have remained *un*translated and, hence, unappreciated in Western psychology. In the canonical literature are various conceptually similar terms, each with subtly different nuances of meaning (Bodhi 2011). These include the two concepts addressed in this chapter, *appamada* and *sampajañña,* as well as terms such as *manasikara* (attention) and *viññāṇa* (consciousness). The danger with the current enthusiasm for mindfulness (as a translation of *sati*) is that the precious insights and teachings bound up with these other concepts may be overlooked. This danger is recognised by Kabat-Zinn himself, who suggested that "the rush to define mindfulness within Western psychology may wind up denaturing it in fundamental ways", and thus there is "the potential for something priceless to be lost" (Williams and Kabat-Zinn 2011, p. 4). So, in addition to exploring the nuances of *sati,* this chapter highlights two further Pali terms—both relating to awareness and both of which could also potentially be translated as mindfulness—that may each have something priceless to offer in terms of psychological development, namely *appamada* and *sampajañña.* Together with *sati*, these two terms offer us three types of awareness: awareness infused with a spirit of recollection *(sati),* awareness infused with an ethos of ethical care *(appamada)*, and awareness infused with a sense of spiritual progress *(sampajañña)*. In part 2 below, we elucidate the meanings embedded within these three terms by exploring their parallels with the other two threads (e.g. stages of the path).

14.2.2 Thread 2: Levels of Conditionality

The second thread concerns a central teaching in Buddhism: *paṭiccasamuppāda*, that is, the law of conditionality. This teaching is absolutely pivotal, being the core insight expressed by the Buddha on attaining enlightenment, a fundamental principle that lies at the heart of Buddhism, upon which other teachings rest (Kang 2009). Essentially, the teaching reflects the insight that all aspects of existence arise dependent upon conditions. As expressed by the Buddha upon his enlightenment (the *Upanisa sutta*): "This being, that exists; through the arising of this, that arises. This not being, that does not exist; through the ceasing of this, that ceases". This insight into the causal operation of the universe—into the general principle of ordered relationships between conditions and their effects—is the central understanding that effectively underpins all other Buddhist teachings, the "meta" law that substantiates all other laws. For example, the Four Noble Truths (e.g. the second truth, that suffering has a cause) are manifestations of this more fundamental insight into *paṭiccasamuppāda*. A further significance of this teaching is that understanding its truth is seen as the key to wellbeing and ultimately to liberation from suffering. As Sangharakshita and Subhuti (2013, p. 49) stated,

> once we have understood and are fully convinced about the nature of reality as *paṭiccasamuppāda*, we align ourselves with those regularities or laws that lead us to liberation.

This law of *paṭiccasamuppāda* has been elaborated upon in various ways in the Buddhist literature. One illuminating elaboration has been the identification of five different levels or orders of conditionality, referred to as the fivefold *niyāmas*. In Keown's (2003) *Dictionary of Buddhism, niyāmas* are defined as, "laws, conditions or constraints that govern processes or phenomena". Collectively then, the fivefold *niyāmas* thus represent "categories of necessary relationship within the principle of conditionality—the five different classes or orders of regularities by which conditioned is bound to conditions" (Sangharakshita and Subhuti 2013, p. 49). It is worth mentioning that the Buddha is only recorded as teaching the *niyāmas* individually; they are not presented together as a fivefold list in the *piṭakas* (Jones 2012). The emphasis on the collective fivefold *niyāmas* only happened in the seminal commentaries of Buddhaghosa in the fifth-century CE. In particular, this can be found in the *Sumaṅgalavilāsinī* (Sv ii.432), Buddhaghosa's commentary on the *Dīgha Nikāya,* where it occurs in the context of a discussion of the meaning of *dhammatā* (i.e. order of events) in the *Mahāpadāna sutta* (DA ii.432). As Jones (2012) elucidates, Buddhaghosa presents this list in the course of commenting on a refrain attributed to the Buddha, namely that "This, in such a case, is the norm" (dhammatā). Buddhaghosa then proceeds to elaborate, as if the Buddha himself was the one speaking, five different laws of nature, each of which provides a sense of the ways in which things necessarily happen. In turn, Sangharakshita embraced Buddhaghosa's teaching and made it central to his own understanding of Buddhism. As such, as to whether the fivefold *niyāmas* are a canonical Buddhist teaching, Sangharakshita and Subhuti (2013, p. 49) argue that although Sangharakshita's presentation of these is "sufficiently different to be regarded in some respects as new", it is nevertheless "not at all inconsistent with the teaching of the Buddha as found in the suttas", nor indeed with "the import of the commentaries themselves".

So, what are these five laws? Essentially, the commentaries recognise five different aspects or domains of life that are subject to law-like principles. First, *utu-niyāma* is the law of the seasons, describing the observable cyclical regularity of certain environmental phenomena (e.g. seasonal and diurnal patterns). Buddhaghosa described this law as "the phenomena of winds and rains". Looked at anachronistically through our contemporary scientific understanding, we might regard this as the domain of physical laws, like the law of gravity. Second, *bīja-niyāma* is the law of seeds, which refers to observable patterns in the realm of living phenomena, such as reproductive continuity in plant and animal species. In Buddhaghosa's commentary, this is explained with reference to "rice produced from rice-seed". Again, regarded anachronistically, this could be seen as the domain of biochemistry, featuring principles such as the genetic inheritance of phenotypes. Third, *citta-niyāma* is the law of the mind, referring to patterns of mental events as described by *abhidhamma* theory. As explained by Buddhaghosa, "Antecedent states of consciousness with their properties stand to posterior states with their properties in the relation of efficient cause". We might view this as the domain of psychology, encompassing phenomena such as the acquisition and manifestation of likes and dislikes. Fourth is *kamma-niyāma,* the law of kamma, which elucidates the idea that actions in the world have consequences. Here, Buddhaghosa refers to "the desirable and undesirable results following good and bad action". We might view this as the domain of ethics and morality, as encapsulated by philosophical and religious teachings. Finally, *dhamma-niyāma* is known as the law of nature, which in this sense refers to the ability or potential of the universe to develop complex qualities such as consciousness and exemplary beings like the Buddha. Buddhaghosa described this as "the order of things concerned with the production by the cosmos of its perfect or norm type [i.e. exemplary individual]". In the context of the mythological worldview present at the time the commentaries were formulated, this law referred partly to supernatural portents accompanying the appearance of a Buddha. From the perspective of modern scientific understanding, we might associate this law with the theory of evolution and, in particular, with emergentist philosophies (e.g. Wilber 1995; Aurobindo 1939–1940) which view the universe as evolving *towards* complex outcomes such as self-consciousness. (That said, Sangharakshita and Subhuti (2013) emphasise that the evolution of qualities such as enlightened consciousness is not an inevitable species-level development. They differentiate between "lower evolution" (i.e. the general emergence of consciousness through the biological evolution of the species) and "higher evolution" (the singular psycho-spiritual development of individual members of the species as a result of personal talent and effort).

The notion of the fivefold *niyāmas* was embraced by pivotal figures responsible for the transmission of Buddhism to the West. Jones (2012) suggested that C. A. F. Rhys Davids, the wife and scholarly partner of T. W. Rhys Davids (introduced above), was particularly enamoured of the concept of the *kamma niyāma,* since this enabled her to argue that a moral law was "woven into the fabric of the universe, as an inescapable immanent process" (Jones 2012, p. 549). As Rhys Davids (1912,

p. 240) stated, the *niyāmas* implied an "organic tendency in the universe" towards "the evolution of a perfect type" (i.e. towards the Buddha, and other exemplary beings). Jones argued that Rhys Davids' enthusiasm for the *niyāma* teaching was partly driven by her keenness to present Buddhism as a type of evolutionary naturalism, consonant with the naturalism of science, yet retaining the moral sensibility of Christianity (which was beginning to lose its hold in the West). However, this critique does not detract from the validity of her interpretation or the concept generally. Consideration of the principle of the fivefold *niyāmas* can be a powerful driver of psychological and spiritual development, and different types of mindfulness might be regarded as being attuned to different *niyāmas*. Briefly, *sati* (i.e. present-moment awareness) could be viewed as focused primarily on the first three *niyāmas* (*utu, bija,* and particularly *citta*). However, it is arguably with the cultivation of *appamada* that a person really becomes cognizant of *kamma niyāma*, that is, starts to become deeply appreciative of the ethical dimensions and consequences of their actions. And it is only with the subsequent development of *sampajañña* that a person develops an understanding of *dhamma niyāma,* that is, begins to enter the stream of spiritual development. Appreciation of these latter two *niyāmas,* which are not necessarily observed through *sati* (i.e. mindfulness as commonly understood in Western psychology), helps further our development in ways that cultivation of *sati* alone may be unable to. As Buddhaghosa suggested, insight into *kamma niyāma* shows us "why we should be good", and insight into *dhamma niyāma* shows us why we should "try to better our good" (Jones 2012, pp. 548–549). Thus, the cultivation of *appamada* and *sampajañña* forms of mindfulness facilitates ongoing spiritual development.

14.2.3 Thread 3: Stages of the Path

Arguably, the overarching point of Buddhism is the possibility of psychological and spiritual *development*. Ultimately, all teachings are about helping people overcome suffering and make progress towards liberation. The metaphor often used for people engaging with Buddhism is that of progressing along a path. Moreover, with their customary precision, Buddhist teachings do not merely assert the existence of a path, but delineate precise stages along it. Various nuanced depictions of this path, with numerous stage-wise teachings, can be found in the canonical literature. For instance, Bucknell (1984) elucidated six different lists of stages within various texts of the *pitakas*. The first of these is the most widely known and taught, namely, the Noble Eightfold Path, featuring right vision, conception, speech, conduct, livelihood, effort, mindfulness, and concentration. Although there is some debate over whether these stages are intended to be understood as sequential, Bucknell suggested that this indeed is the case. For example, the *Mahdcattdrisaka-sutta* stated, "As to this, monks, right view comes first. And how, monks, does right view come first? From right view proceeds right aspiration, from right aspiration proceeds right speech, from right speech proceeds right action ...". On the other hand, Sangharakshita (1998) did not interpret these paths as sequential; rather, he made a distinction between the first limb of the eightfold path—right vision—and the remaining seven limbs, which he refers to collectively as the path of transformation. He argued that right vision involves cultivating insight into reality (e.g. into *paṭiccasamuppāda*) and that the path of transformation involves allowing this insight to permeate and transform one's being.

While the Noble Eightfold Path is the most prominent stage-wise teaching in Buddhism, there are numerous elaborations on the theme of a path, with varying numbers of fine-grained stages (Bucknell 1984). For example, a second stage-wise schema, found in each of the first four *nikayas* and in the *Mahdcattdrisaka sutta,* add two further stages to the eightfold path. Following right concentration, this tenfold path adds right insight *(samma-nana)* and right liberation *(samma-vimutti)*. A third teaching—which occurs in three places in the *Majjhima,* the first being the *Cula-Hatthipadopama sutta* (the Lesser Discourse on the Simile of the Elephant's Footprints)—features 12 distinct stages. These are: *dhamma* (hearing the Buddha teach, and taking ordination as a monk); *sila* (adopting the precepts); *indriyasamvara* (practising guarding the sense doors); *sati-sampajañña* (practising mindfulness and self-possession); the first *jhana* (meditation, that is, purifying one's mind of the hindrances *(nivarana),* and attaining the first *rupa-jhana*); the second *jhana* (attaining the second *jhana*); the third *jhana* (attaining the third *jhana*); the fourth *jhana* (attaining the fourth *jhana*); *pubbenivasdnussati-nana* (recollecting former existences in samsara); *sattanam cutupapata-nana* (observing the death and rebirth of beings according to their *kamma*); *asavakkhaya-nana* (destruction of the *asavas* (mental influences or bias), and profound realisation of the four noble truths); and finally *vimutti* (awareness of being liberated). Even more detailed stage-wise conceptions can be found in the teachings. For example, in the *Maha-Assapura sutta,* in which the Buddha instructs his monks in the "things that are to be done by recluses and brahmans", there is a list of *16* different stages, which includes many of the stages from the 12-fold list articulated above, plus others such as *parisuddha kaya-samaadra* (cultivating pure conduct of body). In addition to these lists in the canonical texts are stage-wise conceptions developed throughout Buddhism's long history of evolution and transmission to other cultures. For example, in Zen we find the path described in terms of the ten ox-herding pictures, initially formulated by Kuo-An Shih-Yuan in the Sung Dynasty (Suzuki 1934; Loori 1999): searching for the ox, finding traces of the ox, seeing the ox, catching the ox, taming the ox, riding the ox home, forgetting the ox, transcending the ox, returning to the source, and entering the marketplace with bliss-bestowing hands.

Thus, we can see that (a) the notion of stage-wise psycho-spiritual development is central to Buddhism, and (b) various conceptions of such development have been conceived within the teachings. Given (b), we focus on one particular developmental model, the Sarvāstivāda Five Path schema, which was first expounded in the Sarvāstivāda *Abhidharma* and later interpreted/reworked by Sangharakshita (1998). (The Sarvāstivāda emerged as a separate Buddhist school, following a schism within the Therevadan tradition, during the reign of Asoka, around 240 BCE, after which they became the main non-Mahayanan Buddhist tradition on the Indian subcontinent (King 1995).) The Sarvāstivāda schema features five stages (Chong 2009).

First, the path of requisites or accumulation *(sambhara-mārga)* is the foundation for development. This involves the accumulation of merits through three primary practices: giving *(dana),* moral observance *(sila),* and the cultivation of meditation *(bhavana)*. Second, the path of preparatory effort *(prayoga-marga)* features the cultivation of meditative practices. This involves a preparatory phase *(mokabhagiya)* of basic practices *(samatha and vipassana),* followed by more advanced practices *(nirvedhabhagiya)*. The third stage, the path of seeing *(darsana-marga),* involves direct comprehension *(abhisamaya)* of the four noble truths, that is, transcendental insight. Beyond this, the fourth stage is the path of cultivation/transformation *(bhavana-marga)*; this refers to the idea that certain defilements cannot be extinguished by insight (the third stage), but only by further cultivation of the mind during this more advanced fourth stage. The final stage is the path of the non-trainee/no more learning *(asaika-marga),* in which the practitioner achieves final liberation. In Sangharakshita's (1998) interpretation of this teaching—described as a "reworking of Mahayana teaching, derived from Sarvāstivādan sources" (Sangharakshita and Subhuti 2013, p. 132)—he reconfigures these five stages under the following terms: integration, skilful intention, spiritual death, spiritual rebirth, and enlightened compassionate activity. It is worth emphasising that although these stages emerge sequentially, progression to a higher stage does not mean that the preceding one is negated or left behind; rather, the stages unfold out of each other, where each emergent stage augments the preceding one. For instance, after the first stage, integration still continues, but in a progressively deeper way, enriched by the developments provided by the subsequent stages. On a point of terminology, it is also worth stating that Sangharakshita sometimes refers to the second stage as one of "positive emotions". However, this label is somewhat ambiguous (i.e. it can imply that this stage centres on pleasant feelings). As such, he has more recently come to prefer the term "skilful intention", since this captures the sense of ethical behaviour that is the hallmark of this stage (as this chapter elucidates); consequently, we use this term here. In addition, Sangharakshita does not always refer to the fifth stage as a separate stage of the path, but rather sometimes presents it as the culmination or completion of the path, that is, as the expression/activity of the enlightened mind. However, in order to preserve the connection with the original Sarvāstivāda Five Path schema, we refer to Sangharakshita's conception of the path as comprising five stages. These stages are elucidated in the second part of this chapter, where we draw out the connections between the threads in terms of three broad phases of practice.

14.3 Part 2: Weaving the Threads

In part 2, we flesh out the three threads by identifying commonalities between these. We do this by the expedient means of identifying three broad phases of practice, which people might ideally move through sequentially. The parallels are not perfect, given that we have identified only three forms of mindfulness (thread 1), but five levels of causality (thread 2) and five stages of the path (thread 3). Thus, there

Table 14.1 Illustration of the connections between the three threads across the three phases of progress

Phase of progress	Type of mindfulness	Awareness of *niyama*	Stage of spiritual path
1	*Sati*	*Utu-niyāma*	I (integration)
		Bija-niyāma	
		Citta-niyāma	
2	*Appamada*	*Kamma-niyāma*	II (skilful intention)
3	*Sampajañña*	*Dhamma-niyāma*	III (spiritual death)
			IV (spiritual rebirth)
			V (compassionate activity)

is not a perfect one-to-one correspondence between aspects of the three threads. Nevertheless, we argue that there are parallels across the threads, which enable us to aggregate these into our broad phases of practice.

Thus, to foreshadow the subsequent discussion, the phases are constituted as follows: the first phase features the first type of mindfulness *(sati),* awareness of the first three *niyāmas* (*utu, bija,* and *citta*), and entry to the first stage of the path (integration). The second phase features *appamada*-mindfulness, awareness of the *kamma niyāma,* and the first (in its fullness) and second stages of the path (integration and skilful intentions). Finally, the third phase encompasses *sampajañña*-mindfulness, appreciation of the *dhamma niyāma,* and the third, fourth, and fifth stages of the path (spiritual death, spiritual rebirth, and enlightened compassionate activity). These connections between the threads are illustrated in Table 14.1 above. It must be emphasised that this framework is just a heuristic device, a generalised model highlighting some interesting common correlations between aspects of spiritual development. In reality, the progression through each of the threads is far more fluid than is implied by this rigid table. Indeed, qualities that are brought out in particular phases are not necessarily absent in earlier phases, but may be only implicit rather than explicit. For example, for some practitioners, *sati*-mindfulness will take them further than this table implies, for example, leading to ethical awareness or spiritual progression. Nevertheless, this framework does help clarify some of the broad patterns of development that can be found in Buddhism.

14.3.1 *Phase 1:* Sati-*Mindfulness, the First Three* Niyāmas, *and Stage I of the Path*

The first of our aggregate phases is characterised by one particular type of mindfulness, *sati*. The term *sati* has connotations of recollection, in the sense of remembering to bring to mind "what is otherwise too easily forgotten: the present moment" (Anālayo 2003, p. 48). As Bodhi (2005, p. 262) stated, *sati*-mindfulness involves "recollection of the present moment, sustained awareness of what is happening to us and within us on each occasion of experience". Readers might be familiar with the mindfulness of breathing, a foundational practice within the MBSR programme. This type of mindfulness is described in the *Satipaṭṭhāna sutta*—the Discourse on the Establishment of Mindfulness—which is regarded as the most influential text in the Pali Canon on the systematic practice of mindfulness (Bhikkhu Bodhi 2011). Its guidance states, "Establishing present-moment recollection right where you are, simply breathe in, simply aware, then breathe out, simply aware. Breathing in long, know directly *I am breathing in long.* Breathing in short, know directly *I am breathing in short*". This type of awareness is reflected in Kabat-Zinn's (2003, p. 145) definition of mindfulness as "the awareness that arises through paying attention on purpose, in the present moment, and nonjudgmentally to the unfolding of experience moment by moment". As such, we submit that contemporary mindfulness-based interventions, influenced as they are by Kabat-Zinn's (1982) formulation of mindfulness, are primarily concerned with *sati*-mindfulness. It is our contention that this type of mindfulness is very useful *as far as it goes,* but that its usefulness is somewhat limited in the context of the other two types of mindfulness presented here; that is, contemporary conceptions of mindfulness do not incorporate the ethical dimensions of *appamada*-mindfulness, nor the sense of spiritual development imbued within *sampajañña*-mindfulness.

Nevertheless, despite these limitations, the cultivation of *sati*-mindfulness is certainly highly valuable and should be encouraged. As has been documented widely in the psychological and clinical literature, helping people to be aware of their present-moment experience can have profound therapeutic consequences. Just to give one example, perhaps the most prominent adaptation of Kabat-Zinn's (1982) MBSR protocol is mindfulness-based cognitive therapy (MBCT), designed to prevent relapse to depression (Zindel et al. 2002). The theoretical basis of MBCT is the differential activation hypothesis: Previously depressed people are susceptible to relapse because even mild dysphoria can reactivate negative thought patterns associated with previous depressive episodes, leading to a consequent "downward spiral" of negative thoughts and worsening negative affect (Teasdale et al. 2000, p. 615). In MBCT, people at risk of relapse are thus taught to pay attention to their current thoughts and feelings, that is, develop *sati*-mindfulness. In doing so, their increased emotional awareness and understanding means people are able to decentre from their negative cognitions, i.e. view these with a degree of detached objectivity, rather than getting caught up in these dysfunctional thinking patterns and then dragged into the kind of downward spiral that might otherwise lead to relapse. Encouraging this kind of mindfulness can be very helpful: MBCT significantly reduces relapse rates in randomised controlled trials for people with three or more previous episodes of depression (Ma and Teasdale 2004). Consequently, in 2004, the UK National Institute for Health and Care Excellence approved MBCT as a treatment for recurrent depression. Aside from depression, interventions based on *sati*-mindfulness have begun to be explored in the context of a range of other clinical conditions, including anxiety (Evans et al. 2008) and bipolar disorder (Weber et al. 2010). More broadly, teaching this kind of mindfulness has been found to engender wellbeing and psychological development in diverse settings, from schools (Erricker and Erricker 2001) to prisons (Samuelson et al. 2007).

It is interesting to reflect upon *sati*-mindfulness in the context of the second thread of this chapter, the *paṭiccasamuppāda* teaching. We contend that *sati* is primarily an awareness of the first three *niyāmas: utu, bīja*, and *citta*. Such awareness can certainly be highly beneficial. To recap, *utu-niyāma* is the law of the seasons, that is, causality operating in the domain of the physical world. This *niyāma* is appraised primarily through attending to our own physicality (i.e. to our own being as a physical object), including any attendant sensations (e.g. how it feels to interact with our surroundings, and how physical laws such as gravity impact upon our body). Additionally, this *niyāma* is appraised secondarily by paying attention to our physical surroundings and to the consequences of actions in this arena. Historically, awareness of this type of causality would have been very important, particularly during epochs when people's existence was highly contingent upon the vagaries of nature (e.g. being able to successfully read weather patterns). A more modern practical example of awareness of *utu-niyāma* might simply be paying close attention while driving a car (e.g. to road conditions), which is associated with positive outcomes like safer driving behaviour (Kass et al. 2008). The second level of conditionality is *bīja-niyāma*, the law of the seeds, that is, causality acting in the domain of living beings. This *niyāma* is appraised primarily through attending to our own organic nature (i.e. to our own being as a living, and not merely inanimate, entity), including any attendant sensations (e.g. how it feels to be formed out of biological processes such as respiration and digestion, and how biological laws such as aging affect our body). Furthermore, this *niyāma* is appraised secondarily by paying attention to the natural environment around us. A salient example of this type of awareness is appreciation of the environmental impact of human behaviour. Cultivation of such mindfulness of nature (Beng 2012) can help kindle our affinity with the natural world, potentially leading to more environmentally friendly behaviour (Amel et al. 2009). Finally, the third level of conditionality is *citta-niyāma*, the law of the mind, i.e. recurrent patterns within one's subjective world. *Sati*-mindfulness of the *citta-niyāma* is arguably *the* predominant type of mindfulness found in contemporary psychological literature. That is, just about all mindfulness-based interventions encourage people to become aware of their cognitions and emotions, and to notice patterns and causal relationships among such phenomena. For example, returning to the example of MBCT, participants are taught to recognise recurrent negative thought patterns that can lead to worsening mood, and to decentre from such thoughts (Teasdale et al. 2000).

The kind of *sati*-mindfulness depicted above—of one's physicality *(utu-niyāma)*, one's biological processes *(bīja-niyāma)*, and one's subjective mind/body *(citta)*—is incredibly valuable and worth cultivating. However, in the context of the wider Buddhist teachings, the value of this kind of mindfulness *alone* is nevertheless limited; for more far-reaching development, the other types of mindfulness must arguably also be developed. This point can be made by considering the third thread, namely, the stages of the spiritual path. In brief, *sati*-mindfulness alone is not *necessarily* indicative of the occurrence of any psycho-spiritual development. That is, in terms of the stages of the path as elucidated by Sangharakshita (1998), the cultivation of *sati*-mindfulness does not *inevitably* mean that a person has embarked upon a spiritual path. (That said, as we discuss below, *sati*-mindfulness practice is often associated with the emergence of the first stage of the path discussed here, i.e. integration). One way to appreciate this point is by considering the fact that many people can and do practice mindfulness in a secular way, without reference to Buddhist teachings (Shapiro 1994), and/or without any consideration of notions like ethics or spiritual development. As Stanley (2012, p. 202) noted, while definitions of *sati* in the Pali canon preserved an ethical dimension, when taken out of this context and understood purely as a technique for training attention, then "mindfulness risks becoming de-ethicised". This de-ethicised form of mindfulness is perhaps revealed most vividly in some of the more contentious ways in which mindfulness interventions have been deployed. For instance, mindfulness-based mind fitness training has been developed as a stress-prevention tool for use with military personnel (Stanley et al. 2011). While this intervention has the laudable goal of addressing the severe mental health risks that soldiers are liable to, it is still the case that one aim of the programme is to help such people perform more effectively on the battlefield, which may include the act of killing other people. Deploying meditative techniques towards military ends is not a new development, as attested to by historical martial arts and warrior traditions within Buddhism, such as the samurai Warrior Zen that flourished in sixteenth to seventeenth century feudal Japan (Johnson 2000, p. 9). Nevertheless, such uses of mindfulness are at the least morally problematic, and show mindfulness *can* be deployed in a decontextualised way simply as an attention training technique, without any necessary reference to ethical or spiritual development.

However, it is also the case that even if people only initially take up mindfulness in a decontextualised, secular way, this engagement may pique their interest in the Buddhist origins of meditation, and/or prompt them to tentatively embark upon a spiritual path. For example, recent qualitative interviews with male meditators revealed that although most interviewees initially just took up meditation as a stress-management technique (Lomas et al. 2013), nearly all developed an interest in exploring the wider Buddhist context of meditation (Lomas et al. 2014b) and many subsequently embraced the notion of a spiritual path (Lomas et al. 2014a). As such, it appears that the practice of *sati*-mindfulness—encouraged by contemporary mindfulness-based interventions—can and does often lead people to enter the first stage of the spiritual path, a stage Sangharakshita (1998) referred to as one of integration. As elucidated by Sangharakshita and Subhuti (2013, p. 128), entering into the stage of integration involves "cultivating ever-more skilful actions of body, speech and mind, so that progressively more satisfying, subtle, flexible, and open states of consciousness emerge as their fruit". Thus, the sense of integration arises from the fact that (a) one begins to develop a nascent sense of the connections between one's subjective experiences (e.g. during mindfulness practice) and one's actions in the wider social world, and (b) one begins to integrate one's actions with one's beliefs and values. It is worth emphasising that while these beliefs and values may well be informed by Buddhist teachings, one can certainly pursue such integration without reference to Buddhism. Indeed, such integration does not necessarily even mean that people conceive of themselves as being spiritual. However, this is only the beginning of the spiritual path. This stage of integration becomes further deepened when people begin to cultivate an awareness of and commitment to ethical behaviour, as the next section explores.

14.3.2 Phase 2: **Appamada**-*Mindfulness,* **Kamma Niyāma,** *and Stages I and II of the Path*

Once practitioners have become adept at *sati*-mindfulness, Sangharakshita's interpretation of Buddhist teachings is that people can make progress along a spiritual path by cultivating other forms of mindfulness, namely *appamada* and *sampajañña.* Phase 2 centres on the former, *appamada.* However, it is perhaps best not to view *appamada* as a distinct type of mindfulness, separate from *sati;* rather than being a different state of mind in its own right, *appamada* might be better seen as a quality with which we would aim to imbue sati (Peacock 2014). Or rather, one might seek to augment the *sati*-mindfulness of phase 1 with a richer form of mindfulness encompassing both *sati* and *appamada.* So, what qualities does *appamada* bring to mindfulness? A helpful way of ascertaining these qualities is to consider the range of ways in which the term *appamada* has been translated. Müller (1881) conceptualised it as earnestness. Other translations found in contemporary literature include vigilant care (Soeng 2006), unremitting alertness (Thera 1941), diligence (Peacock 2014), and heedfulness and carefulness (Nikaya 2008). However, from the perspective of Sangharakshita's interpretation of Buddhism, perhaps the best translation of *appamada* is "moral watchfulness" (Rao 2007, p. 69). This reflects the commentary on the *Dhammapada,* which describes it as "awareness …with regard to the sphere of qualities of good conduct" (Carter 2005, p. 280). As such, our preferred definition here of *appamada* is awareness infused with an ethos of ethical care.

This type of mindfulness moves the concept beyond simply being mindful of what is happening—the predominant *sati*-mindfulness of contemporary interventions—and connects it explicitly to Buddhist teachings on ethics and morality. The teachings are replete with guidance around ethical behaviour. To begin with, three aspects of the Noble Eightfold path are specifically concerned with morality *(sīla),* namely, right speech *(sammā-vācā),* right action *(sammā-kammanta),* and right livelihood *(sammā-ājīva).* Elaborating on these three strands are various lists of precepts within the literature, specifying in more detail what right speech, action, and livelihood consist of. The most widely known set in the Pali canon are the five precepts *(pañca-sīla),* which recommend abstinence from: harming living beings, taking the not given, misconduct concerning sense pleasures (e.g. sexual misconduct), false speech, and unmindful states related to consumption of alcohol or drugs. These five can also be formulated positively, respectively, as cultivating *mettā* (loving-kindness), generosity, contentment, truthfulness, and mindfulness. Sangharakshita (1998) argues that couching these precepts in positive terms is important, as these terms go further when formulated in this way. For instance, expressing *metta* is a far stronger prosocial act than simply refraining from harming; whereas the latter is arguably simply a non-exceptional example of civilised behaviour, *metta* is imbued with a much more active sense of love and care (Ostergaard 1977). Sangharakshita (1998) suggests that this issue of negative versus positive formulations is partly a function of the English language and of the difficulty of retaining the meaning of original Pali/Sanskrit terms when translating these (as also discussed above with respect to mindfulness). For example, in Pali, a term such as *avihimsā* (non-harm), although formulated negatively (*vihimsā* means harm/violence, and the "a" is a negative prefix), retains an actively positive connotation (i.e. relating to the expression of love and care); however, when translated into English as non-harm, this affirmative overtone is not preserved. As such, some scholars have suggested that "love" might be a more encompassing translation of *avihimsā* (Ostergaard 1977).

These five precepts can be seen not as rigid rules governing a monastic Buddhist lifestyle, but as fundamental ethical principles in the Buddha's teaching that are potentially relevant to all people. For more committed Buddhists, these five are supplemented by more rigorous recommendations. For example, in the Triratna movement, ordinants take ten precepts, featuring the phrase "I undertake the item of training which consists in abstention from …", followed by the following proscriptions: killing living beings, taking the not given, sexual misconduct, false speech, harsh speech, frivolous speech, slanderous speech, covetousness, hatred, and false views. At a far more detailed level, the monastic disciplinary code *(pāṭimokkha)* in the monastic rule *(vinaya)* features around 200 rules (versions vary) for monastic life (Keown 2009). In addition to these prescriptions, we find various exhortations to virtuous living in the canonical literature. For example, in the Therevadan tradition, there is an emphasis on the four *brahma-viharas* (divine abidings): loving-kindness *(mettā)*, compassion *(karuṇā)*, sympathetic joy *(muditā)*, and equanimity *(upekkha)*. Similarly, the Mahayanan tradition elucidates six perfections *(pāramitā)*: generosity *(dāna)*, morality *(sīla)*, patience *(khanti)*, perseverance *(viriya)*, concentration *(samādhi)*, and insight *(paññā)*. Thus, broadly speaking, *appamada*-mindfulness involves being aware of one's actions in the light of these ethical guidelines, i.e. reflecting on the extent to which one's actions are in accordance or otherwise with these recommendations.

In reflecting on these prescriptions, a crucial point to consider is *why* these forms of action are recommended. Essentially, Buddhist teachings hold that skilful (i.e. ethical) actions should be pursued because they will result in future positive states of mind, and unskilful (i.e. unethical) actions should be avoided because they will generate future negative states of mind. This fundamental teaching can be explicated by considering our second thread, the teaching of *paṭiccasamuppāda.* We are making the case here that *appamada*-mindfulness means becoming aware and appreciative of the fourth order of conditionality, the *kamma niyāma.* This *niyāma* is the law of *kamma* (Sans. *karma*), that is, the application of the principle of causality with respect to ethics. As Buddhaghosa expressed it, this refers to "the desirable and undesirable results following good and bad action". Although the concept of karma has entered Western discourse, the idea is frequently misrepresented and misunderstood. The term itself simply means action; however, in popular discourse, if people respond to something that happens to them by saying "That's my karma", they are really referring to *vipāka,* meaning the results or fruits of their past actions (Sangharakshita 2003). Nevertheless, this popular usage of the term does capture the central insight of the concept: Actions have consequences. It is vital to differentiate *kamma* from other religious teachings in the realm of ethics, such as Christian notions of sin. The latter teaching may suggest that we are punished *for* our sins by an action of divine retribution (Swinburne 1989). However, the Buddhist notion of *kamma* requires no supernatural agency, but simply proposes that we are rewarded or punished, in a causal sense, *by* our actions. As Kang (2009, p. 73) stated, "the law of karma states that any volitional action rooted in non-greed, non-hatred, and non-delusion (or in positive terms: generosity, love/compassion, and wisdom) gives rise to virtuous or positive imprints in the mind that would subsequently result in experiences of happiness and pleasure". Conversely, "any ethical action rooted in greed, hatred, or delusion gives rise to their opposite non-virtuous/negative mental imprints that later result in experiences of suffering and displeasure".

Given this law, Buddhist teachings state that ethical actions are not only beneficial to other people, but also have direct benefits for the actors themselves. Thus, people have a vested interest in acting ethically and should be motivated to act as such. So, we might say that people enter the second phase of practice when they begin to appreciate the notion of *kamma niyāma* and start to act accordingly. As expressed by Kang (2009, p. 73), "a behavioural guideline that emerges from such an ethical view of causality is that one ought to engage mindfully in positive karma rooted in positive volitions". As such, we can see how *appamada* introduces a further dimension to mindfulness that is not present in *sati*-mindfulness alone: It is no longer simply a question of being aware of our actions and our phenomenal world, but of reflecting on whether our actions are skilful. Such mindfulness also involves tracing the origins of one's mental states "to discover more about their background, so that you can make adjustments to the way you live your life" (Sangharakshita 2003, p. 94). This type of appreciation is simply not found in most modern conceptualisations of mindfulness, based as they are on the concept of *sati,* with its emphasis on present-moment attention. In contemporary mindfulness interventions, if people are experiencing negative cognitions or feelings, they are encouraged to attend to these qualia and ideally decentre from them. Of course, this type of mental response does have great value, and is to be encouraged, since interventions involving this kind of attention training have had profound effects on people's wellbeing in clinical and nonclinical settings. However, what such interventions do *not* do is make any causal connection between such negative qualia and people's actions outside of meditation. This is an omission: While it is useful to learn how to decentre from negative thoughts, a more powerful solution would be to help people learn to live skilfully (i.e. ethically), thus lessening the likelihood of such negative qualia emerging in the first place. It is this type of ethical appreciation that comes into play with the cultivation of *appamada*-mindfulness.

Once people do begin to cultivate this type of mindfulness, we might say that they truly start to make progress along the spiritual path. We saw that *sati*-mindfulness could often lead to a person embarking on the first stage of the path (as elucidated by Sangharakshita), the stage of integration. However, it is perhaps only with the cultivation of *appamada* that this stage is really embraced in its fullness. In particular, Sangharakshita and Subhuti (2013, p. 128) contended that, fundamentally, integration involves "recognising oneself as a moral agent" and allowing this recognition to inform one's actions in the world. Thus, while a person might begin to develop a sense of integration without an explicit commitment to ethics, this stage can only be truly brought to fruition through consciously aligning oneself with some kind of moral awareness. It is when this happens that a person can be said to move into stage II of the spiritual path, referred to by Sangharakshita as one of skilful intention. This essentially refines and builds upon stage I through the "systematic cultivation of skilful intentions and actions that bring the karmic fruit of a more finely tuned mind" (Sangharakshita and Subhuti 2013, p. 133). This might involve a more explicit commitment to practices that help one cultivate skilful intentions, such as the *metta bhavana,* or a more rigorous engagement with the ethical precepts. Moreover, in stage II, one would not only work with what Sangharakshita calls horizontal integration, (i.e. integrating the various aspects of one's life, as per stage I) but also vertical integration, in which one begins to explore and integrate different levels of the self, such as higher states of consciousness. Once this point is reached, a person will be on the threshold of the third phase of practice.

14.3.3 Phase 3: Sampajañña-*Mindfulness,* Dhamma Niyāma, *and Stages III, IV, and V of the Path*

In Sangharakshita's (2003) interpretation of Buddhist teaching, once people have augmented *sati*-mindfulness (phase 1) with *appamada* (phase 2), they may then be ready to open up to a third type of mindfulness: *sampajañña.* As with phase 2, it is better not to view this as a distinct type of mindfulness, separate from the other two, but rather a new quality that one can bring to mindfulness, thereby creating a compound of *sati-appamada-sampajañña* mindfulness.

So, what qualities or abilities are implied by the term *sampajañña*? For some scholars, it refers to the ability to effortlessly sustain *sati.* For example, Śāntideva (2002, verse 33) stated that "*Samprajanya [sampajañña]* comes and, once come, does not go again, if *smṛti* [sati] stands guard at the door of the mind". As explained by Maharaj (2013, p. 67), the "assiduous practice of *sati* ...culminates eventually in the achievement of *samprajanya,* which seems to be a more spontaneous and effortless state of watchfulness of the body and mind". This interpretation would accord with our view of different forms of mindfulness developing sequentially. Likewise, as noted by Maharaj (2013, p. 71), Hariharananda (2008/1892) borrowed the term *samprajanya* to characterise the attainment of *smṛti-sādhan,* which refers to "the active practice of mindfulness that culminates in the establishment of an effortless state of *smṛti*". Beyond this idea of effortless mindfulness, many writers associate the term *sampajañña* specifically with insight. The *Satipaṭṭhāna sutta* features the common refrain *ātāpi sampajāno satimā,* which Bodhi (2011) translated as "ardent, clearly comprehending, and mindful". Thus, each term in the phrase represents a particular mental factor: *ātāpi* (ardent) pertains to energy to engage in practice, *sati* (present-moment mindfulness) refers to watchful awareness, and *sampajāno* (an adjective relating to the noun *sampajañña*) concerns clear comprehension.

So, what type of insight does *sampajañña* imply? One way to approach this question is to consider the second thread, the law of *paṭiccasamuppāda*. According to our interpretation here—which is only one possible exegesis of the original texts—*sampajañña* is associated with awareness of the final *niyāma*, the *dhamma niyāma*. Essentially, this means keeping our spiritual purpose always in mind, that is, aligning our actions with this purpose. As noted above, the *dhamma niyāma* is known as the law of nature, which, following Buddhaghosa, Sangharakshita interpreted as the potential of the universe to develop complex qualities such as consciousness, and exemplary living beings such as the Buddha. From this perspective, the kinds of insights associated with *sampajañña* involve a deep appreciation of the *dhamma-niyāma* and its implications. One such implication is the notion that all living beings also have the potential to become Buddhas and that this is attained through following the spiritual path. Thus, just as *appamada* would endow one with an appreciation of the value of living ethically, *sampajañña* awareness would convince one of the value and indeed necessity of diligently following the spiritual path. This awareness would then necessarily guide and structure our actions, such that we would weigh the utility of all our actions according to whether they served our progress along this path. As Sangharakshita (2003, p. 13) stated, *sampajañña* could be translated as mindfulness of purpose, a state of awareness in which everything we do is "done with a sense of the direction we want to move in and of whether or not our current action will take us in that direction".

Once a practitioner is at this point, then it is likely that they will be firmly committed to Buddhism (or another spiritual system) and to making progress along the path. Thus, bringing in the third thread, according to Sangharakshita's interpretation of the path, here practitioners could be said to be entering stage III, and eventually stage IV and V. In stage III, the stage of spiritual death, we are again speaking about developing insight, and in particular into the three *lakshanas,* the three marks of conditioned existence: *anicca* (impermanence), *anattā* (insubstantiality, or "not-self"), and *dukkha* (frustration or suffering). This teaching is absolutely central to Buddhism, and describes the fundamental nature of reality: All phenomena are seen as being empty of a fixed, enduring, independent nature, but are transitory *(anicca)* and interdependent *(anattā);* as such, it is ignorance or denial of these fundamental aspects of reality, and the consequent attempt to attach to phenomena that are inherently and inevitably subject to change, that causes suffering *(dukkha)*. This conception of the *laskshanas* is a general law covering all aspects of existence; however, spiritual death occurs when this insight is realised experientially with respect to one's self: A deep appreciation of the impermanence and insubstantiality of one's own self. Here, one recognises that "true happiness cannot lie in any particular arrangement of conditioned phenomena", whether in clinging to a sense of self, or attaching to other people and objects (Sangharakshita and Subhuti 2013, p. 133). Thus, spiritual death means "dying, in the sense of loosening our illusions about ourselves and giving up our self-oriented clinging".

However, this is not a nihilistic annihilation of the self, but rather the precursor to a sense of liberating spiritual rebirth, the fourth stage of the spiritual path (as conceived by Sangharakshita). This involves rebirth into a deeper sense of self, one that is coterminous and identified with the *dhamma niyāma,* with the spiritual path itself. That is, Sangharakshita suggested that at this stage, the person's own egoic concerns dissipate, and the *dhamma niyāma* can then work through them, as if the person was a conduit for this deeper supra-personal force. As Sangharakshita and Subhuti (2013, p. 134) stated, "once clinging to the illusion of a separate and enduring self lessens, then the non-egoistic motivations of the *dhamma niyāma* begin arising and it is the function of the stage of Spiritual Rebirth to allow and encourage these to flourish". In this stage, the person connects "more and more deeply with *dhamma niyāma* processes", and learns to "rely on the promptings of the *dhamma* as a living reality rather than one's own narrow self-interest" (p. 134). It is at this point that a person is considered to be a 'stream entrant', i.e. to have achieved sufficient escape velocity that they will inexorably make progress along the spiritual path, and eventually achieve enlightenment. Sangharakshita and Subhuti (2013, p. 134) refer to this culmination of the path as the stage of spontaneous compassionate activity, the naturally compassionate actions of an enlightened being. Here there is no sense of self-agency—in the sense of a volitional, separate self—but simply pure unfolding on the level of the *dhamma niyāma.* At this point, there is no notion of a self that is making progress, but simply the *dhamma niyāma* itself playing itself out through the vehicle of the person, a state that has traditionally been called enlightenment.

14.4 Conclusion

In this chapter, we have attempted to situate mindfulness within the context of Buddhism by identifying three threads within Buddhist teachings and to elucidate the connections between these by weaving them together. The first of these threads is that there are different types of mindfulness in Buddhism, or perhaps expressed more accurately, different *dimensions* to mindfulness, captured by various Pali words. The second thread is the fundamental Buddhist teaching of *Paṭiccasamuppāda,* the law of conditionality, featuring five different *niyāmas* (orders of causality). Finally, the third thread is the idea of the spiritual path, and the notion of there being different stages along this. The key message of this chapter is that our current approach to mindfulness—for example, as a psychological intervention—can be enhanced by considering the various types of awareness within Buddhist teachings. The kind of present-moment awareness that underpins contemporary mindfulness-based interventions, identified here as *sati*-mindfulness, is valuable as far as it goes. However, more far-reaching forms of psychological development may be engendered by considering the other types/dimensions of mindfulness. As one starts to cultivate *appamada*-mindfulness, one begins to appreciate the causality of the *kamma niyāma,* and the value of ethical behaviour. Subsequently, as one develops *sampaja-*

ñña-mindfulness, one gains deeper insight into the nature of spiritual development, and may reach stages of advanced development. It is our contention that this kind of development can be encouraged and facilitated by situating mindfulness within the original Buddhist teachings and harnessing the profound insights and practices encompassed within them.

References

Amel, E. L., Manning, C. M., & Scott, B. A. (2009). Mindfulness and sustainable behavior: Pondering attention and awareness as means for increasing green behavior. *Ecopsychology, 1*(1), 14–25.

Anālayo. (2003). *Satipaṭṭhāna: The direct path to realization*. Birmingham: Windhorse.

Aurobindo, S. (2005). *The life divine/The complete works of Sri Aurobindo* (Vols. 21 and 22). Pondicherry: Sri Aurobindo Ashram.

Batchelor, S. (1987). *Santideva's Bodhicaryavatara: A guide to the Bodhisattva's way of life*. Dharamsala: Library of Tibetan Works and Archives.

Beng, T. S. (2012). *The little handbook of mini-mindfulness meditation*. Pittsburgh: RoseDog Books.

Bishop, S. R., Lau, M., Shapiro, S., Carlson, L., Anderson, N. D., Carmody, J., & Devins, G. (2004). Mindfulness: A proposed operational definition. *Clinical Psychology: Science and Practice, 11*(3), 230–241.

Blackburn, A. M. (1999). Looking for the vinaya: Monastic discipline in the practical canons of the Theravāda. *Journal of the International Association of Buddhist Studies, 22*(2), 281–309.

Bluck, R. (2006). *British Buddhism: Teachings, practice and development*. Oxford: Routledge.

Bodhi, B. (2005). *In the Buddha's words: An anthology of discourses from the pali canon*. Boston: Wisdom.

Bodhi, B. (2011). What does mindfulness really mean? A canonical perspective. *Contemporary Buddhism, 12*(01), 19–39.

Bucknell, R. S. (1984). The Buddhist path to liberation: An analysis of the listing of stages. *Journal of the International Association of Buddhist Studies, 7*(2), 7–40.

Carter, J. R. (2005). Buddhist ethics? In W. Schweiker (Ed.), *The blackwell companion to religious ethics* (pp. 278–285). Oxford: Blackwell.

Chong, L. J. V. D. (2009). *The Sarvāstivāda Doctrine of the Path of Spiritual Progress: A Study based primarily on the Abhidharma-Mahāvibhāsā-śāstra, the Abhidharmakośa-bhāsya and their Chinese and Sanskrit Commentaries*. (PhD), University of Hong Kong.

Conze, E. (2001). *Buddhist wisdom: Containing the diamond sutra and the heart sutra*. London: Random House.

Crowther-Heyck, H. (1999). George A. Miller, language, and the computer metaphor and mind. *History of Psychologu, 2*(1), 37–64.

Erricker, C., & Erricker, J. (2001). *Meditation in schools: A practical guide to calmer classrooms*. New York: Continuum.

Evans, S., Ferrando, S., Findler, M., Stowell, C., Smart, C., & Haglin, D. (2008). Mindfulness-based cognitive therapy for generalized anxiety disorder. *Journal of Anxiety Disorders, 22*(4), 716–721.

National Institute for Clinical Excellence (2004). Depression: Management of depression in primary and secondary care. *Clinical guideline, 23*.

Fortney, L., & Taylor, M. (2010). Meditation in medical practice: A review of the evidence and practice. *Primary Care: Clinics in Office Practice, 37*(1), 81–90.

Gethin, R. (2011). On some definitions of mindfulness. *Contemporary Buddhism, 12*(01), 263–279.

Hariharananda, A. S. (2008/1892). *Yogakārikā*. Madhupur: Kapil Math.

Johnson, N. (2000). *Barefoot Zen: The shaolin roots of kung fu and karate*. York Beach: Samuel Weiser.

Jones, D. T. (2012). The five niyāmas as laws of nature: An assessment of modern Western interpretations of Theravāda Buddhist doctrine. *Journal of Buddhist Ethics, 19,* 545–582.

Kabat-Zinn, J. (1982). An outpatient program in behavioral medicine for chronic pain patients based on the practice of mindfulness meditation: Theoretical considerations and preliminary results. *General Hospital Psychiatry, 4*(1), 33–47.

Kabat-Zinn, J. (2003). Mindfulness-based interventions in context: Past, present, and future. *Clinical Psychology: Science and Practice, 10*(2), 144–156.

Kang, C. (2009). Buddhist and tantric perspectives on causality and society. *Journal of Buddhist Ethics, 16,* 69–103.

Kass, S. J., Cole, K., & Legan, S. (2008). The role of situation awareness in accident prevention. In A. De Smet (Ed.), *Transportation accident analysis and prevention* (pp. 107–122). New York: Nova Science.

Keown, D. (2003). *A Dictionary of Buddhism*. Oxford: Oxford University Press.

Keown, D. (2009). *Buddhism: A brief insight*. New York: Sterling.

King, R. (1995). *Early Advaita Vedanta and Buddhism: The Mahayana context of the Gaudapadiya-Karika*. New York: SUNY.

King, R. (1999). *Orientalism and religion: Post-colonial theory, India and "The Mystic East"*. London: Routledge.

Lomas, T., Cartwright, T., Edginton, T., & Ridge, D. (2013). I was so done in that I just recognized it very plainly, "You need to do something": Men's narratives of struggle, distress and turning to meditation. *Health, 17*(2), 191–208.

Lomas, T., Cartwright, T., Edginton, T., & Ridge, D. (2014a). Engagement with meditation as a positive health trajectory: Divergent narratives of progress in male meditators. *Psychology and Health, 29*(2), 218–236.

Lomas, T., Cartwright, T., Edginton, T., & Ridge, D. (2014). A religion of wellbeing?: The appeal of Buddhism to men in London, UK. *Psychology of Religion and Spirituality, 6*(3), 198–207. doi: 10.1037/a0036420

Loori, J. D. (1999). *Riding the ox home: Stages on the path of enlightenment*. Boston: Shambhala.

Ma, S. H., & Teasdale, J. D. (2004). Mindfulness-based cognitive therapy for depression: Replication and exploration of differential relapse prevention effects. *Journal of Consulting and Clinical Psychology, 72*(1), 31–40.

Maharaj, A. (2013). Yogic mindfulness: Hariharānanda Āraá'ya's quasi-Buddhistic interpretation of smá'ti in Patañjali's yogasūtra. *Journal of Indian Philosophy, 41*(1), 57–78.

McCown, D., Reibel, D., & Micozzi, M. (2010). *Teaching mindfulness*. New York: Springer.

Müller, F. M. (1881). *The Dhammapada*. Oxford: Clarendon.

Nikaya, S. (2008). Right figures of speech. In R. Flores (Ed.), *Buddhist scriptures as literature: Sacred rhetoric and the uses of theory*. Albany: State University of New York Press.

Nyima, K. T., & Gyaltsap, S. (2013). *Vajra wisdom: Deity practice in Tibetan Buddhism*. Boston: Shambhala.

Ostergaard, G. (1977). Duality in non-violence. *Peace News, 48,* 135–138.

Peacock, J. (2014). Sati or mindfulness? Bridging the divide. In M. Mazzano (Ed.), *After mindfulness: New perspectives on psychology and meditation* (pp. 3–22). Basingstoke: Palgrave Macmillan.

Rao, K. R. (2007). Purposeful living. In N. K. Shastree, B. R. Dugar, J. P. N. Mishra, & A. K. Dhar (Eds.), *Value management in professions: Present scenario, future strategies* (pp. 63–71). New Delhi: Ashok Kumar Mittal.

Rhys Davids, C. A. F. (1912). *Buddhism: A study of the Buddhist norm*. London: Williams and Norgate.

Rhys Davids, T. W. (1881). *Buddhist suttas*. Oxford: Clarendon.

Rhys Davids, T. W. (1910). *Dialogues of the Buddha* (Vol. 2). London: Henry Frowde.

Roth, H. (2006). Contemplative studies: Prospects for a new field. *The Teachers College Record, 108*(9), 1787–1815.
Samuelson, M., Carmody, J., Kabat-Zinn, J., & Bratt, M. A. (2007). Mindfulness-based stress reduction in Massachusetts correctional facilities. *The Prison Journal, 87*(2), 254–268.
Sangharakshita, U. (1997). *The rainbow road.* Glasgow: Windhorse.
Sangharakshita, U. (1998). *Know your mind: The psychological dimensions of ethics in Buddhism.* Birmingham: Windhorse.
Sangharakshita, U. (2003). *Living with awareness: A guide to the Satipaṭṭhāna Sutta.* Birmingham: Windhorse.
Sangharakshita, U., & Subhuti, D. (2013). *Seven papers* (2nd ed.). London: Triratna Buddhist Community.
Śāntideva. (2002). *The Bodhicaryāvatāra: A guide to the Buddhist path to awakening.* Birmingham: Windhorse.
Shapiro, D. H. (1994). Examining the content and context of meditation: A challenge for psychology in the areas of stress management, psychotherapy, and religion/values. *Journal of Humanistic Psychology, 34*(4), 101–135.
Shapiro, S. L., Carlson, L. E., Astin, J. A., & Freedman, B. (2006). Mechanisms of mindfulness. *Journal of Clinical Psychology, 62*(3), 373–386.
Shonin, E., Van Gordon, W., & Griffiths, M. D. (2013). Mindfulness-based interventions: Towards mindful clinical integration. *Frontiers in Psychology, 4*, 194.
Soeng, M. (2006). The art of not deceiving yourself. In D. K. Nauriyal, M. S. Drummond, & Y. B. Lal (Eds.), *Buddhist thought and applied psychological research: Transcending the boundaries* (pp. 302–313). Oxford: Routledge.
Stanley, E. A., Schaldach, J. M., Kiyonaga, A., & Jha, A. P. (2011). Mindfulness-based mind fitness training: A case study of a high-stress predeployment military cohort. *Cognitive and Behavioral Practice, 18*(4), 566–576.
Stanley, S. (2012). Intimate distances: William James' introspection, Buddhist mindfulness, and experiential inquiry. *New Ideas in Psychology, 30*(2), 201–211.
Subhuti, D. (1994). *Sangharakshita: A new voice in the buddhist tradition.* Glasgow: Windhorse.
Suzuki, D. T. (1934). *The ten oxherding pictures Manual of Zen Buddhism.* Kyoto: Eastern Buddhist Society.
Swinburne, R. (1989). *Responsibility and atonement.* Oxford: Oxford University Press.
Teasdale, J. D., Segal, Z. V., Williams, J. M. G., Ridgeway, V. A., Soulsby, J. M., & Lau, M. A. (2000). Prevention of relapse/recurrence in major depression by mindfulness-based cognitive therapy. *Journal of Consulting and Clinical Psychology, 68*(4), 615–623.
Thera, S. (1941). *The way of mindfulness: The Satipatthana Sutta and Its commentary.* Kandy: Saccanubodia Samiti.
Vishvapani, D. (2001). Perceptions of the FWBO in British Buddhism. *Western Buddhist Review, 3.*
Weber, B., Jermann, F., Gex-Fabry, M., Nallet, A., Bondolfi, G., & Aubry, J.-M. (2010). Mindfulness-based cognitive therapy for bipolar disorder: A feasibility trial. *European Psychiatry, 25*(6), 334–337.
Wilber, K. (1995). *Sex, ecology, spirituality: The spirit of evolution.* Boston: Shambhala.
Williams, J. M. G., & Kabat-Zinn, J. (2011). Mindfulness: Diverse perspectives on its meaning, origins, and multiple applications at the intersection of science and dharma. *Contemporary Buddhism, 12*(01), 1–18.
Zindel, V., Segal, J., Williams, M. G., & Teasdale, J. D. (2002). *Mindfulness-based cognitive therapy for depression: A new approach to preventing relapse.* New York: Guilford.

Tim Lomas is a lecturer at the University of East London, where he is the programme leader for the MSc in Applied Positive Psychology and Coaching Psychology. After undertaking an MA and MSc in psychology at the University of Edinburgh, Tim completed his PhD at the University of Westminster in 2012. His thesis focused on the impact of meditation on men's mental health, and it was published in 2014 as a monograph by Palgrave Macmillan. Tim is the lead author of numerous books (published by Sage), including a positive psychology textbook (entitled *Applied Positive Psychology: Integrated Positive Practice*), and a six-volume major works in positive psychology series. Tim has also just received two grants to develop mindfulness-based interventions for specific populations (at-risk youth and older adults).

Jnanavaca graduated in physics from Wadham College, Oxford, and worked for Marks & Spencer. His growing interest in Buddhism led him to leave his management career and start working for the London Buddhist Centre (LBC) where he has been working in various capacities since 1997. He was ordained into the Triratna Buddhist Order in 1999 and has been teaching Buddhism and meditation since then, as well as being an active trustee of the LBC. He is also a trustee of Windhorse Trust (an associated Buddhist charity). In 2009, he became the chairman of the LBC—a role that combines leadership in both an organizational and spiritual capacity. Since 2012, he is also a director of Breathing Space—the LBC's secular mindfulness project.

Chapter 15
Mindfulness in an Authentic Transformative Everyday Zen

Spencer A. McWilliams

15.1 Introduction

Over the past several decades, the practice of "mindfulness," derived from concepts of awareness and attention rooted in Buddhism, has expanded into a global movement. Wilson (2014) expounded on the history of this development, describing how it maintains a pattern that Buddhism has historically followed as it has moved into new cultures; people in the new cultures take from Buddhism those elements they believe will address their particular, culture-specific, concerns and problems, generating new versions of Buddhism that fit their needs. This process has historically proven to have practical benefits consistent with Buddhist philosophy by recognizing the ever-changing nature of all phenomena, opening the door to creative adaptation to new circumstances and modifications that made Buddhism relevant to new societies. Wilson explained in detail the history of American interest in Buddhism and the processes that brought mindfulness to America and Western societies.

Wilson (2014) reminded us that the English roots of the term mindfulness make identifying its connection to specific traditional Buddhist meditation techniques difficult. He represented the term mindfulness as derived from the Pali word *sati* (Sanskrit: *smrti*), meaning memory (also implying alertness, attention, and awareness), and related to the seventh step on Buddhism's Eightfold Path, typically referred to as awareness, alertness, or mindfulness, and he elaborated the historical process by which mindfulness evolved as the preferred present-day term. Summarizing and synthesizing a variety of contemporary definitions of the term mindfulness, we could define mindfulness as

> intentionally focusing on evident, sensory experience, which consists of momentary physical sensations and arising thoughts, combined with a willingness to experience these phenomena as they actually appear, with acceptance and curiosity. (McWilliams 2012, p. 239)

S. A. McWilliams (✉)
Psychology Department, California State University San Marcos,
333 S Twin Oaks Valley Rd, San Marcos, CA 92096-0001, USA
e-mail: smcwilli@csusm.edu

E. Shonin et al. (eds.), *Buddhist Foundations of Mindfulness*,
Mindfulness in Behavioral Health, DOI 10.1007/978-3-319-18591-0_15

Wilson (2014) suggested that, historically, ordinary lay practitioners within Asian Buddhist societies did not typically pursue mindfulness practices; such awareness practices took place exclusively within traditional Buddhist monastic practices, with monks seeking transcendent experiences of bliss within the context of a lifelong, strenuous practice of detachment and renunciation. According to Wilson, this theme of mindfulness as rooted in a committed practice in the pursuit of an alternative worldview continued to represent most of the Western Buddhist literature for most of the twentieth century. Subsequently, the rapid growth of interest in Buddhism in the latter third of the twentieth century led many Westerners to adopt meditation practice with transformational goals under the tutelage of Asian masters from Korea, Japan, Thailand, Tibet, Vietnam, Myanmar, Cambodia, Laos, Malaysia, Nepal, Bhutan, and Tibet as well as from Westerners trained in Asian monasteries.

However, as concomitant interest in mindfulness itself has grown, we have seen a decreasing emphasis on the relationship between mindfulness and traditional Buddhist teachings, leading to more emphasis on lay teachers focusing on the practical details of mindfulness by itself, disconnected from its Buddhist roots, and its practical use as a less demanding, easily accessible mode of self-help and self-improvement. This trend raises a serious concern about the extent to which this endeavor has eroded broader traditional Buddhist contexts from which mindfulness arose, leading Wilson to ask how it has evolved

> to this point, where mindfulness apparently can exist entirely outside of Buddhism, and non-Buddhists can teach other non-Buddhists about Buddhist-derived mindfulness to gain control over mental illness, achieve self-fulfillment, and sell books, with nary a mention of the idea of pursuing nirvana? (Wilson 2014, p. 14)

15.2 A Spectrum of Mindfulness: Legitimacy to Authenticity

Many Western Buddhist practitioners and scholars have also raised concerns that the emphasis on mindfulness may obscure the greater benefits of authentic Buddhist teachings for more effective human well-being and functioning (e.g., Heuman 2014; McWilliams 2011, 2014; Kwee 2010; Shonin and Van Gordon 2014), and they have called for the articulation and elaboration of practices accessible to lay Westerners that more fully exemplify these more powerful traditional Buddhist goals. We need not necessarily focus exclusively on the pursuit of transcendent states to acknowledge that the Buddhist teachings from which mindfulness practices derive aspire to a deeper, more radical transformation of human understanding than relaxation and self-improvement.

Perhaps viewing approaches that use mindfulness along a spectrum or a continuum in terms of their explicit relationship to Buddhist teachings would provide a framework for discussion that can respect a variety of methods while acknowledging significant differences. Wilber (1984) sought to formulate a scale that could differentiate a variety of religious and transformative practices in a meaningful manner compatible with his understanding of psychological development in terms of a spectrum of consciousness. Within a particular level of consciousness, he distinguished between its *deep structure,* and the *surface structure,* the elements or components that make up the way the person views the world within that level. He used the term *translation* to describe changes in surface structure that leave the deep structure intact and *transformation* to describe changes in the deep structure that lead to the movement to a higher level. "Any psychosocial institution [e.g., in our case, Buddhist-derived practices] that validates or facilitates translation we call legitimate; any that validates or facilitates transformation we call authentic" (p. 252). Wilber acknowledged the importance and value of both aspects for human and social functioning, so we need not see one as superior to the other, and he suggested that any social institution, in our case Buddhism, requires effectiveness in both.

He described legitimacy as operating along a horizontal scale as "a measure of the degree of integration, organization, meaning, coherence, and stability… within a given level of structural adaptation" (Wilber 1984, p. 252). From this perspective, we could regard mindfulness-based interventions that help individuals find meaning within their current level of development as legitimate ways of assisting them to cope and flourish, and function with greater stability, without necessarily altering their worldview. Authenticity, alternatively, refers to a vertical scale and the degree that a mindfulness-based intervention helps individuals transform their consciousness to a higher level of development, the sort of practices traditionally associated with monastic Buddhist practices. I propose that we might find it useful to adopt Wilber's legitimacy–authenticity model, but view these terms as poles of a continuum along which to understand the function and value of mindfulness-based interventions. Thus, we can see the use of mindfulness techniques to relieve stress and assist people to function more effectively as legitimate Buddhist practices while also recognizing the value of authentic Buddhist practices as supporting people in transforming their way of perceiving themselves and the world.

At the legitimacy end of this spectrum, we could place traditional exoteric religious practices in Buddhist lay communities, in which adherents pray to the Buddha for guidance and priests perform rituals to bring good fortune. Moving along this spectrum to the current mindfulness movement, Shonin and Van Gordon (2014) identified the most commonly used mindfulness approaches as *First Generation Mindfulness-Based Interventions,* which they noted have effectively used "attentional processes to regulate maladaptive cognitive and affective processes" (p. 2), but fail to address the ethical and intentional components of Buddhist teachings. We could view these interventions as primarily addressing issues that characterize the legitimacy portion of the dimension. They then described the early development of *Second Generation Mindfulness-Based Interventions* (SG-MBI) that contain more overt spiritual aspects including the importance of appropriate intention, ethical conduct, and meditational elements such as effort, mindfulness, and concentration, as derived from Buddhism's Noble Eightfold Path. Importantly, they emphasized that the teachers of this SG-MBI practice must have the experience and awareness to authentically convey these teachings. This expansion of mindfulness-based interventions into a wider spectrum that includes more Buddhist content demonstrates a promising development that we may view as nearer to the midpoint of the spectrum, predominantly legitimating, although to the extent that participants experience personal transformation it may cross into authenticity.

Moving further along this spectrum, phasing into the authenticity side of the dimension, we might place Western approaches that aspire to an authentic Buddhist psychology. Kwee (2010, 2012) applied a social constructionist perspective to a Western Buddhist psychology that he called "Relational Buddhism," extending beyond the use of mindfulness-based techniques for relieving symptoms to embrace the broader Buddhist goal of liberating humans from suffering. Drawing on the work of many traditionally trained Asian Buddhists and Western scholars and practitioners representing various schools of Buddhism, he echoed the previous concerns about maintaining the original Buddhist mission. He emphasized the importance of a comprehensive Buddhist psychology that preserves the original teachings using a common paradigm drawn from the Buddha's original teachings, which accentuate impermanence, conditioned existence, unhealthy craving, and an intention toward wisdom, insight, transformation, and liberation. Similarly, constructivist psychology shares Buddhism's core assumptions regarding the nature of phenomena and the understanding of human dysfunction as rooted in mental processes (McWilliams 2009, 2015). A variety of constructivist-oriented therapeutic methods seek to help clients address their concerns by transforming their understanding of themselves and the world (McWilliams 2010, 2012). Both social constructionist and personal constructivist approaches view the traditional Buddhist teachings as provisional concepts that can evolve in an ever-changing social process, in constant dynamic development, while maintaining their original integrity.

We could place the teachings of many fully trained Buddhist teachers throughout the world, including the West, as nearing or anchoring the authentic pole of the dimension. A thoroughly transformational approach to Buddhism, effectively adapted and accessible to the Western lay audience, could demonstrate how we can see an authenticity-oriented mindfulness manifesting within a practice that seeks to get at the roots of human suffering. Such an approach would address the fundamental intentions of Buddhist monastic practices that underlie attentional or mindfulness techniques as a vehicle for human liberation, transforming life experience in a way that sees through both the illusory nature of mental processes and the ambition to attain transcendental states. Later, in the chapter, an example of such an approach is suggested.

15.3 A Common Buddhist Paradigm

First, however, I would like to describe some common elements of authentic Buddhist teachings, disentangled from the various cultural, religious, and ethnic forms that they have taken over the centuries. As an introduction to this topic, it might prove useful to address some commonly held views about Buddhism to provide a general foundation for viewing Buddhism as primarily an approach to human psychology and mental well-being, rather than as a worshipful religion (McWilliams 2010, 2011, 2012, 2014).

15.3.1 Demystifying Buddhism

Most people conventionally regard Buddhism as a religion that includes metaphysical features similar to Western religions. Indeed, many indigenous Buddhist traditions, particularly in various Asian countries, have adopted some of these components and qualities by merging Buddhist teachings with preexisting beliefs and local practices, as described above in relation to the spread of Buddhism, often leading them to treat the Buddha as a deity. Indeed, as a recent traveler to many Asian countries, I have experienced a parallel with tourists' experience in Europe. In Europe, historical Christian cathedrals and churches serve as major tourist attractions, while in Asia Buddhist temples and monasteries occupy that role. (Ironically, although the Chinese annexation of Tibet has attempted to reduce the profile of its Buddhist roots, the remaining Buddhist temples and monasteries serve as the main attractions to which government-approved guides direct foreign visitors.) Thus, the forms (cosmologies, functions, positions, statues, altars, rituals, colors, dress, artifacts, and so on) that appear in Buddhist temples in Myanmar, Thailand, Vietnam, Cambodia, Laos, Malaysia, Nepal, Bhutan, and Tibet, differ, each representing historical characteristics and qualities of the local culture. A review of essential, time-honored principles of Buddhist teachings and thought that we attribute to the historical Buddha and that appear across all major Buddhist traditions shows that it excludes most conventionally understood religious characteristics. Understanding what it does comprise can assist us in viewing Buddhism as an approach to psychological topics and mental well-being without adherence to conventional religious characteristics (Khyentse 2007; Kwee 2010; McWilliams 2011, 2014; Mikulas 2007, 2008, 2010).

The historical Buddha, Siddhartha Gautama, rejected ideas of theism and claimed no divinity himself (Guang 2005, 2010; Khyentse 2007), regarding himself as a fallible, ordinary human being. Buddhist teachings omit the concept of a deity or Supreme Being. They include neither dogmas, creeds, or beliefs taken on faith nor someone to worship (Mikulas 2007, 2008, 2010). Buddha asserted the impossibility of knowing everything, thus denying omniscience (Kariyawasam 2010) and avoided consideration of irresoluble metaphysical concepts (Guang 2005, 2010) and indeterminate questions about the intrinsic nature of the universe, regarding them as irrelevant to his primary concern: eliminating human suffering.

The Buddha addressed the human condition in "the here and now world" rather than on "otherworldly" concerns or the afterlife (Kalupahana 1987, 1992, 2010; Kwee 2010). His way of living focused on personal experience and awakening through one's own efforts, rather than through authority, belief, or faith, and he used a nonauthoritarian teaching approach, directing his students to not *believe* what he taught because he said it, but instead to apply the teachings and examine their utility themselves (Mikulas 2007, 2008, 2010).

15.3.2 Basic Buddhist Assumptions

Buddhist philosophy regards phenomenal reality as "an assemblage of interlocking physical and mental processes that spring up and pass away subject to multifarious causes and conditions and that are always mediated by the cognitive apparatus embodied in the operation of the perceiving person" (Ronkin 2009, p. 14). Buddhist theory emphasizes three interrelated characteristics of this understanding of reality: dependent origination, impermanence, and emptiness, each of which reveals that events do not exhibit their own independent nature (Garfield 1995; Huntington 1989; Luetchford 2002). The identity of occurrences that we label "things" depend on other events or "things." Composite occurrences depend on the assembly of their parts and lose their identity when taken apart. Only the human process of perception and labeling identifies and acknowledges "things," which have no innate, separate identity of their own.

Since phenomena come into existence when conditions supporting their existence occur, when those conditions no longer transpire the phenomena no longer exist. Phenomena have not permanently existed, nor will they always exist, in their current state. Thus, we cannot identify a permanent fundamental nature that defines their identity. Use of the term emptiness means that, since phenomena only exist interdependently and constantly change, we cannot isolate an essence or identity, existing inherently and independently, that constitutes the entity, the thing itself. We can view reality as occurrences emerging within a perpetually mutable process rather than as a container of fixed objects or components.

We may regard the world and the phenomena we experience as indeed real and existing, but created afresh in each instant as a function of the ever-changing conditions of the moment. Khyentse (2007), foregrounded the importance of these perspectives by illustrating that two of them appear in "the four seals," four statements attributed to the historical Buddha that he suggested encompass the essence of traditional Buddhism: the view of all things as impermanent and lacking any essential or permanent substance or content, and the view of phenomena as empty and illusory. Awareness of impermanence reminds us that we do not control the world, and we have no basis for presuming that events will correspond to our hopes and expectations. Further, we have no one to blame when events fail to confirm our desires because of the countless conditions that lead to the occurrence of dependently arisen events.

15.3.3 Buddhism and the Human Situation

Another seal provides a useful transition to the topic of the Buddhist perspective on the human condition and its amelioration. Clarifying that we should not confuse "the four seals" with the Buddha's "four noble truths," which focus on human suffering as a human problem rooted in sensory and mental experience (Khyentse 2007), another seal introduces us to the topic of suffering by proposing that we view all emotions as producing pain and distress and understand that no emotion can produce only pleasure. The first of the noble truths, that life includes suffering, which sets the stage for the remainder of Buddhist teachings, proposes that human mental processes create the unsatisfactory quality of human experience because life fails to correspond to what we want or expect. (Throughout this chapter, use of the first person, singular or plural, in describing these teachings reflects an understanding that they apply universally, to all humans, while varying among individuals in substance, intensity, and duration.) Thus, the root of life's problems lies in the human longing for gratification, the aspiration to be "someone," the craving for self-preservation, attachment to beliefs, expectations, opinions, and self-images. Attachments and cravings appear in the form of the three poisons: greed or passion for what one likes, anger or hatred for what one dislikes, and ignorance or delusion from the failure to understand the mental processes as illusory projections.

The Buddhist view that emotions bring about suffering—the equivalence of suffering and emotion as one and the same—proposes that emotions develop from clinging to the self and to self-centered thoughts (Khyentse 2007). We can thus see emotions as based on ignorance of the illusory, impermanent, essenceless nature of the self, a misunderstanding, a flawed prejudice that contains a judgment about ourselves, and how life should transpire. Emotions, their consequences, and the misunderstandings derive from the source of all ignorance, clinging to a sense of self. We presume that the self actually exists as a separate entity, construct a concept of that self, reinforce its reality and consistency through narrative, all of the time forgetting the Buddha's realization that we can find no independent entity that qualifies as the self. We believe that we "are" the self, but if we closely examine our physical bodies, sensations, perceptions, feelings, actions, and conscious experience, we will see them as different elements of experience but we could not locate where the actual "self" resides:

> Clinging to the fallacy of the self is a ridiculous act of ignorance; it perpetuates ignorance; and it leads to all kinds of pain and disappointment. (Khyentse 2007, p. 45)

We should not underestimate the power and pervasiveness of this created sense of self, imposed upon interdependent assembled phenomena, the importance we place upon it, and the agony that follows our attempt to protect it, all of which lead directly to pain and suffering. Basic fears and insecurities arise and create these emotions, regardless of whether we recognize or name them. We erect our idea of self to protect us from these fears, creating a powerful, greedy, egocentric, vain illusion that controls us like an addiction. We identify ourselves in terms of what we love and what we hate, and we endeavor to validate our self-centered expectations as a way to confirm the existence of the self. Even though events may correspond to our self-centered desires, and we may take these successes as proof that we have truth, security, and well-founded assumptions, this blissful ignorance belies a constant overestimation that events will prove favorable to us. The Buddhist solution to this ignorance requires developing awareness of the emotions as they arise and experiencing them as assembled, dependently arising, impermanent, and empty phenomena (Khyentse 2007). Such awareness characterizes an authentic use of mindfulness to transform our understanding of the illusory self-centered nature of thinking. The following sections of this chapter explore more fully the nature of this self-centered worldview and consider Western lay-oriented approaches to Zen that embrace this transformative manner of mindfulness practice.

15.4 Hubert Benoit's Supreme Doctrine

Hubert Benoit (1904–1992), a French physician and surgeon, spent several years in hospital recovering from wounds suffered in World War II, during which he devoted his time to understanding the human condition and seeking the path of fulfillment, particularly through the study of Zen Buddhism. After his recovery, but unable to conduct surgery, he went into psychiatry and practiced psychotherapy in Paris until his death. The first English translation of his first major work on Zen, *The Supreme Doctrine: Psychological Encounters in Zen Thought* (Benoit 1984) appeared in 1955. A new translation, along with an additional work, *The Realization of the Self,* appeared more recently (Benoit 2004). His dense, rich writing provides a challenging, but rewarding experience for the reader. The following explication summarizes some of his major points; the subsequent section of the chapter may provide a more accessible application of some of Benoit's potentially obscure concepts.

Benoit sought a way to apply Zen teachings to the condition of ordinary human beings and to communicate his understanding to readers who wish to deepen their understanding of the human condition and believe that we can change our functioning in a way that facilitates the enjoyment of our essential nature. Having studied Zen teachings as a Westerner, he believed that Westerners require some intellectual understanding of them, even though traditional Zen teachers avoid intellectualism. Thus, he grounds his approach to understanding the nature of self-centered thinking and its relationship to emotional distress in a decidedly Western voice and in a detailed, well-elaborated manner.

Benoit viewed the human organism as a process, an impermanent fleeting manifestation of the absolute energy of the universe and also an insignificant individual of no particular interest. Inherently, we possess a sense of union with everything, as perfect, eternal, and positive, but this sense remains dormant in us, leading us to believe that we have a problem from which we must achieve deliverance. From the Zen perspective, we need to understand and experience the illusory nature of these beliefs and realize the futility of doing something to liberate ourselves, since we have always been free from the beginning.

He appreciated that people have always experienced dissatisfaction with themselves and that the typical remedies that people have used for this condition, which attempt to relieve symptoms by countering them, which generates a new symptom, fail to address the root cause of suffering:

> We are born feeling fundamentally unsatisfied. Something seems to be lacking. What we are and what we have does not meet our needs. We are waiting for something else to turn up, for real life to begin. We feel that we have a problem and go on looking for a solution.

> We feel we have a right to expect existence to provide us with various different situations. This dissatisfied, demanding attitude of ours is the source of all our suffering, but it has to be fulfilled, not destroyed. (Benoit 2004, p. 213)

Consistent with the essential Buddhist teachings discussed previously, for Benoit the craving for existence as a distinct, separate entity motivates all human activity. We have the illusion that we exist as a separate and distinct being, the fundamental egoistical state. We experience the self as in opposition to not-self, everything not my organism, including other people. I love myself and wish for my own existence to continue, and I hate not-self and wish to get rid of it. I wish for affirmation of myself as a separate entity and to negate not-self, which encroaches on my separate self. In order "to live," I must affirm my separate self and defeat not-self, by acquiring wealth, fame, or glory.

The never-ending debate between existence versus nonexistence or nothingness underlies all human experience. What happens when I feel distressed by some event? Distress evolves from encounter with not-self, raising the fear of defeat of the self, the fear that the outcome will not favor me, raising the specter of facing the nullification of my being. A painful reaction to an event occurs due to the desire to exist. Confusion about "myself" appears as the illusion of identifying with our organism and believing in the reality of our phenomenal experience. When we claim that we exist as separate and distinct entities, it colors our desires, hopes, and beliefs, and it implies that we believe we lack something and the expectation that something will remove our deficiency. This leads to waiting for life to change into the way that completely affirms us. "[W]e all live in the expectation that a day will come when 'true life,' free of all negation, will finally begin" (Benoit 2004, p. 164). We each have our own individual picture of how our life would look with all our imperfections abolished.

15.4.1 Development of the Self-Image

According to Benoit, in the earliest stages of human development, the first 2 years, the brain and the mind remain unfinished and still in development. As children, we experience immersion in the external world without boundaries and have no awareness of a distinction between self and not-self. By the second year of life, the "animal" brain has completed its development, and we begin to develop concrete perceptions similar to the level of nonhuman animals. We then operate on an implicit unconscious conviction that the principles that guide our individual existence correspond to the guiding principles of the universe, so we do not experience any threat to our existence. The distinction between self and not-self, however, begins to emerge as we develop awareness of obstacles in the world, which naturally arise for everyone, and the distress that follows. From these encounters, we learn that we do not bring the world into existence, and that things in the world exist independently of us, leading to a conscious fear of death and the danger to self and the wish to destroy anything outside ourselves that does not favor our own existence. As the sense of self evolves, it consists of everything that supports our existence, with not-self (the other) as anything that serves as a potential threat to that existence. At this stage, our viewpoints remain completely biased and partial to our own individualistic perspective, and the causes of behavior persist from an irrational and emotional base.

As humans develop further, Benoit described the emergence of independent intelligence, the capability for abstract, general, and objective perception, which leads to the possibility of understanding another person's point of view, along with the ability to distinguish between what affirms myself over not-self and the "objective" value or goodness of events independently of how they affect myself. However, although independent intelligence has appeared, the biased and individualistic self-centered approach to life has already established powerful emotional mechanisms, rooted in bodily sensations, from earlier stages of existence. The abstract, mental concerns turn toward pure ideas, devising concepts of the ideal, universal, true, good, and beautiful, which we then project onto the image we form of ourselves, resulting in what we call the ego, an unreal, idealistic, narcissistic self-image that we worship and love. This process leads to a gulf or division within the self, between bodily, sensory, experiences and abstract, mental, thoughts, which exist separately, disuniting our formerly united being and propelling us by two dynamic systems, which sometimes support and sometimes battle each other.

15.4.2 Body (Sensations) and Mind (Thoughts)

The two domains of the physical and mental coexist within us and, although they appear different, they both manifest the same underlying principle. We contact the world through two surfaces, the somatic or physical and the psychological or mental, which have different emotional implications. Impressions occur unconsciously, triggered by interaction with the external world, but felt within the self physically (pleasure–pain) or psychologically (comfort–distress). The sensory level corresponds to the real physical world, but we create the psychological level with our imagination. At the physical level, we respond to sensations, based on actual phenomenal experiences, in a straightforward way, with the particular emotion depending on whether the images affirm the self or negate it. Sensations that we associate with a threat to our existence produce bodily tension or contraction, while those that we associate with maintaining our existence decrease contraction and lead to muscular relaxation. Thus, emotional activity related directly to physical sensations continuously rises and falls in response to impermanent external phenomena. Without a self-concept, we would only experience "negative" experiences as temporary bodily sensations, which quickly pass.

We may feel physical sensations in our body as attraction or repulsion, but we need not attach a sense of the "goodness" or "badness" of the sensory stimuli, which is a mental concept. "My mistake does not lie in thinking of something which affects me as being favorable or unfavorable to my existence; where I go wrong is in considering it 'good' or 'bad,' in other words evaluating it from an affective viewpoint" (Benoit 2004, p. 148). This creates the disease of the mind, according to Zen, of placing what we like against what we dislike. Once we develop a self-image, however, with its ideals, we come to associate "negative" sensations with this more elaborated image of self and not-self, leading to a type of psychological "cramp" as threatening images become connected with contraction of the muscles. This process occurs as events that threaten the imaginary idealized self-image generate the type of physical contraction or tension associated with an existential threat, leading to development of a fixed emotional state, what Benoit called "contracture," a type of chronic tension related to the desire for affirmation and ever-present doubt about the being or the threat of not-being.

Thus, the imaginary psychological level differs from the physical level because, in addition to responding to imaginary images, the chronic emotional state influences the development of physical reactions and thoughts, which leads to further arousal in an escalating emotion–thought spiral. Ultimately, we can view psychological suffering as the result of associations between threatening mental images and a cramped bodily experience.

> Emotions can be positive or negative, joy or suffering; but emotional states are always negative. (Benoit 2004, p. 121)

15.4.3 The Imaginative Cinema

Benoit regarded all thought as imagination and likened it to a film or cinema. As described above, he distinguished between what he called our real, or reactive, imaginative cinema, based on sensory experiences of the external world and our imaginary, or active, imaginative cinema, constructed by mental processes. We use the real imaginative cinema when we solve a problem related to the external world, such as navigating through the city, repairing a broken device, or baking a cake. The imaginary imaginative cinema relates to our mental self-image and plays a useful role early in our lives to help compensate for the trials and tribulations of the human condition. We could not bear what life throws at us without it. Unfortunately, we continue to use the imaginary cinema for its compensatory advantages after we develop independent intelligence, but increasingly it creates more distress and harm. We tend to take the temporary relief that imagination provides from suffering as a real improvement in our condition, but it actually makes the condition worse. Imagination protects the illusory ego, crushes the real body, and turns away from the world, and its obstacles, to take refuge in the imagination.

15.4.4 Imagination as Compensation

As unrealized people, we have a strong need to exist absolutely, as separate entities. Thus, we cannot accept actual existence as it unfolds. We may understand intellectually that the fate of the world does not hinge on our personal existence, but our imagination protects us from actually experiencing this reality by creating a subjective, private world built around us with our self as its center. This imaginary cinema, not based on current reality, provides a compensatory function that manufactures image systems to conceal what we cannot bear, but functions only as long as we keep it running, maintaining its activity. We create these image systems from our sensory experience and mental concepts and organize them uniquely according to our individual personal perspective, based on our values and what gives our life meaning. Compensations have a primary function to create a perspective of the universe that puts us, as a separate individual, at its center. It does not matter whether the compensation affirms or negates us, as long as it maintains our illusory belief of our separate existence.

Compensations function as idols, an attempt to encompass reality in a single fixed, permanent, image. They consist of a depiction of my ego, myself, with a cluster of sub-images, encompassing both positive and negative components. Benoit described several common positive compensations, such as being loved; consuming and enjoying; duty to a moral code or ideal; pleasure from beauty, knowledge, or art; drawing attention to one's self; being admired; being feared; creating world-changing works; developing or realizing myself; material or spiritual ambition; and the adoration compensation that merges all of these compensations together, projects the ego onto an external form, and then imagines itself interacting with that projection.

Benoit described compensations as a "dynamic fixity," consisting of habitual patterns of functioning, a stereotyped way of living, even when they only serve as an ideal tendency and not actively expressed in the person's life. Compensations provide a guiding purpose that gives us a sense of structure and effectiveness in our life, particularly when fully integrated into our organism's functioning. They help to simplify our personality dynamics by finding reality in a particular component and making other aspects dormant, which may provide us with an apparent sense of inner unity. But even well-compensated people practice idolatry by believing that the compensatory image has created the harmonizing qualities of their life and treating their image as real. In this way, people come to treat their idiosyncratic values as objective and believe that others should see things the way they do, leading to proselytizing or intolerance.

15.4.5 The Active Role of Mindfulness

We find ourselves in the circumstance of living in an illusory world that we have created as a way to avoid having to experience the suffering that attends awareness of the possibility of the death of our idealized sense that we constitute a separate being who occupies the center of the universe. How can we find release and liberation from this desperate state of affairs? First, Benoit suggests that we can benefit from his version of what Buddhism refers to as "right understanding," comprehending the illusory nature of our circumstances, seeing the perfection of things as they are, including ourselves, and understanding that we live with the illusion that something is wrong with us that we need to make right. Dissolving an imaginary life involves abandoning the illusory ideal, which we see as sacred; ending anguish ensues when we relinquish the wish for any kind of change.

Benoit proposed a solution that does not require that we attempt to change anything, but he suggested that we shift from the passive way that our attention functions, in which we react to energy that arouses us, and activates the self-centered emotion–thought spiral, particularly when they address our beliefs regarding our "bad" qualities. We might attempt to end these negative thoughts by countering them, replacing them with positive thoughts, or ignoring them, but such a process cannot succeed. We cannot achieve relaxation by trying harder to relax, by counteracting a contracted state with another contraction. A more active form of mindfulness would occur before the mobilization of energy.

We could consider attempting to practice mindfulness by attending to the reactions as they arise. However, although we experience the conscious reaction as occurring instantaneously, it always happens a few milliseconds later, as a reaction. Benoit proposed that we adopt an active approach to mindfulness by alerting ourselves to energy mobilization before it happens. "This will be brought about when, instead of *seeing* the imaginative-emotional processes as they emerge, I *look* at them as they are about to emerge" (Benoit 2004, p. 181, italics in original), by actively directing attention toward perceiving the birth of the energy with a watchfulness that keeps the process "under surveillance." "[A]ctive attention watches out for emerging inner movements of energy…what matters is that formless activity which gives rise to [emotions] subsequent activity…This active functioning of my consciousness…cannot be attained by direct effort or any explicit discipline aiming at Realization" (Benoit 2004, p. 181) .

15.4.6 Spectator to the Spectacle

The method, called Benoit's "Technique of Timeless Realization," requires assuming an attitude of actively watching our imaginative cinema or listening to our own inner soliloquy, giving our imagination permission to do or say whatever it chooses. Doing so, the cinema goes blank or the monologue stops, and they only begin again if we cease the attitude of anticipatory watchfulness. Benoit described the exercise as follows:

> Alone, in a quiet place, muscularly relaxed (lying down or comfortably seated), I watch the emergence within myself of mental images, permitting my imagination to produce *whatever it likes*. It is as though I were saying to my image-making mind, "Do what you please; but I am going to watch you doing it." As long as one maintains this attitude…the imagination produces nothing and its screen remains blank, free of all images…. As soon as there is a weakening of my voluntary effort of pure attention, thoughts (images) make

> their appearance.... I discover that I have started to think of this and that. The moment I make this discovery, I say to my imagination, “So you want to talk to me about that. Go ahead; I’m listening.” Immediately everything stops again, and I become conscious of the stoppage. (Benoit 2004, p. 300, italics in original)

Thus, the way to triumph over our automatic imagination occurs, not by trying to stop it, but by consciously, actively, allowing it to play freely. This approach to inner work attempts to see our own nature, particularly the place where emotions arise. We can carry out this inner work on a daily basis without the need for spiritual concepts, morals, desire to do “good,” or intellectual analysis. By employing a direct, active scrutiny of this imaginary emotional–mental activity, authentic emotional activity remains, corresponding to the direct bodily experience at the sensory plane. This “animal” level, existing in us before we had words or ideals, consists of the only real experience we ever have. Returning to this organismic experience, we embrace the muscular contractions, fear, nausea, worry, sadness—the profound bodily unease of suffering. Beneath the imaginary cinema, we seek this deep, paralyzing grip, immobilizing cold, cramp-like feeling, and rest in this hard, immobile layer of experience. Without attending to any corresponding imaginary cinema, we endure in bodily stillness, the somatic contracture loses its emotional character, and we experience true suffering without perpetuating more false suffering.

15.4.7 The Inner Work of Realization

We will not find any recipes for attaining realization; understanding our illusory imaginings and attending to physical experience provides the means to dissipate our present state of illusion. This understanding finds practical expression in the form of a special kind of real-world inner work suitable for daily life, a mindfulness embracing active attention. This inner work does not attempt to change our lives, nor does it involve an intervention, which modifies or disturbs our organization. It does not directly change the mental cinema; it interrupts it without triggering any other image to intercede. If it “does” anything, it consists of “not doing” what we usually do. It does not focus directly on a mental image of relaxation, but releases the contracting process indirectly by requiring us to relinquish control over the active perceptual functions of consciousness. If we actively authorize consciousness to engage in its autonomous functions, completely, impartially, and unconditionally, we open ourselves to the unchanging presence of our very existence, with no preference for any object nor preconceptions, an alertness to everything.

Benoit acknowledged the difficult, challenging nature of the type of inner work that brings us into direct contact with our physical being, and requires a long, dedicated, gradual practice of self-realization. Each interruption of the imaginative cinema lasts only for a moment. Over time, experiencing present-moment reality slowly annihilates our imaginings about our past and our future, all of which lack present reality. Perfect joy awaits us in the total elimination of our hopes.

15.5 Jōko Beck's Ordinary Mind Zen

The teachings of the late Charlotte Jōko Beck (1917–2011), founder of the Ordinary Mind School of Zen, exemplify how an American Zen teacher, trained by Japanese Zen masters (Hakuyu Taizan Maezumi, Sōen Nakagawa, and Hakuun Yasutani) in both Soto and Rinzai traditions, has evolved and adapted the authentic qualities of traditional Zen teachings using innovative methods that have made them more accessible to Western lay students. She received formal dharma transmission from Maezumi Roshi of the Zen Center of Los Angeles in 1982 and served as the resident teacher at the Zen Center of San Diego from 1983 to 2006 and the Prescott, Arizona, Zen Center from 2006 to 2011. I had the good fortune of studying and practicing with her from 1983 until her death. In describing her approach, I draw upon my personal experiences as her student, her two published books (Beck 1989, 1993), numerous transcripts and recordings of her talks, and books written by her dharma successors and students (Bayda 2002, 2003, 2009, 2014; Block 2005; Hamilton 2007; Magid 2002, 2008, 2013; Rizzetto 2006; Smith 2012). With gratitude to all, I take full responsibility for my understanding and interpretation of these sources.

I laid much of the groundwork for my deliberation of Jōko's teachings with the foregoing consideration of Benoit's work because of its influence on her. Jōko described Benoit's *The Supreme Doctrine* (Benoit 1984) as "the main teacher I've had all of my life," and "the best book on Zen ever written" (Beck 1993, p. 124). She recommended it to me early in my work with her, and I have come to see much of the foundation for her teachings in it. Although Jōko articulated her viewpoint in simple language and emphasized ordinary daily living as the context for Zen practice, her perspective grew out of the insights of classic Zen teaching. This view differs from some popular perspectives on meditation that focus on attaining special states of consciousness. It emphasizes, instead, awareness of how we respond to ordinary daily life experience.

15.5.1 Origin of the Self-Image

Similar to Benoit's perspective, Jōko regarded the basic essence of a person as a "true self," open to life, encompassing love, security, worthiness, justice, and compassion as our very nature. We naturally consist of all of these things at birth. She did not view this true self as something transcendent or esoteric; rather, it corresponds to our actual genuine selves when free of conditioned responses to life, with receptivity to, and no reservations about, life. However, early in life we lose sense of true self. She suggested that at birth human babies remain essentially in a fetal stage for the first 9 months, due to the narrowness of the birth canal that requires babies to continue to develop outside the womb. She pointed out the pleasant characteristics of life in the womb. The baby has constant access to food, warmth, peace, and a nonspecific sense of total love where it gets everything it wants, with total satisfaction, all of the time. Even with the most careful and effective parenting, however, the baby begins to see the impossibility of this desire. No baby will avoid meeting innumerable occurrences of experiences it does not like. Even something as common as a 2-year-old with a new sibling brings terror to the child; from the baby's point of view, its love has shrunk from 100 to less than 50 %, which seems absolutely in the wrong to the baby.

The baby cannot consider the god-like parents as imperfect, so can only imagine a fault in itself, "something's wrong with me, I'm unworthy, worthless, don't amount to anything." This basic psychological situation, in which the parents cannot meet the child's every desire, leads to the development of a self-image as a way of handling this sense of defectiveness. The true self's sense of total love gives way to a feeling that I am lacking something that I need to get somewhere, somehow. So the child begins to erect an elaborated image, similar to Benoit's imaginative cinema, in order to replace the missing sense of love, security, worthiness, and justice, to build an idealized version of self, unique to the individual, and accompanied by various strategies designed to obtain what they believe they lack. Jōko asserts that we all build an image to obtain things that we feel we lack; it is neither good nor bad, just something that humans inevitably do. However, these images come to run our lives. We can know if we operate from this self-image if we ever get emotionally upset by anything.

15.5.2 Sensations and Thoughts

This description of the origin of the self-image omits a very important component. The experience of this shocking loss of total love generates a feeling of terror for the child, who has not developed language and concepts to understand the situation. The child experiences this terror in the form of bodily sensations, such as the contractures that Benoit described. As the compensatory self-image evolves, an association develops among its images and the bodily sensations, leading to the chronic bodily experience that Benoit referred to as an emotional state. Similar to Benoit's understanding of an emotional state, this self-image and its related beliefs is always negative, since it relates to the child's sense of something wrong with itself.

Here, we also see another parallel between Jōko's and Benoit's perspective. For Jōko, present life experience consists only of two basic elements: bodily sensations and thoughts. Bodily sensations constitute the most important, most real, life experiences, while thoughts, which can operate independently of actual sensory experience, while very useful, can create problems. Jōko distinguished between two categories of thoughts, paralleling Benoit's similar distinction. She described technical or functional thinking, similar to Benoit's "real imaginative cinema," as responding to sensory experiences in the service of concrete planning and implementation of daily tasks or solving problems. She contrasted this with self-centered thinking, which responds to the self-image, similar to Benoit's "imaginary imaginative cinema." We will see the importance of these distinctions as we consider Jōko's methods for practicing with the self-image.

15.5.3 The Purpose of Practice

Jōko expressed the essence of Zen practice as paying attention to this very moment, our entire experience of the "right now" occurrence. This seems simple and straightforward except that we do not want to pay attention because we do not always find the experience pleasant. It does not correspond to what we want:

> We constantly dream about the future, about the nice things we're going to have, or that are going to happen to us. So we filter anything happening in the present through all that: "I don't like that. I don't have to listen to that." This goes on constantly: spinning, spinning, spinning, always trying to create life in a way that will be pleasant, that will make us feel safe and secure, so that we "feel good."
>
> But when we do that we never see this right-here-now, this very moment. We can't see it because we're filtering what it says. And when we do that, this moment is clouded over. Just ask any ten people who read this page. You'll find they all tell you something different. They'll forget the parts that don't quite catch them; they'll pick up something else, and they'll even block out the parts they don't like. Even when they go to a spiritual teacher they hear only what they want to hear. Being open to a teacher means not just hearing what you want to hear, but hearing the whole thing. And the teacher is not there simply to be nice to you.
>
> So the crux of meditation is this: we must constantly create a little shift from the spinning world we've got in our heads to right-here-now. That's our practice. The intensity and ability to be right-here-now is what we have to develop. We have to be able to develop the ability to say, "No, I won't spin off here"—to make that choice. Moment by moment, our practice is like a choice, a fork in the road: we can go this way, we can go that way. It's always a choice, moment by moment, between the nice world that we want to set up in our heads and what really is.... Zen training is designed to enable us to live comfortable, beneficial lives. But the only people who live comfortably are those who learn not to dream their lives away, and instead to be with what's right-here-now, no matter what it is: good, bad, nice, not nice, having a headache, being ill, being happy. It doesn't make any difference. Did you think it did? (Beck 1999, p. 1)

The essence of Ordinary Mind Zen meditation practice thus lies in the willingness to accept and experience life "as it is" regardless of whether it meets our expectations, desires, or convenience. If we manifest the right-here-now awareness that Jōko describes, we would act flexibly and effectively. For most of us, however, right-here-now awareness remains a continuing challenge and requires a disciplined methodology like Zen practice.

Jōko viewed such practice as a lifelong activity. "Our practice is about our life, and we practice forever" (Beck 1996, p. 1). She regularly emphasizes that, while most people experience some immediate effects, the benefits begin to manifest more fully after about 20 years of disciplined daily practice, regular intensive practice retreats, and working directly with a capable teacher. Additionally, Zen practice focuses on the conduct of daily life as well as the specific activities involved in formal sitting meditation. When students ask her, "How is my practice going?" Jōko responds, "How is your life going?"

Regular daily sitting forms the fundamental base of Zen practice. The proper physical form of formal sitting meditation provides an essential foundation of an effective practice. Whether sitting cross legged on a cushion or on a chair, the body should feel balanced and at ease, erect but not stiff. Regular practice requires daily sitting, not missing more than 1 day per week. Sitting practice provides a formal time to develop awareness of the two basic elements of life experience: present bodily sensations and mental process and thoughts. Clarity, calmness, or insight may occur during sitting, but they do not represent its goal; rather the process should focus on observing and attending to the reality of the moment, including and embracing feelings of confusion, discouragement, anxiety, and so on.

15.5.4 Three Planes of Mindfulness

Three interrelated mindfulness techniques support Ordinary Mind practice: (1) focusing or concentrating, (2) labeling thoughts and experiencing bodily sensations, and (3) attending to emotional reactivity. Focusing or concentrating provides a ground for practice and serves as a means to settle our speedy "monkey mind." By focusing on a specific stimulus, concentration practice enables us to quiet the mind and develop stable sitting. It might consist of attending to the in-and-out movement of the breath or counting each breath from one to ten and then starting at one again. As the mind wanders away from the breath, attention gently returns to the practice. Concentration practice by itself, however, tends to shut out life experience, instead of opening ourselves to it, so while serving as an important step in practice this technique alone has limitations.

As focusing or concentrating helps to settle sitting, we can then move to "wide open awareness," observing thoughts as they continuously arise and fall away while attending to the variety of bodily sensations. To a great extent, this mode of practice forms the core of everyday sitting and daily life awareness. In the beginning of practice, and typically the beginning of a sitting period, after concentration enables the mind to slow down, we may become aware of the constant flow of thoughts that arise, and we begin to see recurrent patterns and themes in these thoughts. We do not have to "do anything" about these thoughts; rather, we may take the position of a witness or observer to the thoughts. We benefit from labeling or categorizing the type of thoughts as they arise, which assists us in seeing their recurrent nature. Although thoughts continue to arise, after time we begin to see them from a more distant perspective, and they lose their sense of importance or urgency. At some point, we may find that we become bored with the repetitive nature of these self-centered thoughts, and we begin to lose interest in many of our cherished opinions and ideas.

As we slowly decrease interest in thoughts, we may become more acutely aware of bodily sensations, particularly noticing areas of the body where we tend to hold tension (e.g., stomach, shoulders, neck, face). Again, rather than trying to change or relax these sensations, Ordinary Mind Zen practice directs awareness toward these entrenched bodily sensations, allowing ourselves to fully experience the sensations. In doing so, we may experience change in the quality of the sensations and the tension.

The third aspect of practice emphasizes attending to emotional reactions to experiences and events and the thoughts that create the emotional reactivity. By recognizing that we create the emotion through attachment to a self-centered belief, we can observe the emotion–thought spiral. We see that emotional sensations lead to thoughts that, due to our attachment to them, generate more sensations of physical tension. In attending to emotions and thoughts, and examining what we gain from holding to the beliefs, we understand more fully the core beliefs, requirements, patterns, and strategies we have developed to avoid awareness of them, which we will consider further below. This third aspect of practice consists of attending to the total experience of our distress, particularly in terms of the physical, bodily sensations, so that we can see directly how the core beliefs reside in the body itself.

A description of the methods does not convey the extent of the challenge of actual practice. Resistance, turbulence, and emotional upset may follow an initial "honeymoon" period. Meditators often experience fatigue, boredom, and leg pain. These experiences provide more opportunity to gain awareness of thoughts, emotions, and bodily sensations. Beck (1996) cautioned against avoiding sitting during times of emotional upset and noted the particular value of sitting when difficulties arise. Further, she suggested that once a week we should sit 10–15 min longer than we wish to as a way of enhancing reactivity. As Jōko stated:

> What we learn from having to sit quietly with that discomfort is so valuable that if it didn't exist, it should. When you're in pain, you can't spin off. You have to stay with it. There's no place to go. So pain can be really valuable. (Beck 1999, p. 1)

Bayda (2002) described how Ordinary Mind Zen practice emphasized illuminating our tendency to believe in the "truth" of our thoughts about ourselves and focused on the direct physical experience of the present moment, including recalcitrant emotional reactions:

> As we clarify our believed thoughts, no longer taking them as truth, and as we reside in the bodily component of our experience, we begin to see that our experience of these little holes is actually nothing more than a combination of deeply believed thoughts and a complex of subtle and not-so-subtle uncomfortable bodily sensations. Seeing this—and I mean seeing it in the way that fosters real understanding—is a taste of freedom. (p. 21)

15.5.5 Practicing with the Self-Image

We now see the purpose and function of Jōko's Ordinary Mind Zen practice and its emphasis on mindfully focusing awareness on the immediate experience of bodily sensations and developing familiarity with recurrent patterns of thoughts. Although Jōko spoke and wrote about these issues, her primary concern rested with assisting individual student practitioners in developing a mature, fruitful practice. She recurrently saw that her students experienced great challenge in working with the way self-image operates and its relation to emotional experience. She devoted most of her energy as a teacher to devising ways to facilitate more effective practice with the self-image. We will next discuss three approaches that she developed for this purpose, working with systems, lists, and core beliefs.

Systems As you will recall, Jōko suggested that the self-image derives from the loss of the true self's unconditional response to life, due to the childhood experience of loss. We develop the self-image to attempt to replace out natural experience of total love, security, worthiness, justice, and compassion. The self-image that we build evolves into artificial systems that we use to get things we think we lost from the outside world. These systems end up running our life, and we feel shattered when we feel that something threatens or attacks them. What does Jōko mean by a system?

Systems consist of requirements that we believe life or ourselves must meet in order for us to obtain or maintain love and security. The world, of course, does not care about our artificial set of requirements. We can come to see the system and its requirements when we sit and notice the thoughts that arise, particularly the recurrent patterns about how we try to get something we feel lacking from life. These requirements have their roots in childhood experiences, and may have proved useful for us at the time, but we forget their origin and make them the laws of our life. We demand the maintenance of these systems and that events affirm them. If we have a system related to having others love us, we require others to behave a certain way, according to our system's criteria, and we will feel hurt or threatened if the person behaves differently. We expect others to conform to our requirements, but of course, they do whatever they do, so we have difficulty maintaining our system.

Systems usually consist of two sides: the things we go after, like love, power, freedom, recognition, and the opposite side that we experience when we do not get it, such as depression, disappointment, guilt. When we feel good, we think our system is working well. We get praised, promoted, a good job, a new lover, and we feel good for a time. However, eventually, we find that we cannot rely on any of these successes, so we feel attacked, and we descend into the negative side of the system.

The systems consist of totally invented thoughts, with no intrinsic reality, and typically contain 2 or 3 major systems and 5–15 minor ones. Over the years, Jōko worked with students using various methods to help them identify and get acquainted with their own unique, individual systems. Recognizing their individuality, we can identify major themes of patterns of personality systems that may help individuals in perceiving and articulating their personal version. Useful examples occur in classic psychological literature, such as Rogers' (1951, 1959, 1961) ideal self, Horney's (1950) three solutions, the expansive appeal of mastery, the self-effacing appeal of love, and the resigning appeal of freedom, and Angyal's (1965) patterns of vicarious living and noncommitment.

At one time, Jōko used the Enneagram, an ancient Sufi-based personality typology system (Hurley and Dobson 1991; Keyes 1992; Naranjo 1990; Palmer 1988, 1995; Riso 1990) to help her students' identify their systems. As an academic clinical psychologist, I held a skeptical view of the enneagram for several years until a time when I traveled to San Diego and stayed at the home of fellow Zen students. Next to the bed, I saw Palmer's (1988) book and started to peruse it. As I read the description of the first type, Point One, the Perfectionist, I experienced a growing shock of recognition, thinking to myself, "How could anyone know these intimate things about me." This experience powerfully assisted me in understanding and working with my own system. The value of these system models does not lie in intellectual understanding, however, but in coming to see how they actually manifest themselves in our daily life.

We can test whether an experience has attacked our system by seeing when we get upset, and everyone gets upset. When upset, we normally turn our attention to the situation or the person who upsets us and project blame and criticism, but, if we mindfully practice with the situation, we turn our attention to the systems itself. By seeing the systems, and how they work, patiently, over time, the attention itself and going back to the physical place where the systems began will tend to weaken them. Watching them carefully, we return to the original trauma, the bodily contraction, and by residing in the contracting and leaving it alone, it will slowly fade.

Working with the system this way, a shift occurs from our previous pattern of trying to get the system to work effectively (which life will always defy) to observing the system, not attempting to change it or get rid of it. Jōko also encouraged students to weaken the system by consciously going against it and see how they react. For example, if you have a system of not getting noticed, you might choose to actively speak up, to see what you do not want to do and go ahead and do it, and then experience the fear, attend to the bodily sensation, and feel the original terror. This experience may sound terrible, but through it we see that we only experience a bodily sensation, a tightness in the neck or abdomen, overall bodily tension, nausea, that does not actually threaten us.

Eventually, we see that we cannot get satisfaction living out of our systems. Although practice may address psychological problems of life, it aims to weaken these systems, not perfect them, or replace them with an alternate system. Only weakening the system and seeing through it, seeing its lack of reality, gives lasting help. As another benefit of work with systems, we come to see that no person or no event can threaten or upset us. Our tendency to focus on the world and cast blame when injured diminishes with practice.

Lists Jōko implemented another approach to systems where she asked her students to construct three lists that help to articulate and clarify the origins of the self-image system, their current adult form, and how they create suffering. Although still somewhat psychological, she designed it to help make clear how the requirements and systems relate directly to experiential practice and using that for release into freedom. She also suggested that through this exercise we can come to experience deeply that "I am enough just as I am," as is everyone else, even if I do awful things sometimes, and decrease our judgmental approach to the world. She wanted students to see that our interactions with the people we spend time with, particularly as children, but also our particular culture, quickly mold most of how we come to think of ourself. The three lists consist of:

1. How I was trained to be as a child. This derives from my personal temperament and tendencies, feedback from parents, relatives, and friends, the culture we live in, the time frame of our generation, our socioeconomic status, etc.
2. What I require of myself as an adult. This consists of things like the decisions I make, the strategies I employ, how I relate to various situations, how I differ in what I do from others.
3. My current false suffering. This list consists of the emotional reactions and accompanying thoughts that I experience in the present that relate to and corroborate the items on list #2.

For example, I might have an item on list #1 regarding being punished or berated as a child for making minor mistakes and the pressure that I to do things perfectly in order to avoid this castigation. I might have a related item on list #2 that describes how I believe that I must always do everything perfectly. On list #3, this might appear as experiences of emotional upset, defensiveness, or self-berating thoughts when criticized. This exercise helps us see more clearly where we came from, what we learned from others and from the social and physical environment when we were young, and how we go about living our life at present. The activity helps make it clearer what we do and to see that we do not need to view the things we cling to as good or bad, but, if we make them a requirement that we or others behave in a certain way, we create an experience of false suffering.

We benefit from seeing that if we have requirements that we behave in a certain way, see ourselves, for example, as bright, friendly, self-sufficient, fastidious, or studious, we have no freedom. We hold ourselves to these requirements and so we have no choice about how we must act. If we do not live up to the requirements on the list, our false suffering occurs, in the form of, for example, guilt, anger, depression, and we fail to attend to what life actually presents to us. We even turn qualities that we believe an ideal Zen student has into further requirements, such as being serene, or practicing correctly.

The first list has unconscious roots that observing and the labeling and listing process opens up to awareness, so whatever we do or think will show up as we create the list, particularly by labeling thoughts as they arise. The second list may consist of very positive qualities, like kindness, patience, humility, or good worker, but the value of the list comes from experiencing the suffering that occurs because we make them requirements. The third list actually shows up in the irritations of daily life, in the form of annoyance, frustration, and thoughts about the wrongness of the world and how it abuses us. If we learn to practice with experiencing the third list items in the body, without attending to the thought elements, eventually the list #3 reactions disappear, along with the list #2 requirements, due to the connection between the two lists.

Work with the lists, if fruitful, leads to the awareness of the unreality of all of the lists. Since the first list only derives from memories, we should not take them as truthful. Thus, we can view the first list as an unreal fantasy, along with the second list, since it derives from the unreal first list. The experiences of the third list derive from the second, consisting only of unreal thoughts, too. When we purge list #3 of its accompanying sentences and only attend to the bodily experiences, healing occurs, and we experience freedom, joy, and compassion for others, who remain stuck in their own lists.

Core Beliefs Working with our core beliefs, descriptions of our self in terms of an image or idol provides yet another related method for working mindfully with the self-image system. Jōko describes how our self-centered anger arises when something threatens the image of our self. She describes examples of positive images we might hold of ourselves: a kind person, a good parent, someone with meaningful accomplishments, or an authority on a particular subject. Or we can have a negative image: a mean person, a mediocre person, someone who never accomplishes anything. We love our deeply rooted images, and they run our lives. We may attempt to replace a negative image with a positive one, but our attachment to any image maintains it as an idol that we will defend and leaves us in a state of bondage.

A defended image always obstructs the open awareness necessary for effective action. Even a spiritual image, that "I am awakened" obstructs genuine seeing because awakening means existing without image, without defense, and open to life as it unfolds. Since we develop life strategies based on core decisions that we make early in life,

> we believe that this thought-based picture of reality is who we are and what life is. The more we believe in this artificial life, the more we move away from "life as it is." (Bayda 2002, p. 49)

Ordinary Mind Zen emphasizes how we tend to accept as real the negative self-image that we construct around these decisions and the narratives that support it. Effective Zen practice includes learning to observe the all-pervasive nature of these decisions and the expectations and requirements of our self and others that they engender. It also emphasizes developing awareness of the strategies that we use to protect ourselves. Once we learn to see clearly our core decisions and interrupt our strategies, we can experience directly the emotional reactions that we avoid feeling. "Only by uncovering and entering this dreaded part of ourselves can we see through the artificial construct of our substitute life and ultimately reconnect with awareness of our basic wholeness" (Bayda 2002, p. 54). Effective practice of this approach requires careful, disciplined, mindful, self-observation, which includes watching everything going on "within" us and around us almost as if it was happening to another person (de Mello 1990).

15.5.6 The Four Practice Principles

Jōko continuously sought ways to convey Buddhist ideas in forms more accessible and meaningful to current, Western students. In collaboration with her student Allan Kaprow, Jōko (Beck 1993) reformulated the Buddha's Four Noble Truths, the existence of suffering, the cause of suffering, an end to suffering, and a way to end suffering, which provide the foundation of the basic teachings of Buddhism, along with the principles underlying the vows taken in traditional Japanese Zen Practice. Ordinary Mind Zen practitioners call these the Four Practice Principles. These four principles remind us why and how we practice (Smith 2012), and they succinctly capture and summarize the preceding discussion of Ordinary Mind Zen practice.

> Caught in the self-centered dream, only suffering.
> Holding to self-centered thoughts, exactly the dream.
> Each moment, life as it is, the only teacher.
> Being just this moment, compassion's way. (Beck 1993, p. 275)

We create dissatisfaction, unhappiness, and suffering by separating ourselves from the experience of the moment by functioning within a self-centered world of our own creation, with its beliefs and requirements. We hold to this view, not seeing it as a dream, focusing on seeking what we want, avoiding what we do not want, and blaming others for our dissatisfaction. "Life as it is" refers to the right-here-now, actual events as they unfold, and practicing with "life as it is" means seeing the requirements we place on life, experiencing the emotions and thoughts, residing in the bodily experience of the moment, and responding flexibly to the current situation. Through this process, we gain awareness of the transparent nature of the self-centered dream, and we act without the hindrance of dualistic thinking. We can see what life needs and we act appropriately. "Not doing anything special, our life is revealed as the compassionate activity that it truly is. In this compassionate life, suffering has been resolved" (Smith 2012, p. 10), and we can perceive more clearly and serve the world and others more effectively.

15.6 What about Nirvana?

Other than in Wilson's (2014) reference to the absence of Nirvana in much of the mindfulness literature, the term has received nary a mention. How might we view this seemingly important Buddhist topic from the standpoint of the perspectives presented in this chapter, a consideration of an authentic approach to Zen accessible to lay, Western practitioners?

Benoit frequently referred to satori (the Japanese Zen term for awakening or seeing one's true nature) as an ultimate Zen attainment and viewed the mindfulness practice he described, understanding and seeing through the illusory nature of self-image and dwelling in bodily experience, as a gradual, evolving form of preparation that might lead to an experience of satori, which, if it did occur, came on its own with nothing we could do to bring it about.

Jōko did not like to talk about enlightenment, nirvana, or satori because she believed that (1) people already come to Zen practice with impractical ideas of achieving a transcendental state from their ambitious spiritual practice, (2) achievement of such a state would serve as yet another self-image with a goal to attain and its accompanying requirements, and (3) even with her vast experience with experienced

Buddhist practitioners and Zen roshis, she had never met a fully enlightened person. She emphasized the value of a slow, deliberate, lifelong approach to a transformative practice rather than attaining a sudden dramatic flash of insight.

To explore this topic further, we return to Khyentse's (2007) consideration of Buddhism's four seals. You may have noticed that we have only discussed three of them. Khyentse describes the fourth seal of Buddhism as: "Nirvana is beyond concepts" (2007, p. 3). He means that enlightenment does not consist of a blissful perfect heaven that transcends normal human experience, but instead it refers to liberation from delusion. He described how the Buddha regarded as fantasies versions of nirvana as a perfect, trouble-free, heavenly afterlife (what Khyentse called "the ultimate vacation"). He also regarded the goal of perpetual happiness as an illusion. For the Buddha, nirvana does not refer to a place and certainly not one that transcends normal human life.

Tilakaratne (1993, 2010) effectively articulated this non-transcendental interpretation of nirvana as a positive healthy psychological experience characterized by freedom and an undefiled mind, rather than a metaphysical state achieved after death: "The idea of transcendence relevant to the Buddhist concept of nirvana has to be understood as referring to the moral quality of the state of mind that has realized nirvana" (1993, p. 149). The transcendence or cessation to which the concept applies refers to the end of grasping or clinging. The Buddha viewed it as release of the shackles of delusion, something that occurs right here and now in this very human life.

> Nirvana can indeed be understood as a joyful state, because having no confusion and no ignorance, no happiness and no unhappiness, is bliss…bliss is not the same as happiness. Siddhartha emphasized…the futility of seeking peace and happiness in this world or in the afterlife. (Khyentse 2007, p. 88)

Seeking peace and happiness proves futile, and eliminating our hopes brings joy and bliss. Jōko explained this paradoxical nature of the consequences of Zen practice in variety of ways, over the course of her teaching. Drawing on many of her comments and statements, I summarized and synthesized the following example, presented in the first person singular to emphasize the very personal nature of the course of a committed practice.

A very subtle, slow change occurs in the way I see my life. There comes a point when I begin to see that I just do what I do. I feel amenable to being myself "as I am." The great ambition, the enthusiasm for attainment, weakens over time, disillusionment sets in, and my drive to get something for myself fades. Not needing to get something evolves into a genuine understanding that "I am as I am," which includes firmness and determination, the intelligence to know that when I do not like something at the moment that is "who I am" and I have to experience it fully with mind and body. I do not figure this out in my head, and I cannot write it down in a paragraph; the realization soaks into my whole life.

I have responsibility for awakening, with awareness of life as it happens, which consists of what I sense: seeing, hearing, touching, tasting, and smelling. Experiencing life also means being aware of my inner world, including my thoughts, knowing that otherwise the thoughts take over, and I will have no awareness of anything real. Things are as they are, and always have been, and I see that my desire for them to be otherwise is the problem. The only thing I can do is try to see when I live life from a self-centered viewpoint. I do not expect results, because that would imply something I could fix, and I less frequently assume that anything that does not please me needs fixing.

My everyday life goes better. I feel more trust, more willingness to join the flow of life. I have less desire to push the world around to make it the way that suits me. More clarity and kindness than before, of a more genuine nature, begin to show. I emotionally react less to events and experience more openness and appreciation for everything around me. These changes look inconspicuous and subtle, not showy. Practice is simply my life. Life just flows along. When no separate "me" to defend exists, no problem exists. I do my best with what turns up.

Acknowledgment I wish to express my gratitude to Dr. Al Zolynas, Ordinary Mind Zen teacher in Escondido, California, for his helpful suggestions during the preparation of this chapter.

References

Angyal, A. (1965). *Neurosis and treatment: A holistic theory*. New York: Wiley.

Bayda, E. (2002). *Being Zen: Bringing meditation to life*. Boston: Shambhala.

Bayda, E. (2003). *At home in the muddy water: A guide to finding peace within everyday chaos*. Boston: Shambhala.

Bayda, E. (2009). *Zen heart: Simple advice for living with mindfulness and compassion*. Boston: Shambhala.

Bayda, E. (2014). *The authentic life: Zen wisdom for living free from complacency and fear*. Boston: Shambhala.

Beck, C. J. (1989). *Everyday Zen: Love and work*. San Francisco: Harper & Row.

Beck, C. J. (1993). *Nothing special: Living Zen*. San Francisco: Harper & Row.

Beck, C. J. (1996). *Some suggestions on practice*. Unpublished manuscript, Zen Center of San Diego.

Beck, C. J. (1999). *Right-here-now*. Unpublished manuscript, Zen Center of San Diego.

Benoit, H. (1984). *The supreme doctrine: Psychological encounters in Zen thought*. New York: Inner Traditions International.

Benoit, H. (2004). *The light of Zen in the west*. Portland: Sussex Academic.

Block, S. H. (2005). *Come to your senses: Demystifying the mind-body connection*. Hillsboro: Beyond Words.

de Mello, A. (1990). *Awareness*. New York: Doubleday.

Garfield, J. (1995). *The fundamental wisdom of the Middle Way*. New York: Oxford.

Guang, X. (2005). *The concept of the Buddha: Its evolution from early Buddhism to the* trikāya *theory*. New York: RoutledgeCurzon.

Guang, X. (2010). The historical Buddha: A psychological analysis. In M. G. T. Kwee (Ed.), *New horizons in Buddhist psychology: Relational Buddhism for collaborative practitioners* (pp. 53–78). Chagrin Falls: Taos Institute.

Hamilton, E. (2007). *Untrain your parrot and other no-nonsense instructions on the path of Zen*. Boston: Shambhala.

Heuman, L. (2014). The embodied mind: An interview with philosopher Evan Thompson. *Tricycle*. http://www.tricycle.com/interview/embodied-mind. Accessed 27 Oct 2014.

Horney, K. (1950). *Neurosis and human growth: The struggle toward self-realization*. New York: Norton.

Huntington, C. W. (1989). *The emptiness of emptiness: An introduction to early Indian Mādhyamika*. Honolulu: University of Hawaii.

Hurley, K. V., & Dobson, T. E. (1991). *What's my type?: Use of the enneagram system of nine personality types to discover your best self.* San Francisco: Harper.

Kalupahana, D. J. (1987). *The principles of Buddhist psychology*. Albany: State University of New York Press.

Kalupaha, D. J. (1992). A history of Buddhist philosophy: Continuities and discontinuities. Honolulu, HI: University of Hawaii Press.

Kalupahana, D. J. (2010). Miracles: An early Buddhist view. In M. G. T. Kwee (Ed.), *New horizons in Buddhist psychology: Relational Buddhism for collaborative practitioners* (pp. 173–184). Chagrin Falls: Taos Institute.

Kariyawasam, T. (2010). Omniscience: The Buddhist point of view. In M. G. T. Kwee (Ed.), *New horizons in Buddhist psychology: Relational Buddhism for collaborative practitioners* (pp. 153–171). Chagrin Falls: Taos Institute.

Keyes, M. F. (1992). *Emotions and the enneagram: Working through your shadow life script*. Muir Beach: Molysdatur.

Khyentse, D. J. (2007). *What makes you not a Buddhist*. New Delhi: Timeless.

Kwee, M. G. T. (2010). *New horizons in Buddhist psychology: Relational Buddhism for collaborative practitioners*. Chagrin Falls: Taos Institute.

Kwee, M. G. T. (2012). Relational Buddhism: Wedding K. J. Gergen's relational being and Buddhism to create harmony in-between-selves. *Psychological Studies, 57*(2), 203–210.

Luetchford, M. E. (2002). *Between heaven and earth: A translation of Nāgārjuna's Mūlamadhyamakakārikā*. Bristol: Windbell.

Magid, B. (2002). *Ordinary mind: Exploring the common ground of Zen and psychotherapy*. Boston: Wisdom.

Magid, B. (2008). *Ending the pursuit of happiness: A Zen guide*. Boston: Wisdom.

Magid, B. (2013). *Nothing is hidden: The psychology of Zen Koans*. Boston: Wisdom.

McWilliams, S. A. (2009). Interdependence, essence, and conventional reality: Middle way Buddhist and constructivist perspectives. In L. M. Lightner & J. C. Thomas (Eds.), *Personal constructivism: Theory and applications* (pp. 365–383). New York: Pace University Press.

McWilliams, S. A. (2010). Inherent self, invented self, empty self: Constructivism, Buddhism, and psychotherapy. *Counseling and Values, 55,* 79–100.

McWilliams, S. A. (2011). Contemplating a contemporary constructivist Buddhist psychology. *Journal of Constructivist Psychology, 24,* 268–276.

McWilliams, S. A. (2012). Mindfulness and extending constructivist psychotherapy integration. *Journal of Constructivist Psychology, 25*(3), 230–250.

McWilliams, S. A. (2014). Foundations of mindfulness and contemplation: Traditional and contemporary perspectives. *International Journal of Mental Health and Addiction, 12*(2), 116–128.

McWilliams, S. A. (2015). Personal construct psychology and Buddhism. In D. A. Winter & N. Reed (Eds.), *The Wiley-Blackwell handbook of personal construct psychology*. Chichester: Wiley-Blackwell.

Mikulas, W. (2007). Buddhism and western psychology: Fundamentals of integration. *Journal of Consciousness Studies, 14*(4), 4–49.

Mikulas, W. (2008). Buddhist psychology: A western interpretation. In K. R. Rao, A. Paranjpe, A. K. Dalal (Eds.), *Handbook of Indian psychology* (pp. 142–162). New Delhi: Foundation.

Mikulas, W. L. (2010). Integrating western psychology and Buddhist psychology. In M. G. T. Kwee (Ed.), *New horizons in Buddhist psychology: Relational Buddhism for collaborative practitioners* (pp. 271–287). Chagrin Falls: Taos Institute.

Naranjo, C. (1990). *Ennea-type structures: Self-analysis for the seeker*. Nevada City: Gateways/IDHHB.

Palmer, H. (1988). *The enneagram: Understanding yourself and the others in your life*. San Francisco: Harper.

Palmer, H. (1995). *The enneagram in love and work: Understanding your intimate and business relationships*. San Francisco: Harper.
Riso, D. R. (1990). *Understanding the enneagram: The practical guide to personality types*. Boston: Houghton Mifflin.
Rizzetto, D. E. (2006). *Waking up to what you do: A Zen practice for meeting every situation with intelligence and compassion*. Boston: Shambhala.
Rogers, C. R. (1951). *Client-centered therapy*. Boston: Houghton-Mifflin.
Rogers, C. R. (1959). A theory of therapy, personality, and interpersonal relationships, as developed in the client-centered framework. In S. Koch (Ed.), *Psychology: A study of a science: Vol. 3. Formulations of the person and the social context* (pp. 184–256). New York: McGraw-Hill.
Rogers, C. R. (1961). *On becoming a person*. Boston: Houghton-Mifflin.
Ronkin, N. (2009). Theravada metaphysics and ontology. In W. Edelglass & J. Garfield (Eds.), *Buddhist philosophy: Essential readings* (pp. 13–25). New York: Oxford University Press.
Shonin, E., & Van Gordon, W. (2014). Managers' experiences of meditation awareness training. *Mindfulness, 5*(4), 351–470.
Smith, E. G. (2012). *Everything is the way: Ordinary mind Zen*. Boston: Shambhala.
Tilakaratne, A. (1993). *Nirvana and ineffability: A study of the Buddhist theory of reality and language*. Colombo: Postgraduate Institute of Pali and Buddhist Studies, University of Kelaniya, Sri Lanka.
Tilakaratne, A. (2010). Nirvana of the healthy mind. In M. G. T. Kwee (Ed.), *New horizons in Buddhist psychology: Relational Buddhism for collaborative practitioners* (pp. 185–202). Chagrin Falls: Taos Institute.
Wilber, K. (1984). *Eye to eye: The quest for the new paradigm*. Garden City: Anchor.
Wilson, J. (2014). *Mindful America: The mutual transformation of Buddhist meditation and American culture*. New York: Oxford University Press.

Spencer A. McWilliams is a professor emeritus of psychology at California State University San Marcos. He earned a doctoral degree in clinical psychology from the University of Rochester, and served as the director of clinical psychology training at the University of Arizona in the 1970s. His scholarly work addresses the implications of the active role of human processes in creating phenomenal experience, with an emphasis on constructivist psychology and Buddhist psychology. He is the former president of the constructivist psychology network and a member of the editorial board of the Journal of Constructivist Psychology. He studied with Zen master Charlotte Jōko Beck from 1983 until 2011.

Chapter 16
Pristine Mindfulness: Heartfulness and Beyond

G. T. Maurits Kwee

16.1 Introduction

This chapter expands my work on Relational Buddhism which comprises Karma Transformation: conversations and meditations. It offers an alternative practice and view on "mindfulness meditation" in the context of a remodeled Buddhist teaching which is founded on ancient Greek Buddhism and pan-Buddhism whose basic tenets are congruent with what the Buddha (sixth century BCE), Nagarjuna (second century), and Asanga/Vasubandhu (fourth century) had taught. Relational Buddhism may differ from traditional accounts as it radically discards all other-worldly/metaphysical views. Thus, Relational Buddhism eschews ideas on the Buddha's divinity, deification, omniscience, transcendentalism, mysticism, authoritarianism, worship, dogma, creed, belief, magic, miracles (except the "miracle of education"), and views any such allusion as metaphoric (Kwee 2010; McWilliams 2014). It is not my intent to eliminate the long-standing traditions but bring into focus a more promising demystified alternative which suits twenty-first-century rational beings and secular societies. The objective of this chapter is to delineate the practice and theory of pristine mindfulness or "heartfulness," which follows eight states/steps. Pristine mindfulness is also called heartfulness because the experience is in essence a love affair of "me" and "self" which leads to a vanishing of the lover and the beloved.

Western fascination for *sati* by psychologists already began with William James (1842–1910), founding father of American psychology. He broke new ground by addressing the functional value of *sati* that operates in the space of "pure" (preconceptual) perception. It seems that James (1890) was aware that Buddhist meditation is not to be isolated from the whole teaching of Buddhism as he had Anagarika Dharmapala teach during one of his lectures at Harvard in 1904, on which occasion he allegedly said to the man from Sri Lanka "to take his chair." After the lecture

G. T. Maurits Kwee (✉)
Karma Transformation by Conversation & Meditation,
Teunisbloemlaan 24, 2116 TD Bentveld, The Netherlands
e-mail: mauritskwee@gmail.com

E. Shonin et al. (eds.), *Buddhist Foundations of Mindfulness*,
Mindfulness in Behavioral Health, DOI 10.1007/978-3-319-18591-0_16

(apparently on the modalities), James declared that this is the psychology everybody will be studying 25 years from then on (Sangharakshita 1964). Although this prediction did not pay off, the basic elements for a Buddhist psychology "on cognitive behavioral lines" were initiated in the vanguard work of three clinical psychologists in the past decades: Mikulas (1978), De Silva (1984), and Kwee (1990). A congress in Gothenburg, Sweden, confluencing Buddhism and cognitive behavior therapy embedded a conferential series of eight symposia was convened by this author in 2005. This event was likely the historical milestone James was talking about one century ago (Kwee et al. 2006).

Nowadays, mindfulness meditation is enjoying mushrooming interest after its inception in the medical setting in 1979 through the work of J. Kabat-Zinn in the USA. Since his introduction of an eight-week outpatient program, called mindfulness-based stress reduction (MBSR), other mindfulness-based interventions (MBIs) followed suit. Having entered the field of health care, the meditation has become a hot topic among psychologists and therapists as well as among the public at large. Kabat-Zinn (1994, p. 4) defined mindfulness as, "paying attention in a particular way: on purpose, in the present moment, and non-judgmentally." He further emphasized that his take of mindfulness is just a human capacity, thus seemingly excluding the Buddhist wisdom inherent in the practice by framing mindfulness by the Hippocratic oath (Kabat-Zinn 2009a, b) instead, rather than fairly declaring allegiance to Buddhism. Psychologists with a Buddhist background have harshly criticized this Buddhist-lite rendition at various conferences as these programs deny the undeniable Buddhist roots of mindfulness meditation (e.g., Kwee 2010, 2012a, b, 2013a, b, c; Kwee et al. 2006). Most importantly, the mindfulness-based mindfulness (e.g., Segal et al. 2002; Shapiro and Carlson 2009) isolates the training from the "12 Buddhist meditations" that embeds the Four Ennobling Realities and the Eightfold Balancing Practice. Discarding eurocentric and (post)colonial views on Buddhism, we rather speak about realities than truths. Realities in and of itself cannot be noble; nobility, like becoming an earl or a duchess, is not at stake. Viewing life and its vicissitudes via these four "Buddhist realities" ennobles/purifies the heart. Likewise, balancing and practice are more appropriate as the path is rather an equilibrating training toward a noble heart. Moreover, as a psychological approach Relational Buddhism avoids religious wording as used by the early Christian translators of Buddhism, because this will inevitably lead to a "Wittgensteinian language game" of religion. The use of secular wording provides a common ground of Relational Buddhism with the mindfulness in the MBI offering; the only difference is that in the latter case, Buddhism was (seemingly) taken out altogether prompting Buddhist watchers think of a *chutzpah*.

Fully Buddhist is pristine mindfulness, which refers to meditation training, a practice of self-compassion, love, and healing integrated in a pan-Buddhist context and which makes use of the best of all Buddhist teachings down the centuries, hence pan-Buddhism. This mindfulness, called heartfulness, is a core process for clearing the mind and a springboard to practice a family of 12 meditations (themes of awareness and attention) that include: (1) Breathing (of air passing the nostrils as an anchor for concentration); (2) Behaviors (the four dignities of sitting, standing, walking, lying, and their varieties); (3) Repulsiveness (the body is a skin bag enveloping organs, liquids, and digested food); (4) Elements (dis-identifying from disintegrating body of water, fire, earth, and wind); (5) Decomposing (the body eventually rots, stinks, and turns into bones and dust); (6) Feelings (can be positive, negative, or neutral and skin deep or heartfelt); (7) Hindrances (human pleasures, ill will, sloth, torpor, agitation, and worry); (8) Modalities (or BASIC-I *skandhas* of clinging, an acronym of Behavior–Affect–Sensation–Imagery–Cognition–Interactions); (9) Senses (eyes, ears, nose, tongue, skin, and the mind's eye); (10) Awakening (includes being analytical, forbearing, serene, enthusiastic, focused, even minded and aware); (11) the Four Ennobling Realities (there is emotional suffering which is dependently originated through greed and hatred; craving for and grasping/clinging to these states require eradication by countering ignorance and traversing a balancing path, an eightfold practice clearing ignorance, delusions, and illusions); and (12) the Eightfold Balancing Practice which aims at attaining Nirvana (extinction of disturbing emotional arousal).

This practice, comprising awareness and attention (i.e., heartfulness), forms an inseparable part of one's: (1) views (how the mind/emotions work); (2) intentions (discerning its wholesomeness vs. unwholesomeness); (3) speech (meaningful talk and self-talk); (4) actions (karmic intentional conduct and its consequences); (5) living (constructive daily life); (6) efforts (zeal, diligence, forbearance); (7) awareness (witnessing one's own sensing/feeling, thought, and action); and (8) attention (focused concentration). The self-quest investigates: Is there a balance in our "view-understanding, intention-thought, speech-communication, action-behavior, living-habitude, effort-commitment, attention-concentration, awareness-introspection?"

To be sure, heartfulness is embedded in a holistic framework, not only of the 12 meditations, but also of pan-Buddhism (comprising 15 principles endorsed in all schools and denominations of Buddhism), an effort to move toward one basic Buddhism. As an overarching process, heartfulness constitutes both the general and central factor for clearing the mind to practice these meditations, which the Buddha offered humanity as a gift of compassion some 2600 years ago. Ingrained in the Eightfold Balancing Practice, *sati* (Pali) or *smriti* (Sanskrit), the proper terms for heartfulness (and mindfulness for that matter), is a scaffold for a meditative *modus vivendi* implying the balancing of attention–concentration (meta-perception of the mind's eye) and awareness–introspection (bare attention from now to now).

16.2 On the Smallest Units of Experience (*dhammas*)

The first step in the Buddhist discipline of meditation training is the taming of the restless mind toward tranquilizing by first relaxing the body by sitting. This can be done in any position as long as the back is held in an upright posture, not slouched forward. Psychophysiological research findings suggest that holding the back and head straight strengthens confidence in the emitted thoughts, whether negative or positive (Brinol et al. 2009), and that this posture boosts positive mood, while a doubtful posture invites or worsens a dejected mood (Haruki et al. 2001). In the Buddhist discipline, this sitting is called *Jhāna*. It uses breathing as an anchor, which aims at sharpening concentration leading to immersion–absorption *(Jhāna)* in four steps (the four *jhāna*s). These steps are first *Jhāna* (one pointedness/pleasure–joy), second *Jhāna* (one pointedness/joy–happiness), third *Jhāna* (one pointedness/contentment), and fourth *Jhāna* (one pointedness/equanimity–stillness). One-pointed concentration is a run up to fully developed *sati* and to awakening in emptiness: An experience prompted by the insight and understanding that the ever-changing nature of impermanence regarding the experience of things, persons, and self implies a pervasive and omnipresent emptiness at the ultimate level of reality.

Pristine mindfulness fine-tunes attention–concentration (to discipline a wandering mind) and awareness–introspection (to understand karma as intentional action and not-self). It operates through the mind's eye in sensorium and refers to the process and outcome, and it is a tool that enables seeing and experiencing emptiness as an ultimate reality and inner liberation. The mind's eye is the sixth perceptual organ discerned by the Buddha which is inferred here as the neuroplastic brain with infinite synaptic interconnections which is able to perceive and integrate internal stimuli. Pristine mindfulness can be a process (perceiving and observing) or an outcome (being consciously aware). It is an inward or outward concentration of attention (swiftly changeable foreground presence) and introspective awareness (slowly changeable backdrop presence), which illuminate consciousness (constant backdrop presence in wakeful states) and enable the alert monitoring and luminous comprehending of *dhammas,* a technical term which refers to the smallest units of BASIC-I experience, that is, the arising and subsiding of emotion, cognition, and action in dependent origination *(pratitycasamutpada).*

A major factor in the Buddhist training toward awakening to karma, emptiness, and not-self, the Buddha ascribed *sati* a central place in his *dhamma* as designated in the *Mahasatipatthana Sutta* and the *Satipatthana Sutta* on the four frames of reference of *sati.* These frames are (1) the body (i.e., action and feelings: sensations and emotions), (2) the body's behaviors (i.e., motions of internal/external physique), (3) the mind (i.e., thinking: visualizing imagery and conceiving cognition, and (4) the mind's behaviors (i.e., motions of images and cognition). The first six meditations refer to mindfulness of the body and bodily feelings and the second six to mindfulness of the mind and brainy thoughts. Inseparably belonging to the Buddha's liberating system of ceasing *duhkha,* these exercises comprise the 12 themes summarized previously. There are many more meditations. Well known are the *Brahmaviharas:* contemplations on loving kindness, empathic compassion, sympathetic joy, and relational equanimity. Because the Buddhist teachings imply a *modus vivendi,* life is preferably spent in a meditative way. Informal meditative exercises can be done on all simple daily experiencing, like looking, watching, laughing, smiling, singing, drinking, eating, chewing, savoring, or silencing.

The body/speech/mind connection requires some explanation. The Buddha had a tripartite view, which includes life's social aspect—speech; thus, body/speech/mind. Put in this order, it reflects that the mind is constructed through speech and inter-mind, which was prior to the individual mind. The Buddhist proposition is that mind's activity involves speech through language in talk with others and that it emits self-speech or self-talk. The mind's voices are in a continuing dialogue with significant others even though these persons are not physically present. Viewed this

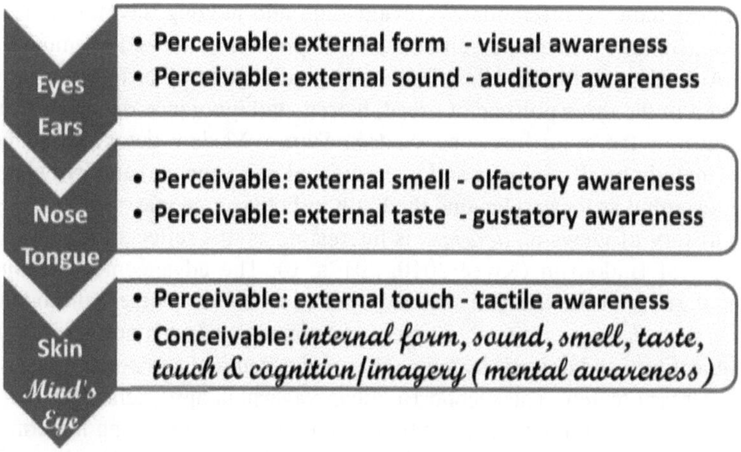

Fig. 16.1 The Buddha's sixth sense or the mind's eye able to be aware and attentive to anything conceivable based on what is perceived (externally and internally)

way, one is never alone and indeed constantly together with self in conversation internally with others. Hence, the term inter-mind (or inter-self) rather than (the single) mind is used here to emphasize the psychology of mind's interconnectedness in life. Inter-mind leaves the meaning of mind as in the perceptual function of the mind's eye unimpeded as inter-mind includes the single minds of individuals.

In order to fully understand pristine mindfulness, it is imperative to comprehend the mind's eye with the brain as the "eye organ" (see Fig. 16.1). The mind's eye is able to apperceive what takes place in a split of a second, post-perceptual but preconceptual. Thus, apperception is a preconceptual perception that excludes preconceived ideas, which are by definition conceptual and judgmental. Nonetheless puzzling, this sixth sense, usually translated as "mind" is not something metaphysical as it functions within the sensory modality. Still, mind sounds "airy" and does not parallel the other "fleshy" organs: eyes, ears, nose, tongue, and skin. Nowhere in the literature can an account for this sense be found (Austin 2010).

What is the mind's eye? Could the Buddha's sixth sense be the brain as an organ able to scan *dharmas*, which come about in dependent origination of body/speech/mind, that is, the modalities of feeling (sensation–affect/emotion), thinking (cognition–imagery/thinking), and doing (behavior/conduct–action) in interaction with others? Thus, the acronym BASIC-I of clinging is formed. The mind's eye notices what is experienced, which encompasses what is innovatively called "perceivables" varying from neutral sensations to charged emotions. They comprise the visualization of perceived external input and the immediate experience in body/feelings linked to the object (*nimitta*; Kuan 2012) in combination with knowables, like conceivables or thinkables. These are internal events comprising the cognitions, which are covert and appear in the mind and experienced as thinking (*sanna*; Kuan 2012). Indeed, gray matter is able to integrate perceptions of external as well as internal stimuli that might contain everything that is conceivable or thinkable and imaginable, which include memories, dreams, illusions, and delusions. In essence, pristine mindfulness aims at differentiating, evaluating, and judging unwholesome versus wholesome *dharmas* in the pursuit of karmic happiness or the end of emotional suffering. According to the Buddha, the human predicament of suffering is relational and rooted in the three poisons of greed, hatred, and ignorance/delusions–illusions regarding how the mind functions *(Sedaka Sutta).* Wisdom detoxifies by healing speech (including self-dialogue and interpersonal performance) and by being heedful of inter-mind as located beyond the brain in-between people.

The history of views on *dharmas* is interesting as this reflects the scholarly development of Buddhism (Kwee 2010, 2012a, b). The advancement of Buddhist thought starts with the Buddha who expounded in his discourses (throughout the *Nikayas*) that *dharmas* are neither empty nor not empty. In his non-theistic middle way, subjectivity and objectivity are neither real nor unreal and not-self is basic and complementary to self. The second Buddha, Nagarjuna approached the emptiness of *dharmas* as something that is empty of emptiness: ever-changing impermanence implies emptiness. Subjectivity and objectivity are both unreal due to the total emptiness of self. Thus, he spoke about nonself of everything rather than the not-self of persons. His comments on the perfection of wisdom sutras *(Prajnaparamita Sutras)* is a *via negativa* which negates the selfness of things ad infinitum. Nonetheless, one might consider his philosophical "emptiness of emptiness of emptiness" as still somethingness. This insight was taken up by Vasubandhu who countered with a *via positiva,* an antithesis which views *dharmas* as empty of duality, thus as non-dual experiences. Subjective inner experiences are real, but empty, while objective things are considered to be unreal and also empty. It is therefore sanctioned to fill them with empty projections. His commentaries on the Buddha Womb sutras *(Samdhinirmocana Sutras)* make the proliferation of Mahayana cosmology, which is basically empty, understandable as skillful means *(upayakaushalya)* of Buddhism's reaching out to cater the masses and quench their thirst for the beyond. The reverse is now happening in the contemporary world where a call for secularity and scientific evidence can be loudly heard.

One might ask whether other approaches to the emptiness experience is possible. Social constructionism as championed by Gergen (2009a, b) posits that things are empty of transcendental truths as experiences are fed by meanings that are only valid in relational context, social groups, and communities. Subjective and objective experiences are only real as social constructions. Having discovered social constructionism, and its striking correspondence with the Dharma, a dilemma arises whether to take the bold step to involve it or not? The quest resulted in postulating a daring confluence of a traditional teaching and a postmodern psychology that was coined Relational Buddhism.

In effect, the merging of ideas meandered in a meta-vision which views reality from a relational perspective and which proposes *dharmas* as "ontologically-mute-social-constructions-empty-of-Transcendental-Truths." Moreover, thinking is a relational activity executed as covert–private verbalized/visualized speech. This relational stance has lead to the co-creation of inter-mind as *interdependent being in between selves* and of a non-foundational morality of collaborative action, which renders a team spirit for humanity with congenial bonds as lifeline. To paraphrase

Gergen (2009a, b), truth and morality can only be found within community; beyond community, there is silence. Thus, the practice of mindfulness toward emptiness is enriched by a fourth exercise, a postmodern provision which likely deepens the experience of *dharmas* as empty social constructions comprising empty perceivables and knowables and recognizes their illusory and delusional qualities. Entering the Western world, Buddhism is in dire need for scholarly innovation. Relational Buddhism functions as a nexus for integrating the views of Theravada, Mahayana, psychology/therapy, and social constructionism.

16.3 Heartfulness: Mindfulness in Relational Perspective

While *sati* has traditionally been viewed as individually bound, the present view transcends this understanding by adopting a relational perspective to this seemingly solipsistic exercise. Many practitioners' first encounter with meditation is to do it the *Bodhidharma* way by sitting in front of a wall. Grappling with the meaning of sitting alone (with self), the question arises whether this suggests that one cuts oneself off from the world in solitary confinement. Is total isolation feasible and desirable on the road to awakening (toward realizing not-self)?

From a Chinese Mahayana perspective, the term mindfulness as a translation of *sati,* feels like a misnomer as the "strifeless striving" is toward being "mind empty" and "full of heart" while remembering to be constantly watchful in full attention and awareness on whatever appears in the stream of body/speech/mind consciousness, in order to awaken. Although the term *sati* is preferred, the term mindfulness will be maintained because of its vested usage. For those who prefer to see the mind located in interconnected loving hearts (like in the Chinese term *nian*) heartfulness is a more appropriate designation to reflect the practice ("lovefulness" might be an alternative translation for it is about loving self via buddhanature toward a buddha-within/not-self). In the Buddhist languages of Asia, mind accounts for the emotional realm as affect feels like inhabiting the heart. The heart as a location of mind is not an outlandish idea if one considers how love and infatuation are experienced and depicted in European culture. Hence, heartfulness is an appealing alternative and the more so because it associates with a resonating heart rather than mind (*Vimalakirtinirdesa Sutra*). The notion that mind is located in the heart implies that it is "neither within nor without, nor is it to be apprehended between the two" (*Vimalakirtinirdesa Sutra*). As in the *Gandhavyuha Sutra,* mind is not locked up between the ears but operates as interdependent mind in-between people, which is equivalent to inter-mind, the main proposition of Relational Buddhism.

Heartfulness is a general factor sustaining meditation, including concentration and contemplation toward wholesome intentional action (karma), which at any initial time works like a metonym. This implies that there is no grand aim to pursue at the start of the exercise: What one does in the moment is means and goal at the same time. During heartfulness, one perceives sensory experience by an effortless effort of a beginner's mind with no aim and no gain. Thus, there is no way to mindfulness, mindfulness is the way, which is realizing that we are not going anywhere for we are already there; therefore, nothing needs to be done: the grass will grow by itself. The relational practice of pristine mindfulness as heartfulness refers to cultivating (affective) memory not to forget to neutrally focus, observe, or note every moment to guard or protect against unwholesomeness, to introspect, to inquire intelligently, and to form wholesome karma in relational (intrapersonal and interpersonal) context (Kuan 2012; Kwee 2013c). The chapter title "Heartfulness and Beyond" refers to a karmic metaphorical "law of magic": Cause is effect and effect is cause in a chain of causality; thus, a seed accrues a tree and a tree ensues seeds. Hence, the advice abounds: If effect is cause, create the effect. In daily life: Be genuinely happy and luck will follow suit (Kwee 2013a).

Aiming no less than the accomplishment of *Buddhahood,* pristine mindfulness is presented here in contrast with the Buddhist-lite mindfulness, which has progressively imbued the psychological literature in the past decades. The present comprehension of heartfulness is constructed on the pillars erected by the Buddha, Nagarjuna, Vasubandhu, Chan/Zen, and Relational Buddhism. Based on these integrating views and grounded in almost a half century of exercise in encountering *dharmas*, I came to the following differentiation of two phases, four stages, and eight states of awareness and attention cultivation. The cyclical spans are based on psychological understanding and (relational) insights regarding heartfulness. Even though cycles suggest strict categories, the phases, stages, and states do have some overlap as they are not static terms, but fluid processes of discernible but inseparable stretches. Table 16.1 encapsulates the two phases (A and B), four stages (I–IV) and eight states (1–8) .

In Mahayana terms, phase A (stages I and II, states 1–4) is a gradual journey of absolute *bodhicitta,* the spirit of heartfelt diligence to awaken along introvert experiences which traverse a process of socially deconstructing self via insight and understanding (or aha experiences) while sitting in front of a wall in order to gain

Table 16.1 Pristine mindfulness in four stages and eight states/steps

Context: the Eightfold Balancing Practice	Attention Verbal/speech (description)	Awareness Nonverbal/no speech (acquaintance)
Stage I (gradual) Heedfulness of a one-point concentration with zeal and diligence(*appamada* /vigilance)	1 *Samatha* targets calm and tranquillizing (serenity)	2 *Samadhi* targets flame extinction: *Nirvana* (flow)
Stage II (gradual) Wise reflection: aims at wholesome karmic action (*yoniso manasikara*/focusing)	3 *Vipassana:* insight in Dependent Origination (The Buddha)	4 *Sunyata* as wisdom of nonself/emptiness (Nagarjuna)
Stage III (sudden) Wisdom through an alert and clear comprehension (*sampajanna*/spying)	5 *Non-duality* of subject–object/ emptiness–form (Vasubandhu)	6 *Kill the Buddha:* the last of hindrances (Chan/Zen)
Stage IV (sudden) Accomplishing benevolence of Inter-being (*antaratman*/inter-mind)	7 *Brahmaviharas:* social meditations-in-action (Mahayana)	8 *dharmas*: empty social constructions (Relational Buddhism)

full insight into self's emptiness (*anatman*). Balancing and fine-tuning heartfulness during stage I, the student, in watching and witnessing, develops the composure of self-control by calm tranquillizing and stress-free/undisturbed serenity amid adversity (*Samatha*), leading to Nirvana (the extinction of emotional arousal flames which is a momentary state that might become an enduring trait) via a stable/firm concentrative but gentle focus, receptive immersion/absorption of the object and non-suppressing quiescence during the activity which could be any. This state is also known as flow or the zone (*Samadhi*), being one with ever-changing impermanence and emptiness. Having thus tamed emotional afflictions, the practice advances into cleansing the doors of perception enabling the seeing of things as they are. This introspective insight comes about by remembering to be heedful regarding the unwholesomeness/wholesomeness of karma. Speech, thought, and self-dialogue arise toward insight in the dependent origination of body/speech/mind and karma (*Vipassana*) leading to the highest wisdom of *Sunyata* (not-self/emptiness), a state of luminous suchness or vast zeroness, a reset point in the total absence of emotional flames and the pinnacle of self-inquiry. The witness disappears in oblivion and emptiness.

Shifting to phase B (stages III and IV, states 5–8), a deepening of phase I, one is ready for sudden insight when travelling in relative *bodhicitta*, the dedication to awaken along extravert or joyful haha experiences which reflect a process of (re) constructing inter-mind via delightful affect while fully functioning in the marketplace. Inter-mind is depicted as Indra's net in the *Gandavyuha Sutra;* this is a jewel net with a gem at each crossing which reflects every other gem mirroring infinite interpenetration. Emptiness is deepened by practicing and experiencing the silencing state of non-duality (i.e., *mahamudra*) which transcends and eradicates Yin–Yang dualities created by speech, language, and inhering concepts (Dunne 2011). Thus, cause = effect, emptiness = form, beginning = end, left = right, up = down, heaven = hell, beautiful = ugly, good = bad, yes = no, and so on, which usually culminates in a mind-expanding humor.

In this non-dual spirit, *Kill the Buddha* is a Chan anarchistic practical instruction of the genius Lin-chi (died 866) who eradicated awakening–hindering concepts like "the Buddha" and progress-impeding dependency. The Buddha often used Brahmanistic terms like *Brahmaviharas* to which he alluded a different meaning. Thus, for Buddhists the term is a metaphor for sublime places of benevolent dwelling in one's heart that embodies kindness, compassion, joy, and equanimity. Many more exercises boosting positive affect can be practiced, for example, mirth-laughing, joy-smiling, delight-singing, savoring-eating, and so on. These meditations in action are applied most solidly post emptiness. Lastly, there is the experiencing of *dharmas* as neither empty nor not empty, empty of emptiness, empty non-duality, and as ontologically mute social constructions empty of Transcendental Truths. Thus, telescoping and encountering *dharmas* in inner galaxies, insight dawns that things and thoughts are empty on the ultimate level and socially constructed on the provisional level. The whole process is a track of social deconstruction. Point zero of emptiness is not a goal in itself. A blank mind is a resetting or rebooting point and a scaffold for jumpstarting the collaborative practice of social reconstruction via joyful experience while fully functioning in the marketplace in the pivotal tenor of what we already are: inter-mind/inter-self. As Dogen (1200–1253) said:

> To study Buddhism is to study the self, to study the self is to forget the self, to forget the self is to be one with others and be able to help others.

Each stage requires a particular mental investment. The four phases and eight states require in stage I of gradual progress during the heartfulness states 1 and 2: heedfulness of a one-point concentration with zeal, diligence, and vigilance (*appamada*) while training toward Nirvana (emotional flame extinction). Note that states 1 and 2 parallel the four *jhāna*s discussed earlier as these *jhāna*s also result in immersion and absorption, thus to Nirvana; they are equivalent to the Buddhist-lite mindfulness-based approaches. Understandably and as a matter of course, heartfulness continues in the remaining stages II, III, and IV. Stage II of gradual progress during states 3 and 4 requires wise reflection on karma and dependent origination (including the functional links of BASIC-I, i.e., *pathanas*), while focusing (*yoniso manasikara*) toward the highest wisdom: the emptiness of self. Stage III provides sudden experiences of insight during states 5 and 6: an alert and clear comprehension while working toward autonomy (freedom of dependency) by non-clinging to the last hindrance, the Buddha concept by spying (*sampajanna*) or witnessing and by understanding the *dharma's* Tao of Yin–Yang, the non-dual nature of things and thoughts. Stage IV provides sudden experiences of insight during states 7 and 8 by accomplishing benevolence toward understanding inter-mind, mind in-between selves (*antaratman*), while exercising and applying kindness, compassion, joy, and equanimity, based on a deep understanding of the empty nature of *dharma's* reality as a social construction (Kwee 2013a, b, c).

The eight states or steps specify as follows:

1. *Samatha*: a stress-free serenity amid adversity state subsequent to the 12 meditations and preceded by concentration and immersion of the *jhāna*s, and consecutive calming as a basis for serenity during sensing, perceiving, and metacognizing. Apex is absorption (neither perception nor non-perception), taught to the Bodhisattva Gautama by gurus Kalama and Ramaputta at the start of his quest.
2. *Samadhi*: a deep concentrative awareness state quenching all flames of emotional arousal, that is, Nirvana, experienced in firm focus/receptive absorption (also in action, for instance, when painting, making music, or writing) called flow in psychology (Csikszentmihalyi 1990). As a child, Siddharta spontaneously slipped into a state of flow while focusing on a plow pulled by an ox.
3. *Vipasanna*: a state of insight on emotions. The mind and karma works in dependent origination, a process which refers to body/speech/mind: feeling, thinking, behaving, and interacting, BASIC-I modalities of karmic clinging which arise/subside in conjunction, while feeling greed (or underlying fear of loss or sadness of the lost) or hatred (or underlying other-hate/aggression or self-hate/depression).
4. *Sunyata*: a state of emptiness, a reset/reboot point after discerning–cleansing unwholesomeness and constituting the highest wisdom as opposed to believing

in a god, metaphysics or supernatural powers, which would imply the end of seeking self and self-inquiry, and missing the Buddhist wisdom on emptiness, not-self, and the nonself nature of things.

5. *Yogacara's* non-duality (*advaya*) is a state requiring heartfulness of speech and self-speech, which inheres in dualities as a trap. The practice transcends cyclical (*samsaric*) suffering and Nirvana.
6. "If you meet The Buddha on the road, kill him" is an expression by Chan master Lin-chi whose anarchistic/iconoclastic genius is still impressive for those who are eradicating binding concepts in favor of the freedom of emptiness by insight and understanding. As the Buddha is already dead, liquidation alludes to the hampering, progress-impeding psychological dependency on a guru.
7. *Brahmaviharas*: This refers to values that the Buddha and Buddhists revere. It does not mean a residence where the gods dwell literally, thus not some other-worldly place, but a this-worldly heartfelt heaven or paradise inhabited by the affect of loving kindness, empathic compassion, shared joy, and meditative equanimity. These metaphoric sublime feelings are to be immeasurably multiplied.
8. The *dharmas: dharma* is a scholastic term for the smallest unit of experience and is conceivable as neither empty nor not empty (the Buddha), empty of emptiness (Nagarjuna), and empty non-duality (Vasubandhu). It is here now fathomed as ontologically mute social construction empty of transcendental truths (Relational Buddhism).

Transitional conditions or feeling states might transform over time into relative stable personality traits. Note that the mindfulness-based Buddhist-lite approach only covers the first two states, which do not deal with self/not-self and preserves the illusion of self, which pristine mindfulness aims to dispel.

16.4 Contrasting Buddhist-lite and Pristine Mindfulness

Reviewing the literature leads to the conclusion that the salubrious outcome evidence of the Buddhist-lite MBI approaches are limited to the four *jhāna*s and heartfulness: the first two states of stress-free serenity (*Shamatha*) and concentrative absorption (Samadhi) leading to a state of Nirvana. The *Bahiya Sutta* includes an instruction toward *Samadhi* by the Buddha in a seemingly urgent situation. Bahiya was a man who was stressed, hurried, and was apparently going to die. It reads as follows:

> Bahiya, in the seen, there is only the seen, in the heard, there is only the heard, in the sensed, there is only the sensed, in the cognized, there is only the cognized. Thus you should see that indeed there is no thing here; this Bahiya is how you should train yourself. Since Bahiya there is for you in the seen, only the seen, in the heard, only the heard, in the sensed, only the sensed, in the cognized, only the cognized, and you see that there is no thing here, you will therefore see that indeed there is no thing there. As you see that there is no thing there, you will see that you are therefore located neither in the world of this, nor in the world of that, nor in any place betwixt the two. This alone is the end of suffering. (Udāna, 1.10)

Compared to Buddhist-lite mindfulness, pristine mindfulness offers a practice that inherently includes a judgmental aspect *(vikappa)* by differentiating and cultivating beneficial karma. Pristine mindfulness offers a practice that explicitly includes judgment as an inherent part of the exercise by discerning wholesome and unwholesome karma and cultivating beneficial karma as an inseparable part of training. In a book from circa 150 BCE, the paracanonical *Milindapanha,* The Questions of King Menandros (an ancient Greek king of the Indo-Greek kingdom who reigned in 155–130 BCE), the rationale of *sati* is presented. This work reports on a Socratic dialogue between King Menandros and the Hermit Nagasena comprising 304 questions and answers. *Basileos Soteros Menandrou* of Taxila (stretching from Afghanistan to Northern Pakistan and India) was called Dharma follower. After him, 27 Indo-Greek kings were all (but one) Buddhist until the demise of the kingdom in about the year 0 (http://en.wikipedia.org/wiki/Indo-Greek_Kingdom) at about the same time when ancient Greece in the West was taken over by the Romans. Take note of the following passage (as, e.g., in www.sacred-texts.com/bud/milinda.htm):

> What, Nagasena, is the characteristic mark of mindfulness? Noting and keeping in mind: as mindfulness springs up in the mind of the recluse, he repeatedly notes the wholesome and unwholesome, blameless and blameworthy, insignificant and important, dark and light qualities and those that resemble them thinking…
> How is keeping in mind a mark of mindfulness? As mindfulness springs up in the mind, he searches out the categories of good qualities and their opposites thinking, "Such and such qualities are beneficial and such are harmful." Thus does he make what is unwholesome in himself disappear and maintain what is good (takes possession of it)…

Besides being part and parcel of the 12 meditations and the Eightfold Balancing Practice, *sati* was also pointed at as a factor, out of seven factors, which are conducive for awakening (*bojjhanga*). This practice is indicated as a chord holding awareness and attention in place, that is, it corrects distraction and guards against the intrusion of unwholesome thoughts. This involves a distinctive capacity of what is wholesome and unwholesome, and the retention of what is beneficial and what is not in the pursuit of salubrious karma. The purpose is then to remove the unhelpful thoughts/feelings/actions and to retain the helpful thoughts/feelings/actions. Although *sati* starts in bare attention (Gunaratana 1992) and with a choiceless of awareness (Krishnamurti, 1895–1986) as in the first two states of pristine mindfulness, it is clearly not nonjudgmental. A choiceless awareness implies that there is no prejudice, sympathy, or antipathy for what appears in the spaces of body/speech/mind while apperceiving *dharmas*. Being nonjudgmental is confined initially when the trainee learns to respond rather than react automatically. The key is that one learns to see a thought or feeling as a thought or feeling, which is a distancing and dis-attaching leading to, for example, stopping to believe in the content of self-sabotaging thoughts (e.g., Segal et al. 2002). From a Buddhist perspective, these arguments make Kabat-Zinn's (2003a, p. 145) phrase "the awareness that emerges through paying attention on purpose, in the present moment, and non-judgmentally to the unfolding of experience, moment to moment" a training comprising "attention," "on purpose," "present moment," and "nonjudgmentally" a constrained exercise, that is, partly valid and incomplete vis-à-vis *sati*. Besides, the Buddhist purpose of *sati* is the end of suffering by awakening to emptiness; however, it is not clear what "on purpose" exactly means in Kabat-Zinn's phrase. It does seem to refer to the purpose of health and healing, but not to awakening and not-self/nonself in the Buddhist sense. For Buddhist practitioners who aim for the end of suffering by *sati* and a complete understanding of the *dharma,* the Buddhist-lite definition seems ill-founded.

Contrasting Buddhist-lite and pristine mindfulness further, the latter practice does not forget to be judgmental as the training in presence of mind, that is, not being absentminded, regards the most central notion of Buddhism: the formation of karmic intentional action. Body/speech/mind is judged vis-à-vis virtuousness in present and future intentions and actions. The grappling question what is meant by nonjudgmental in the MBI was also noted by Gethin (2011, p. 273), who aptly remarked: "Yet…an unqualified emphasis on mindfulness as 'non-judgmental' might be seen as implying that being nonjudgmental is an end in itself and that all states of mind are somehow of equal value, that greed is as good as non-attachment, or anger as friendliness." Furthermore, he surmised: "Yet…by saying that although—or precisely because—the aim is to rid ourselves of greed, hatred and delusion, getting angry with and hating our own greed, hatred and delusion when they arise, or conversely, becoming pleased with and attached to our own nonattachment, friendliness and wisdom when they arise, is clearly something of a trap. And it is perhaps precisely this kind of practical approach that…[is] intended to highlight by characterizing mindfulness as 'non-judgmental'" (p. 274).

However, this conjecture seems far-fetched as many aspects of the full-fledged Buddhist mindfulness/heartfulness effort as reviewed above are neglected or purposefully not included for political reasons to get it accepted in a non-receptive world of physicians where it was initially presented. Reinstalling the full meaning of *sati* seems to be a logical step now that the times are changing. Mind that Buddhist-lite mindfulness does not cover insight in the dependent origination of karma, neither does it include an understanding of not-self/emptiness. Kabat-Zinn (2011, p. 19) noted that, "Non-judgmental does not mean to imply to the novice practitioner that there is some ideal state in which judgments no longer arise. Rather, it points out that there will be many many judgments and opinions arising from moment to moment, but that we do not have to judge or evaluate or react to any of what arises, other than perhaps recognizing it in the moment of arising as pleasant, unpleasant, or neutral…"

Moreover, the Buddhist-lite MBIs do not take a relational perspective into account. Ever since the Buddha's time, there have been several conceptualizations of and approaches to the practice of *sati.* According to the *Sedaka Sutta,* the Buddha expounded a relational perspective on *sati* that evolved onto a Mahayana variant of realizing inter-mind (*Gandhavyuha Sutra*). This discourse addresses the relational aspect of mindfulness by narrating a simile on two balancing acrobats: a master acrobat and his young female apprentice. Their act is that the man holds a bamboo pole on which the girl climbs via his shoulder. While she climbs the man says: "you watch me, while I watch you, and thus we will both be safe." Her response: "No, master it is better if I watch myself and you watch you and by watching ourselves we protect each other; that's the safest way to show our act." The clue of this story is that we practice *sati* in order to protect each other and that being older or a master or famous does not necessarily mean being wise. Analayo (2003) corroborated the point that *sati* is a way to protect oneself and protect others. This reciprocal process will eventually be beneficial for human relationships and the society at large.

Much different from Buddhist-lite mindfulness, confined to an individual view, pristine mindfulness' relational perspective encompasses a social psychology. Buddhism not only deals with processes of how people perceive, imagine, conceive, feel, emote, behave, but equally so with how we relate and live with each other. Unlike most psychologies which consider the mind located and confined in the brain, pristine mindfulness endorses a psychology of Relational Buddhism which views mind as originated in-between people, that is, as located outside rather than inside the skull. It deals with karma as intentional interactivity and with inter-mind/inter-self rather than with mind/self. Based on the psychology of social construction, Relational Buddhism states that mind is not only lurking behind the eyeballs and locked up between the ears, but operates foremost between people. The basic idea of Relational Buddhism is that human beings live in an ocean of relationships from the cradle to the grave. Born into a space of linguistic meanings in-between selves, inter-mind denounces the delusion of sinful souls and the illusion of bounded self cut off from others. Post parental lustful intercourse (*kamadathu*), sensing–emoting/thinking–talking capability is embodied. Speech is formed by the syllable (*mantra*) during meaning-making exchange (*rupadathu*). As "languaging" progresses, formless thoughts transform into fickle mind (*arupadathu*) and self-organize illusory independent self that fails to see inseparable selves spaced in-between people embedded in culture (*Gandavyuha Sutra*).

In order to cultivate gluing relationships in-between minds, it is helpful to apprehend the Buddha's view that everyone is embedded in a network of interconnected relationships (*Sigalovada Sutta*). Using a compass metaphor, there are six relational types each of which requires specific responsibilities and complementary conduct (kids/parents-East, siblings/friends-North, partner/spouse-West, teacher/student-South, disciple/guru-Upward, employee/employer-Downward). This template offers guidance to find the way in defining stances in relationships whose balance and harmony depend on *how* you say things rather than *what*. It is therefore pivotal to soak speech in vernacular reflecting interpersonal significance of "binding we" in full understanding of our human condition which is "relational being in dependent origination" (cf. Gergen 2009b). As a Buddhist practice, pristine mindfulness also deals with the three poisons that arise in interpersonal context. The human predicament is rooted in greed, hatred, and ignorance on how the mind works. Its realization corrects the illusion of self/soul and cures the delusion of the metaphysics of god(s) and the supernatural. The psychology of greed inheres in the fear/anxiety about losing a loved object and the sadness/grief for having lost a loved object. The psychology of hatred inheres in the anger toward oneself leading to depression and the anger toward someone that might lead to aggression. By lifting the karmic causes of these self-sabotaging emotions, one is liberated to freely move toward the *Brahmaviharas* (*Brahmavihara Sutta*).

Thus, seven relational scenarios of basic emotions are discerned: depression, fear, anger, sadness, joy, love, and silence–serenity–emptiness. In effect, "I am linked, therefore I am" (Gergen): to be is to be related or inter-be and to act is to interact. Intelligible thinking is relational activity executed as covert verbalized or visualized speech much in the same vein that emotions are relational scenarios according to the culture one lives by. Thus, the karmic result of intentional action, which usually appears unbeknownst, affects body/speech/mind. Embedded in a web of interpersonal relationships, the individual's psychological malaise cannot but inhere in relational meaning. *Duhkha,* the whole gamut of emotional suffering and dissatisfaction linked to birth, aging, illness, and death is interpersonal. They are relational performances of affect, creative scenarios expressing sociocultural meaning. Meaning is anchored in speech, a prime interest in Relational Buddhism and pristine mindfulness. Speech is the shared common ground in the pursuit of the real, the rational, and the good. It submits that anything conceivable is an interpretation emanating from a particular social group or community that owes intelligibility to sociocultural values. In other words: There is no reality unless the majority agrees on its truthfulness.

In search for meaning, Relational Buddhism leans on Wittgenstein's heritage regarding the relationship between speech/language and reality. Referring to metaphysical questions, Wittgenstein (1922, p. 90) came up with the proposition, "Whereof one cannot speak, thereof one must be silent," which sounds Buddhist. In the human sciences, where absolute synonymy between words and objects does not exist, reality can only be approached, not exacted. Therefore, there are no unilateral definitions of rationality or goodness. A definition is only valid in a particular context and in certain circumstances and societies. Speech reflects interconnectedness and is effective whenever people of the same language group understand each other. In order to secure sane interaction and healthy interrelatedness, one is heedful of intelligible speech. Meaning and reality are social constructions that come about through communal use.

If pristine mindfulness is a psychological experience, Nirvana is not a paradise beyond, a destiny for reincarnation of the soul, but a psychological (re)birth of liberation on the level of affect after extinguishing negative emotions. To arrive at this level, one empties from self by un-defiling, un-afflicting, and un-fermenting unwholesome karma of I–me–mine/self or ego. The psychological inference of karma as intentional interaction reflects a secular view that does not refer to retribution or tallying good and evil deeds. Rather than using ethical terms like god or devil, which mold the user into a religious blueprint, the terms wholesome and unwholesome, which might differ from person to person, are preferred to qualify and judge the type of karma pursued in *sati*. What is more, karma is considered not located in the head separated from others but as embodied action born in relationship and in dependent origination with thought/reason, feeling/emotion, and volition/motivation. Few are prepared for such wrenching dislocation, but for the practitioner of pristine mindfulness the horizons are exciting. The acumen of pristine mindfulness depends on clinical and relational experience based on a demystified and metaphorical but secular interpretation of Buddhism.

16.5 Mindfulness-Based Approaches: A Critical–Constructive Review

MBIs have become a hot topic among health-care workers who base their work on empirical evidence (Didonna 2009). The prototype is MBSR, an 8-week outpatient intensive course, comprising body scan visualization, hatha yoga, sitting, walking, CD-guided homework, and self-monitored practice. This practice has sparked hype among adherents who have developed similar programs like mindfulness-based cognitive therapy (MBCT), mindfulness-based relapse prevention, and mindfulness-based eating awareness training. For instance, MBCT is effective in preventing relapse into depression for up to 60 weeks for those who have suffered three or more depressive episodes (Kenny and Williams 2007; Ma and Teasdale 2004) and could reduce the use of antidepressant maintenance medication (Kuyken et al. 2008). Shown to be more effective than a waiting list or treatment as usual control group in heterogeneous samples, MBIs meet the American Psychological Association's designation as probably efficacious (Baer 2003; Grossman et al. 2004; Shigaki et al. 2006) and the National Institute for Clinical Excellence approval for its use in the National Health Service in the UK. Since 2004, it is indicated by the British National Health Service for depression and as a prophylaxis against stress, anxiety, and depression.

Studies of what might be the mechanisms of action of mindfulness-based mindfulness have mushroomed. Despite promising results, suggesting the intervention is beneficial for treating psychological and physical disorders, the findings are inconclusive. For example, in a review of 15 controlled studies, Toneatto and Nguyen (2007) found that MBSR does not have a reliable effect on clinical symptoms of anxiety and depression. It seems to me that the state of the art of MBIs is statistically efficacious rather than clinically effective. The jury is still out.

One systematic review and meta-analysis of the effects of MBCT was based on six randomized controlled trials, with a total of 593 participants (Piet and Hougaard 2011). Compared to treatment as usual or placebo controls, MBCT significantly reduced the risk of relapse with a risk ratio of 0.66, corresponding to a relative risk reduction of 34 %. Participants with three or more previous episodes had a relative risk reduction of 43 %. There was no risk reduction for participants with only two episodes. In two studies, the intervention was at least as effective as maintenance antidepressant medication. Thus, the results indicated that MBCT is an effective intervention for relapse prevention in patients with recurrent major depressive disorders in remission with three or more previous depressive episodes. This finding was substantiated in a more recent meta-analysis by Khoury et al. (2013) who reported that MBIs are effective for a variety of psychological problems and especially for reducing anxiety, depression, and stress.

In the most recent meta-analysis of 47 MBI studies (Goyal et al. 2014), randomized clinical trials with active controls for placebo effects were graded in terms of the strength of evidence based on effect sizes. MBIs had moderate evidence of improved anxiety (effect size = 0.38 at 8 weeks; 0.22 at 3–6 months), depression

(0.30 at 8 weeks and 0.23 at 3–6 months), and pain (0.33), with low evidence of improved stress and mental health-related quality of life. There was low evidence (no effect or insufficient evidence of any effect) of these programs on mood, attention, substance use, eating habits, sleep, and weight. The authors conclude that there was "insufficient evidence of any effect of meditation programs on positive mood, attention, substance use, eating habits, sleep, and weight…no evidence that meditation programs were better than any active treatment (i.e., drugs, exercise, and other behavioral therapies)…[they]… result in small to moderate reductions of multiple negative dimensions of psychological stress" (p. 357).

One needs to bear in mind that the populations targeted in *sati,* Buddhist psychology/therapy and mindfulness-based mindfulness differ as their aims differ: awakening, personality change, coping with stress and other disorders. Quantitative outcome evidence endorsing Buddhist practice as a whole and pristine mindfulness/heartfulness in particular is lacking. The question is whether the qualitative evidence down the ages on the salubrious outcome of Buddhism suffices, that is, sufficiently corroborates Dharma's boon, considering its surviving the ravages of time during 2600 years and with hundreds of million people who claim its benefits. In this framework, the statistical evidence on mindfulness-based mindfulness, how little favorable it may be, contributes to pristine mindfulness' effectiveness even though Buddhist-lite mindfulness only covers calming serenity (*Samatha*) and concentrative absorption (*Samadhi*). Buddhism's mature state in human history asks for adjustment to the information age and psychological guidelines. Developments in this direction are already underway. Recently, Theravada Buddhist theory based on interpretations of the *Abhidhamma* (an abstraction of the Buddha's discourses) entered the space of mainstream psychology in a quest to account for the effectiveness of MBI (Grabovac et al. 2011).

The positive research data on MBIs are embraced as an important ingredient by clinicians in various treatments (Shapiro et al. 2006). This is in spite of the fact that the definition of the mindfulness-based mindfulness concept is a subject of continuous debate: What exactly constitutes this mindfulness? Which factors are involved? Kabat-Zinn's (1990) early definition includes: (1) nonjudging, (2) nonstriving, (3) acceptance, (4) patience, (5) trust, (6) openness, and (7) letting go. Kabat-Zinn (2003b) further added (8) compassion, (9) interest, (10) friendliness, and (11) openheartedness toward the experience observed regardless of its quality. Kabat-Zinn (2005) added (12) nonreactivity, and (13) intentionality. However, this intentionality does not seem to refer to karmic intentionality, but rather to mindfulness' deliberate and effortless practice. The most recent addition is (14) memory as "one natural function of present moment awareness [is] to remember the immediate past" (Kabat-Zinn 2011, p. 19). The rationale is that "the element of retention… did not seem either necessary or useful to feature in a working definition of mindfulness in the West, given how cognitive we tend to be already" (p. 19). Finally, Kabat-Zinn (2011, p. 20) added (15) non-duality as an element as well, "as per the teaching of the Heart Sutra"…"thus, on non-doing, non-striving, not-knowing, non-attachment to outcomes" which reflects a Chan/Zen influence. Others have added further characteristics, such as: gentleness, generosity, empathy, gratitude, loving kindness (Shapiro et al. 1998); and self-regulation, values clarification, cognitive–emotional–behavioral flexibility, and exposure (Shapiro et al. 2006). Furthermore, Shapiro and colleagues postulated that "re-perceiving" is the meta-mechanism of change and that "on purpose" can be interpreted as "intentional", that is, a personal view why one practices (e.g., to reduce hypertension). Acknowledging intention as the investigative effort to observe thoughts and feelings, a consensus explanation emphasizes acceptance. Meanwhile, we may conclude that the term intention as used by these authors does not reflect the Dharma's meaning of intention as karmic willful activity meant to pursue a wholesome life. It is safe to state that there is no consensus about what exactly constitutes either mindfulness or intention in the MBI approaches.

A consensus panel proposed a two-component definition: "the self-regulation of attention so that it is maintained on immediate experience, thereby allowing for increased recognition of mental events in the present moment"and "adopting a particular orientation toward one's experiences in the present moment, an orientation that is characterized by curiosity, openness, and acceptance" (Bishop et al. 2004, p. 232). According to Siegel et al. (2008), nonjudgment, compassion, and acceptance are clinical expansions of the original meaning of *sati,* which only includes the basic elements of attention, awareness, and remembering. Therapists embrace the acceptance component as one needs first to be aware of the problem to be able to change it. Indeed, according to Mikulas (2011), most definitions of mindfulness formulated by Western authors refer to concentration rather than *insight.* This corroborates pristine mindfulness' proposition that the salutary outcome of Buddhist-lite mindfulness refers to *Samatha* and *Samadhi.* Most importantly, MBI mindfulness conspicuously lacks Buddhist psychology as a framework of its practice (DelMonte 2011; Kwee 2010; McWilliams 2011).

A review of questionnaires reveals the psychometric potential of five factors: (1) nonreactivity to experience, (2) observing inner experience, (3) acting with awareness, (4) describing with words, and (5) nonjudgmental about experience (Baer et al. 2006). Whether mindfulness is a state or trait, process or outcome, cure or care remains the subject of ongoing study. Mindfulness as conceived and dispensed in health care is floating adrift not only from *sati* from which it has been wrest but also from its avowed purpose as it is missing crucial Dharma basics. Mindfulness in the MBI approaches like dialectical behavior therapy (DBT) and acceptance and commitment therapy (ACT), advertently exclude the Dharma as well. Although it is emphasized that mindfulness as intervention is not a quick fix, the Buddhist psychological underpinning is evidently absent. The question arises: Can MBIs be invoked without subscribing to the Dharma? Traditionally, *sati* is not a goal in itself, but a tool with an inextricable function in the Buddha's project to liberate humanity from *duhkha*. This is a larger aim than alleviating patients' stress. The tactics behind abating MBI's mindfulness from its Buddhist roots is to not burden clients with Buddhism and to not repel mainstream professionals (e.g., Grepmair et al. 2008). This leaves MBI professionals and clients with a procedure decontextualized from Dharma.

No one is obliged to master the Dharma and Buddhist psychology (e.g., Shapiro and Carlson 2009, p. 9), but is it justifiable to privilege "universal values" due to skittishness to embrace Buddhist values? As Kabat-Zinn (2003b) stated:

> [Dharma] is at its core truly universal, not exclusively Buddhist…*a coherent phenomenological description of the nature of mind, emotion, and suffering and its potential release…* mindfulness…being about attention, is also of necessity universal. There is nothing particularly Buddhist about it (italics added, p. 145)…. It is an inherent human capacity…received its most explicit and systematic articulation and development within the Buddhist tradition…although its essence lies at the heart of other ancient and contemporary…teachings as well (p. 146)…[Mindfulness-Based Stress Reduction] needed to be free of the Buddhist origins…the objective was not to teach Buddhism…but to…experiment with…novel…methods…. At the same time, the program needed to remain faithful…to the universal dharma dimension alluded to, which…lies at the very core of…mindfulness. The task…is to translate the meditative challenges and context into…the lives of the participants, yet without denaturing the dharma dimension…. This requires…understanding of that dimension… through…personal engagement…meditation retreats at Buddhist centers…. (p. 149)

Thus, there is the bewildering impression that the Dharma is diluted to some universal lawfulness. Also Davidson and Kabat-Zinn (2004, pp. 150–152) dismiss Buddhist psychology by stating that mindfulness, defined as a moment-to-moment nonjudgmental awareness, "does not include Buddhist psychology"; it is an isomorphic translation "for greater awareness,self-knowledge, equanimity, and self-compassion" practiced "across all activities of daily living" aimed at "the cultivation of insight and understanding of self and self-in-relationship" "the cultivation of openhearted presence [has] nothing particularly Buddhist." Revisiting these issues, Kabat-Zinn (2009b, pp. xxviii–xxix) seemed to obfuscate the above by contriving that his use of the mindfulness concept is also:

> [A]n umbrella term that subsumes…the Eightfold Noble Path, and…the dharma itself…. We never limit our use of mindfulness to its most narrow technical sense…. I offered an *operational* definition…[which] leaves the full dimensionality and impact of mindfulness…implicit and available for ongoing inquiry…. [T]he word *mindfulness* does double-duty as a comprehensive but tacit umbrella term that included other essential aspects of dharma, [the choice] was made as a potential skilful means to facilitate introducing what Nyanaponika Thera referred to as *the heart of Buddhist meditation* into the mainstream of medicine…and the wider society in a wholly universal rather than Buddhist formulation and vocabulary…[His] inclusive and non-dual formulation offered both validation and permission to trust and act on my own direct experience of the meditation practice and the dharma…even if…it was glossing over…Buddhist psychology…that I felt could be differentiated and clarified later….

If this post hoc rationalization is acceptable, disgruntled Asian psychologists with a Buddhist background, who expressed their worry about Buddhist-lite mindfulness, cannot but feel relieved. Buddhist meditation without Buddhism is not a *chutzpah* after all?! (For instance at the Second Asian Cognitive Behaviour Therapy conference, Bangkok, 2008; reported in Kwee 2009.)

Mindfulness is indeed just a human quality, that is nothing new (Shapiro and Carlson 2009). Do something dangerous and *sati* will arise in a natural way. However, by excluding the Eightfold Balancing Practice, one deforms and cripples the Dharma from where mindfulness is taken. Besides, by making an appeal to the

Hippocratic oath (Kabat-Zinn 2009a) to call on ethics is a creative move, although most MBI practitioners are not MDs, but no guarantee to prevent mindfulness-based sniping and raping? What's more, substituting the Four Ennobling Realities by a universal Dharma is in a way disparaging and mind boggling. Is there more behind the move than the politics of getting mindfulness accepted in the medical ranks? As Gethin formulated (Williams and Kabat-Zinn 2011, p. 14; italics added):

> …the abstraction of mindfulness from its context within a broad range of Buddhist meditative practices might seem like an appropriation and distortion of traditional Buddhism that loses sight of the Buddhist goal of rooting out greed, hatred and delusion. From a different Buddhist perspective, it might seem to be an example of "skill in means"…it provides a way of giving beings the opportunity to make a first and important initial step on the path that leads to the cessation of suffering. From yet another perhaps still Buddhist perspective that might be characterized as "modernist," it strips Buddhism of some of its unnecessary historical and cultural baggage, focusing on what is essential and useful. A non-Buddhist perspective might regard the removal of the unnecessary historical and cultural baggage as finally revealing the useful essence that had hitherto been obscured by the Buddhist religion. *Finally we might regard the coming together of practices derived from Buddhism with the methods of modern western cognitive science as affording a true advance that supersedes and renders redundant the traditional Buddhist practices.*

Is it appropriation after all which will lead to pushing Buddhism into oblivion? One might think so, but in a laudable special issue of *Contemporary Buddhism* (2011) mindfulness is reinstalled in the larger Buddhist context by acknowledging its provenance. Williams and Kabat-Zinn (2011) declared that the introduction of mindfulness into mainstream medicine was a matter of politics to get the Trojan horse inside and conjecture that employing Buddhist traditional language would have led to its rejection by physicians and psychologists. Whether that would be the case remains obscure. After the fact, nobody knows how and what: was it appropriation, exploitation, fragmentation, decontextualization, or recontextualization? No MBI professional seems to be unappreciative toward Buddhism and one cannot but be struck by the openness the *Contemporary Buddhism* issue radiates considering its breadth and scope of bringing back mindfulness in the bosom of the Dharma. That anthology reinstalls and reinstates the Buddhist caliber of mindfulness. No doubt is left about the Buddhist roots of mindfulness in the MBI approaches.

16.6 Discussion

The "beyond" in this chapter's title is dealt with next. Mindfulness as in MBI has begun a march in Western culture initially as a healing panacea for various ills. It has reached not only seekers but also a whole gamut of people: therapists, patients, doctors, celebrities, executives, prisoners, soldiers, and politicians. Buddhists who have studied Buddhism and practiced *sati* will support the health and healing efforts of MBI, but do not certify the stealth Buddhist offering of a universal quality as Buddhist authentic (www.tricycle.com/blog/10-misconceptions-about-buddhism). The flip side is that the mushrooming courses heighten the risk of malignant practice. While it requires basic psychological knowledge and clinical experience as well as sufficient personal training and Buddhist wisdom, most MBI trainers in the open market seem to lack proper education in these areas. Overclaiming the effects may lead to blindness for adverse side-effects. Considering the potential drawbacks (like psychosis, depersonalization, panic, headache, or trauma reliving) and the pseudo-competence of many providers, clients might become victimized. The self-occupation by taking a step back to only watch thoughts and feelings go by and keep a wandering mind focused requires hard work with an expert guide. Not surprisingly, even quacks show up in a booming business. Low or non-qualified teachers, like individuals who followed the program once, present themselves as an MBI expert for a quick fix. As among the courses' attendants are likely susceptible people with mental health problems, the training is advisably done by mental health workers. MBI is not a magic bullet: Will a register help prevent McCompassion?

The growing numbers of trainers and trainees makes mindfulness as in MBI a mainstream practice that is still frenzied and which is perhaps, according to Kabat-Zinn (2014; www.youtube.com/watch?v=5y8ARA6yDrA), making headway from revolution to movement to renaissance. It has "the potential to ignite a universal or global renaissance on this planet that would put even the European and Italian Renaissance into the shade…[and] may actually be the only promise the species and the planet have for making it through the next couple hundred years." The secret is science. Not so much the outcome studies as discussed above, but rather the neuroscientific data on the brain as a plastic organ of experience able to alter its structure and function, and shape skills. To date, reports were on the selective structural thickening (of the neocortex, hippocampus, and insula), the shrinking of the amygdale and the functional quieting of default mode networks (Davidson 2013). These findings seem to have impressed the public at large, even if the significance is yet unclear. In effect, mindfulness as in MBI is not a passing fad. From a Buddhist perspective Buddhist-lite mindfulness is not inadequate, but incomplete; thus, completion is recommended. Relational Buddhism's pristine mindfulness offers links, fills gaps, and recontextualizes. The art of heartfulness and the science behind the MBI do not bite each other. Pristine mindfulness' eight states are appealing to people who seek awakening, while people who participate in Buddhist-lite mindfulness target the alleviation of health problems by "nirvanic calming." It would be exciting to see hardwired studies on pristine mindfulness, Relational Buddhism, Buddhist psychology/therapy and Karma Transformation. To date, there is growing evidence that various "Buddhist-derived interventions" applied to mood spectrum disorders, substance use disorders, and schizophrenia accrue promising results (Shonin et al. 2014).

The heart of heartfulness is the emptiness experience, clearly described by the Buddha (*Maha Sunnata Sutta* and *Cula Sunnata Sutta*). Relational Buddhism is about relational living and heartfulness of speech based on a social constructioning perspective which reflects the spirit of Buddhist liberating emptiness and not-self. Aiming at merging Western psychology/therapy and Buddhism, Relational Buddhism proposes to be mindful of inter-mind. At the bottom, Relational Buddhism may be viewed as the "Fourth Turning of the Dharma Wheel" after the Buddha's first turning *(Dharmachakra),* Nagarjuna's "middle way" turning *(Madhyamaka)* and Vasubandhu's "practice only" turning *(Yogacara)*. Indeed, Relational Buddhism's aspiration is realizing a fourth turning (www.taosinstitute.net/psychotherapy-kwee) by moving toward a paradigm shift to establish cutting-edge psychology/therapy as a vehicle for disseminating a twenty-first-century secular Dharma in a non-Buddhist world. This sounds like there is another current which synchronically works alongside the mindfulness movement toward realizing a renaissance: the renaissance of Buddhism as a Way *(Magga)* for humanity's serenity, contentment, and happiness http://relationalbuddhism.org).

References

Analayo (2003). Satipatthana: the direct path to realization. Kandy, Buddhist Publication Society.

Austin, J. (2010). Meditating selflessly. In M. G. T. Kwee (Ed.), *New horizons in buddhist psychology: Relational Buddhism for collaborative practitioners* (pp. 417–432). Chagrin Falls: Taos Institute.

Baer, R. A. (2003). Mindfulness training as a clinical intervention: A conceptual and empirical review. *Clinical Psychology: Science & Practice, 10,* 125–143.

Baer, R. A., Hopkins, J., Krietemeyer, J., Smith, G. T., & Toney, L. (2006). Using self-report assessment methods to explore facets of mindfulness. *Assessment, 13,* 27–45.

Bishop, S. R., Lau, M., Shapiro, S., Carlson, L., Anderson, N. D., Carmody, J., Segal, Z. V., Abbey, S., Speca, M., Velting, D., & Devins, G. (2004). Mindfulness: A proposed operational definition. *Clinical Psychology: Science & Practice, 11,* 230–241.

Brinol, P., Petty, R. E., & Wagner, B. (2009). Body posture effects on self-evaluation: a self-validation approach. *European Journal of Social Psychology, 39,* 1053–1064.

Csikszentmihalyi, M. (1990). *Flow: Thepsychology of optimal experience.* New York: Harper & Row.

Davidson, R. (2013). *The emotional life of your brain.* New York: Penguin.

Davidson, R., & Kabat-Zinn, J. (2004). Response to J. C. Smith. *Psychosomatic Medicine, 66,* 148–152.

De Silva, P. (1984). Buddhism and behaviour modification. *Behaviour Research & Therapy, 22,* 661–678.

DelMonte, M. M. (2011). Mindfulness: Psychodynamic perspectives. *Paradoxia: Journal of Nondual Psychology, 3,* 1–26.

Didonna, F. (Ed.). (2009). *Clinical handbook of mindfulness.* New York: Springer.

Dunne, J. (2011). Toward an understanding of non-dual mindfulness. *Contemporary Buddhism, 12,* 71–88.

Gergen, K. J. (2009a). *An invitation to social construction* (2nd ed.). London: Sage.

Gergen, K. J. (2009b). *Relational being: Beyond the individual and community.* Oxford: Oxford University Press.

Gethin, R. (2011). On some definitions of mindfulness. *Contemporary Buddhism, 12,* 263–279.

Goyal, M., Singh, S., Sibinga, E. M. S., Gould, N. F., Rowland-Seymour, A., Sharma, R., Berger, Z., Sleicher, D., Maron, D. D., Shibab, H. M., Ranasinghe, P. D., Linn, S., Saha, S., Bass, E. B., Haythornthwaite, J. A. (2014). Meditation programs for psychological stress and well-being: A systematic review and meta-analysis. *JAMA Internal Medicine, 174,* 357–368.

Grabovac, A. D., Lau, M. A., & Willet, B. R. (2011). Mechanisms of mindfulness: A Buddhist psychological model. *Mindfulness, 2,* 154–166.

Grepmair, L., Mitterlehner, F., & Nickel, M. (2008). Promotion of mindfulness in psychotherapists in training. *Psychiatry Reserch, 185,* 265.

Grossman, P., Niemann, L., Schmidt, S., & Walach, H. (2004). Mindfulness-based stress reduction and health benefits. A meta-analysis. *Journal of Psychosomatic Research, 57,* 35–43.

Gunaratana, H. (1992). Mindfulness in plain English. Boston: Wisdom.

Haruki, Y., Homma, I., Umezawa, A., & Masaoka, Y. (2001). *Respiration and emotion.* Tokyo: Springer.

James, W. (1890). *Principles of psychology.* New York: Holt.

Kabat-Zinn, J. (1990). *Full catastrophe living: Using the wisdom of your body and mind to face stress, pain, and illness.* New York: Delacourt.

Kabat-Zinn, J. (1994). *Wherever you go, there you are: Mindfulness meditation in everyday life.* New York: Hyperion.

Kabat-Zinn, J. (2003a). Mindfulness-based stress reduction (MBSR). In M. G. T. Kwee, & M. K. Taams (Eds.), Special issue: A tribute to Yutaka Haruki. *Constructivism in the Human Sciences, 2,* 73–106.

Kabat-Zinn, J. (2003b). Mindfulness-based interventions in context: Past, present and future. *Clinical Psychology: Science & Practice, 10,* 144–156.

Kabat-Zinn, J. (2005). *Coming to our senses.* New York: Hyperion.

Kabat-Zinn, J. (2009a). Foreword. In S. L. Shapiro, & L. Carlson (Eds.), *The art and science of mindfulness* (pp. ix–xii). Washington: American Psychological Association.

Kabat-Zinn, J. (2009b). Foreword. In F. Didonna (Ed.), *Clinical handbook of mindfulness* (pp. xxv–xxxiii). New York: Springer.

Kenny, M. A., & Williams, J. M. G. (2007). Treatment-resistant depressed patients show a good response to mindfulness-based cognitive therapy. *Behaviour Research & Therapy, 45,* 617–625.

Khoury, B., Lecomte, T., Fortin, G., Masse, M., Therien, P., Bouchard, V., Chapleau, M. A., Paquin, K., & Hofmann, S. G. (2013). Mindfulness-based therapy: A comprehensive meta-analysis. *Clinical Psychology Review, 33,* 763–771.

Kuan, T. (2012): Cognitive operations in Buddhist meditation: Interface with western psychology. *Contemporary Buddhism, 13,* 35–60.

Kuyken, W., Byford, S., Taylor, R. S., Watkins, E., Holden, E., White, K., Barrett, B., Byng, R., Evans, A., Mullan, E., & Teasdale, J. D. (2008). Mindfulness-based cognitive therapy to prevent relapse in recurrent depression. *Journal of Consulting & Clinical Psychology, 76,* 966–978.

Kwee, G. T. M. (2012a). Relational Buddhism: Wedding K.J. Gergen's relational being and Buddhism to create harmony in-between-selves. *Psychological Studies, 57,* 203–210.

Kwee, G. T. M. (2012b). Relational Buddhism: A psychological quest for meaning and sustainable happiness. In P. T. P. Wong (Ed.), *The human quest for meaning: Theories, research and applications* (2nd edn., pp. 249–274). New York: Routledge.

Kwee, G. T. M. (2013a). Relational Buddhism: An integrative psychology of happiness amidst existential suffering. In S. A. David, I. Boniwell, & A. Conley Ayers (Eds.), *The Oxford handbook of happiness* (pp. 357–370). Oxford: Oxford University Press.

Kwee, G. T. M. (2013b). Psychology in buddhism. In A. Runehov, & L. Oviedo (Eds.), *Encyclopedia of sciences and religions* (Vol. 3, Ch. 159; pp. 1892–1901). Dordrecht: Springer.

Kwee, G. T. M. (2013c). Psychotherapy by karma transformation: Relational buddhism and rational practice. Downloadable @ www.taosinstitute.net/psychotherapy-kwee (free accessible as from 2013).

Kwee, G. T. M., Gergen, K. J., & Koshikawa, F. (Eds.). (2006). *Horizons in Buddhist psychology: Practice, research & theory.* Chagrin Falls: Taos Institute.

Kwee, M. G. T. (1990). (Ed.), *Psychotherapy, meditation, and health: A cognititive-behavioural perspective.* London: East-West.

Kwee, M. G. T. (2009). A cognitive-behavioural approach to karma modification. In T. P. S. Oei, & C. S. Tang (Eds.), *Current research & practices on cognitive behaviour therapy in Asia* (pp. 89–111). Brisbane: CBT Unit Toowong Private Hospital.

Kwee, M. G. T. (Ed.). (2010). *New horizons in Buddhist psychology: Relational Buddhism for collaborative practitioners.* Chagrin Falls: Taos Institute.

Ma, H. S. W., & Teasdale, J. D. (2004). Mindfulness-based cognitive therapy for depression: Replication and exploration of differential relapse-prevention effects. *Journal of Consulting & Clinical Psychology, 72,* 31–40.
McWilliams, S. A. (2011). Contemplating a contemporary constructivist Buddhist psychology. *Journal of Constructivist Psychology, 24,* 268–276.
McWilliams, S. A. (2014). Foundations of mindfulness and contemplation: Traditional and contemporary perspectives. *International Journal of Mental Health and Addiction, 12,* 116–128.
Mikulas, W. L. (1978). Four noble truths of Buddhism related to behavior therapy. *Psychological Record, 28,* 59–67.
Mikulas, W. L. (2011). Mindfulness: Significant common confusions. *Mindfulness, 2,* 1–7.
Piet, J., & Hougaard, E. (2011). The effect of mindfulness-based cognitive therapy for prevention of relapse in recurrent major depressive disorder: A systematic review and meta-analysis. *Clinical Psychology Review, 31,* 1032–1040.
Sangharakshita. (1964). *Anagarika Dharmapala: a biographical sketch.* Kandy: Buddhist Publication Society.
Segal, Z. V., Williams, J. M. G., & Teasdale, J. D. (2002). *Mindfulness-based cognitive therapy for depression: A new approach to preventing relapse.* New York: Guilford.
Shapiro, S. L., & Carlson, L. E. (2009). *The art and science of mindfulness: Integrating mindfulness into psychology and the helping professions.* Washington: American Psychological Association.
Shapiro, S. L., Schwartz, G. E., & Bonner, G. (1998). Effects of mindfulness-based stress reduction on medical and pre-medical students. *Journal of Behavioral Medicine, 21,* 581–599.
Shapiro, S. L., Carlson, L., Astin, J. A., & Freedman, B. (2006). Mechanisms of mindfulness. *Journal of Clinical Psychology, 62,* 373–386.
Shigaki, C. L., Glass, B., Schopp, L. (2006). Mindfulness-based stress reduction in medical settings. *Journal of Clinical Psychology in Medical Settings, 13,* 209–216.
Shonin, E., Van Gordon, W., & Griffiths. M. D. (2014). The emerging role of Buddhism in clinical psychology: Toward effective integration. *Psychology of Religion and Spirituality, 2,* 123–137.
Siegel, R. D., Germer, C. K., & Olendzki, A. (2008), Mindfulness: What is it? Where does it come from? In: F. Didonna (Ed.), *Handbook of mindfulness* (pp. 17–35). New York: Springer.
Toneatto, T., & Nguyen, L. (2007). Does mindfulness meditation improve anxiety and mood symptoms? A review of the controlled research. *Canadian Journal of Psychiatry, 52,* 260–266.
Williams, J. M. G., & J. Kabat-Zinn (2011). Mindfulness: diverse perspectives on its meaning, origins, and multiple applications at the intersection of science and dharma. *Contemporary Buddhism: An Interdisciplinary Journal 12,* 1–18.
Wittgenstein, L. (1922). *Tractatus logico-philosophicus.* London: Kegan Paul.

G. T. Maurits Kwee a clinical psychologist, is a faculty member of the Taos Institute (USA)—Tilburg University (Netherlands) and founder of the Institute for Relational Buddhism & Karma Transformation, Netherlands (http://relationalbuddhism.org). Dr. Kwee earned his doctorate in Medicine at Erasmus University, Rotterdam, and was a clinical director of an inpatient psychiatric facility for two decades as well as a research fellow at Waseda University, Tokyo, and honorary professor at the University of Flores, Buenos Aires. Dr. Kwee promulgates a cutting-edge secular Buddhist psychotherapy based on what he coined "Ancient Greek Buddhism." His latest books: New Horizons in Buddhist Psychology (2010; Taos Institute Publications, USA), Psychotherapy by Karma Transformation (2013; downloaded in 51 countries) and Buddha as Therapist: Meditations (2015; download @ www.taosinstitute.net/psychotherapy-kwee)

Index

E. Shonin et al. (eds.), *Buddhist Foundations of Mindfulness*,
Mindfulness in Behavioral Health, DOI 10.1007/978-3-319-18591-0

MIX
Papier aus verantwortungsvollen Quellen
Paper from responsible sources
FSC® C105338

If you have any concerns about our products,
you can contact us on
ProductSafety@springernature.com

In case Publisher is established outside the EU,
the EU authorized representative is:
Springer Nature Customer Service Center GmbH
Europaplatz 3, 69115 Heidelberg, Germany

Printed by Libri Plureos GmbH
in Hamburg, Germany